HANDBOOK OF COMPLEX PERCUTANEOUS CAROTID INTERVENTION

CONTEMPORARY CARDIOLOGY

CHRISTOPHER P. CANNON, MD
SERIES EDITOR
ANNEMARIE M. ARMANI, MD
EXECUTIVE EDITOR

Handbook of Complex Percutaneous Carotid Intervention

Edited by

Jacqueline Saw, MD
Division of Cardiology, University of British Columbia, Vancouver, BC, Canada

J. Emilio Exaire, MD
Department of Interventional Cardiology, Instituto Nacional de Cardiología "Ignacio Chávez," Mexico City, Mexico

David S. Lee, MD
Interventional Cardiology, Hillsboro Cardiology, Hillsboro, OR

Jay S. Yadav, MD
Department of Cardiovascular Medicine, The Cleveland Clinic Foundation, Cleveland, OH

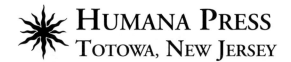

Humana Press
Totowa, New Jersey

© 2007 Humana Press Inc.
999 Riverview Drive, Suite 208
Totowa, New Jersey 07512

www.humanapress.com

Cover design by Patricia F. Cleary.

Cover illustration: Figure 6 from Chapter 7, "Cerebrovascular Angiography," by J. Emilio Exaire, Jacqueline Saw, and Christopher Bajzer.

For additional copies, pricing for bulk purchases, and/or information about other Humana titles, contact Humana at the above address or at any of the following numbers: Tel.: 973-256-1699; Fax: 973-256-8341, E-mail: orders@humanapr.com; or visit our Website: www.humanapress.com

This publication is printed on acid-free paper. ∞
ANSI Z39.48-1984 (American National Standards Institute) Permanence of Paper for Printed Library Materials.

Printed in the United States of America. 10 9 8 7 6 5 4 3 2 1

eISBN 1-59745-002-2   ISBN13 978-1-59745-002-7
Library of Congress Cataloging-in-Publication Data
Handbook of complex percutaneous carotid intervention / edited by Jacqueline Saw ... [et al.].
            p. ; cm. — (Contemporary cardiology)
        Includes bibliographical references and index.
        ISBN 1-58829-605-9 (alk. paper)
        1. Carotid artery—Surgery. 2. Carotid artery—Stenosis. 3. Stents (Surgery) I. Saw, Jacqueline. II. Series:
    Contemporary cardiology (Totowa, N.J. : Unnumbered)
        [DNLM: 1. Carotid Stenosis—surgery—Case Reports. 2. Angioplasty,Balloon—methods—Case Reports.
    3. Stents—Case Reports.WL 355 H2356 2007]
        RD598.6.H36 2007
        617.4'13—dc22   2006004982

DEDICATIONS

To my husband, David, and our son, Evan, and my family, who make my life endeavors worthwhile. And to my mentors in Interventional and General Cardiology (Drs. Donald Beanlands, Deepak Bhatt, Irvine Franco, John Jue, David Moliterno, Eric Topol, and Jay Yadav), for their guidance and support through my training, and for inspiring me to excel.

Jacqueline Saw, MD

To my wife, Karin, and my parents, Cristina and Emilio, with all my love and gratitude. This book would not be possible without the teachings of Dr. Jay Yadav and the remarkable Peripheral Intervention Staff at the Cleveland Clinic Foundation.

J. Emilio Exaire, MD

To Megan and my family for their love, support, and encouragement, and to the interventional cardiologists at the Cleveland Clinic (especially Drs. Yadav, Franco, Whitlow, Topol, and Bajzer) for their mentorship, friendship, time, and investment in me. I would not be who I am and where I am without you.

David S. Lee, MD

To my family for their unfailing support and understanding, and to the interventional cardiology fellows at the Cleveland Clinic for their curiosity and inspiration.

Jay S. Yadav, MD

PREFACE

Since the first carotid angioplasty that was performed in 1980, this technique has undergone tremendous modifications and improvements. Stents for the carotid artery were utilized in the early 1990s, and emboli protection devices were introduced about 2000. Advances in equipment (guidewires, catheters, balloons, stents, and emboli protection devices) have improved the technical success and safety of carotid stenting. With the recent SAPPHIRE publication revealing non-inferiority of carotid stenting compared with carotid endarterectomy for high-risk surgical patients, this percutaneous procedure is now considered a viable alternative to endarterectomy for these patients. In fact, the FDA has approved carotid stenting for high-risk patients using the AccuLink™ stent and AccuNet™ device (Guidant Corporation, Santa Clara, CA) in August 2004, and the Xact™ and EmboShield™ system (Abbott Vascular Devices, Redwood City, CA) in September 2005.

Increasing numbers of carotid stenting are being performed around the world, and established interventionalists and trainees alike are seeking to be instructed in performing this meticulous procedure. Unfortunately, there are insufficient well-established peripheral vascular training programs to meet this increasing demand. Only a small proportion of current trainees are enrolled in fellowship programs with dedicated carotid interventional training that perform high-volume extracranial carotid stenting; even fewer are enrolled in programs that also partake in intracranial and acute stroke interventions. In North America, this shortage of dedicated training programs leaves interested interventionalists pursuing carotid stent training through short educational courses, and often haphazard and limited "hands-on" experience in other institutions.

The purpose of our *Handbook of Complex Percutaneous Carotid Intervention* is to provide a learning resource to complement the "hands-on" training of established interventionalists and trainees. This handbook is intended for various disciplines participating in the management of patients with carotid and vertebral artery stenosis, including interventional cardiologists, vascular surgeons, interventional radiologists, and interventional neurologists. The focus of this handbook is on percutaneous intervention of patients with extracranial carotid artery stenosis. As interventionalists of the cerebrovasculature are often faced with stenosis involving other cerebral vessels, we complemented our handbook with sections on percutaneous interventions of intracranial stenosis, vertebral artery stenosis, and acute stroke.

We have provided a detailed introduction to the techniques of extracranial and intracranial, carotid, and vertebral interventions. We reviewed the indications, approaches, equipment, and potential complications of these percutaneous interventions. As many patients undergoing such procedures are elderly and high-risk with challenging anatomy, we also provided some useful pearls and troubleshooting of technically difficult cases. In addition, our section on challenging cases illustrates our approach to frequently encountered challenges at the Cleveland Clinic.

The *Handbook of Complex Percutaneous Carotid Intervention* is also meant to provide a comprehensive review of the management of carotid artery stenosis. Thus, we have included chapters reviewing the epidemiology and significance of carotid stenosis, medical therapy, noninvasive and invasive imaging of the carotid artery, and carotid endarterectomy. In this current era of evidence-based medicine, we have also included chapters reviewing sentinel studies supporting carotid endarterectomy and carotid stenting.

Carotid stenting is an exciting and burgeoning field. It is often a challenging procedure, which may expose patients to life-threatening complications. Its success as the preferred revascularization therapy of high-risk patients is contingent upon low periprocedural complications, which in turn is highly dependent on operator skills. As studies comparing carotid stenting and endarterectomy for low-risk patients are completed, we may see a further increase in the volume of carotid stenting. We hope that our *Handbook of Complex Percutaneous Carotid Intervention* will provide a useful resource to guide interventionalists through this challenging and important revascularization procedure of the 21st century.

Jacqueline Saw, MD
J. Emilio Exaire, MD
David S. Lee, MD
Jay S. Yadav, MD

CONTENTS

PART III CHALLENGING CASE ILLUSTRATIONS AND PEARLS

CONTRIBUTORS

ALEX ABOU-CHEBL, MD • *Section of Stroke and Neurological Critical Care, Department of Neurology, Cleveland Clinic Foundation, Cleveland, Ohio*

CHRISTOPHER BAJZER, MD • *Department of Cardiovascular Medicine, Cleveland Clinic Foundation, Cleveland, Ohio*

QASIM BASHIR, MD • *Neurology Fellow, Department of Neurology, Cleveland Clinic Foundation, Cleveland, Ohio*

DEEPAK L. BHATT, MD, FACC • *Staff, Cardiac, Peripheral, and Carotid Intervention, Associate Professor of Medicine, Department of Cardiovascular Medicine, Cleveland Clinic Foundation, Cleveland, Ohio*

IVAN P. CASSERLY, MB, BCH • *Director of Interventional Cardiology, Denver Veterans Affairs Medical Center, Cardiology Section, Denver, Colorado*

J. EMILIO EXAIRE, MD • *Department of Interventional Cardiology, Instituto Nacional de Cardiología "Ignacio Chávez," Tlalpan, Mexico City, Mexico*

ANTHONY Y. FUNG, MBBS • *Division of Cardiology, Vancouver General Hospital, Vancouver, BC, Canada*

JOËL GAGNON, MD • *Vascular Surgery Fellow, Division of Vascular Surgery, University of British Columbia, Vancouver, BC, Canada*

CAMERON HAERY, MD • *Director, Interventional Cardiology, Illinois Masonic Medical Center, West Suburban Cardiologists, L.L.C., Chicago, Illinois*

YORK N. HSIANG, MD • *Professor of Surgery, University of British Columbia, Division of Vascular Surgery, Vancouver General Hospital, Vancouver, BC, Canada*

SAMIR KAPADIA, MD, FACC • *Associate Professor of Medicine, Director, Interventional Cardiology Fellowship, Department of Cardiovascular Medicine, Cleveland Clinic Foundation, Cleveland, Ohio*

SHARAT KOUL, DO • *Cardiovascular Diseases Fellow, Illinois Masonic Medical Center, Chicago, Illinois*

DAVID S. LEE, MD • *Interventional Cardiology, Hillsboro Cardiology, Hillsboro, Oregon*

MIKHAEL MAZIGHI, MD • *Neurology Fellow, Department of Neurology, Cleveland Clinic Foundation, Cleveland, Ohio*

RAVISH SACHAR, MD • *Interventional Cardiologist, Wake Heart and Vascular, Raleigh, North Carolina*

JACQUELINE SAW, MD, FRCPC • *Clinical Assistant Professor of Medicine, University of British Columbia, Division of Cardiology, Vancouver General Hospital, Vancouver, BC, Canada*

JAY S. YADAV, MD • *Director, Peripheral Vascular Intervention, Department of Cardiovascular Medicine, The Cleveland Clinic Foundation, Cleveland, Ohio*

COMPANION CD

The accompanying CD ROM contains the movies associated with Part III, Challenging Case Illustrations and Pearls, and all color illustrations from the book.

The following hardware and software are the minimum required to use this CD-ROM:

- For Microsoft Windows: An Intel Pentium II with 64 MB of available RAM running Windows 98, or an Intel Pentium III with 128 MB of available RAM running Windows 2000 or Windows XP. A monitor set to 832 × 624 or higher resolution.
- For Macintosh OS X: A Power Macintosh G3 with 128 MB of available RAM running Mac OS X 10.1.5, 10.2.6 or higher. A monitor set to 832 × 624 or higher resolution.
- For Macintosh Classic: A Power Macintosh G3 with 64 MB of available RAM running System 9.2. A monitor set to 832 × 624 or higher resolution.

I CLINICAL EXPERIENCE

1

Epidemiology and Significance of Carotid Artery Stenosis

Anthony Y. Fung, MBBS
and Jacqueline Saw, MD

CONTENTS

Summary

Carotid artery stenosis is a prevalent disease, caused predominantly by atherosclerosis. The reported prevalence is dependent on the population screened, investigative tool used, and the criteria employed. The presence of carotid artery stenosis is associated with an increased risk of stroke and other ischemic manifestations of systemic atherosclerosis (e.g., myocardial infarctions and vascular deaths). Thus, carotid revascularization strategies for stroke prevention had been aggressively pursued over the past five decades. This chapter reviews the epidemiology and prevalence of carotid artery stenosis.

Key Words: Carotid artery stenosis, carotid artery stenting, carotid endarterectomy, epidemiology, stroke.

INTRODUCTION

Carotid artery stenosis is a prevalent disease, caused predominantly by atherosclerosis. Other causes are rare and include fibromuscular dysplasia, trauma, and carotid dissection. The reported prevalence of carotid artery stenosis is dependent on the population screened, investigative tool used, and criteria employed. In the Framingham Study cohort, the prevalence of significant carotid artery stenosis (carotid ultrasound stenosis >50%) was 7% in women and 9% in men (1). The prevalence is higher among individuals at risk for atherosclerosis (11%), those who have underlying cardiac disease (18%), and those presenting with acute stroke (60%) (2). It is clear that age and the presence of atherosclerotic risk factors increase the prevalence of disease. Not surprisingly, the presence of carotid artery stenosis is associated with an increased risk of

From: *Contemporary Cardiology: Handbook of Complex Percutaneous Carotid Intervention*
Edited by: J. Saw, J. E. Exaire, D. S. Lee, and S. Yadav © Humana Press Inc., Totowa, NJ

stroke and other ischemic manifestations of systemic atherosclerosis (e.g., myocardial infarctions and vascular deaths). Thus, carotid revascularization strategies for stroke prevention had been aggressively pursued over the past five decades.

STROKE

Prevalence of Stroke and Economic Burden

The primary goal of revascularization of significant carotid artery stenosis is to prevent strokes. Strokes can have major impact on both the individual and the society, incurring disability and draining the healthcare system and the economy. Each year, approx 750,000 Americans and 50,000 Canadians experience a new or recurrent stroke *(3)*. Stroke is the third leading cause of death, and the principal cause of long-term disability. Approximately one third of patients die within 30 d, and one third are left with permanent disability. The economic burden in North America is astounding, costing the healthcare system more than 50 billion dollars annually in the United States and approx 3 billion dollars annually in Canada *(3)*.

Stroke Etiology

More than 80% of all strokes are ischemic in origin (Fig. 1), while 20% are due to intracerebral hemorrhage (Fig. 2). Three quarters of ischemic strokes involve the anterior circulation, and one quarter involve the posterior vertebrobasilar system *(4)*. Overall, 20–30% of all strokes are accounted for by extracranial carotid artery stenosis *(5)*, whereas intracranial atherosclerosis account for roughly 5–10% of strokes *(6,7)*. However, most of these data are based on a predominantly Caucasian population, and epidemiologic studies have also shown ethnicity to affect stroke etiology. For instance, in the Northern Manhattan Stroke study, intracranial atherosclerosis was shown to account for 6–10% of ischemic strokes of white patients, but up to 29% among African Americans and Hispanics *(8)*. Among patients with lacunar infarcts, the prevalence of extracranial carotid artery disease (>50% stenosis) is approx 10% (which is likely an incidental finding). Whereas among patients with nonlacunar hemispheric stroke, 41% had ipsilateral carotid artery disease (>50% stenosis) *(9)*.

CAROTID ARTERY STENOSIS

Location of Carotid Artery Stenosis

Atherosclerotic plaques tend to accumulate at branch ostia and bifurcations due to the disturbance of laminar flow. Thus, in the carotid circulation, there is a predilection of plaque accumulation at the carotid bifurcation into the internal carotid artery (ICA) and external carotid artery (ECA). The ostium of the ICA is most often affected, involving the outer posterior wall of the carotid sinus, and often extending into the distal common carotid artery (CCA). Atherosclerosis of the intracranial ICA and its branches is much less common (described in Chapter 13).

Prevalence of Concomitant Intracranial Atherosclerosis

Although uncommon, a small proportion of patients with extracranial carotid stenosis have concomitant intracranial involvement. In a series of 100 consecutive patients with severe extracranial carotid disease being considered for carotid endarterectomy, cerebral angiography showed significant intracranial disease in 15% of patients *(10)*. In

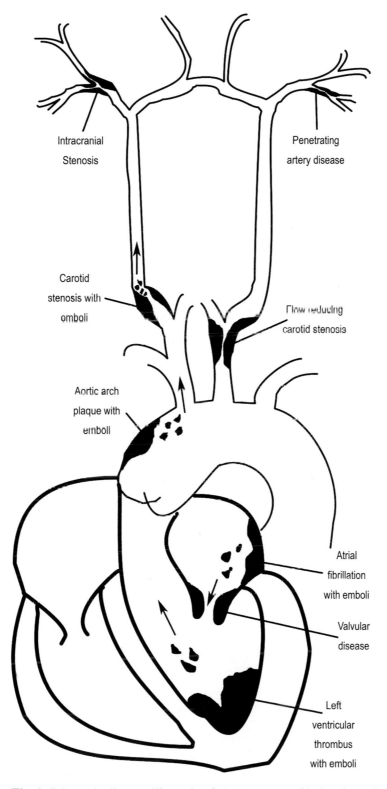

Fig. 1. Schematic diagram illustrating frequent causes of ischemic strokes.

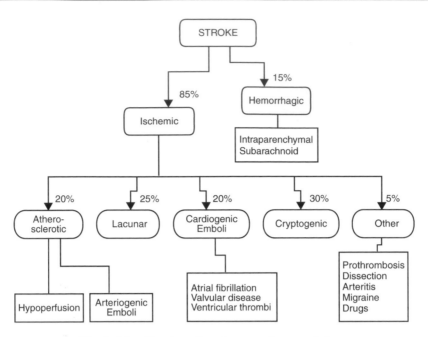

Fig. 2. Classification of stroke according to etiology.

the NASCET (North American Symptomatic Carotid Endarterectomy) study of symptomatic patients with extracranial carotid disease, mild intracranial disease was found in 33% patients. However, by protocol design, patients with severe intracranial disease were excluded *(11)*.

Significance of Carotid Bruit

Carotid disease may be discovered as patients are worked up for carotid bruit. However, the presence of carotid bruit is poorly specific for carotid stenosis. In fact, the prevalence of significant carotid stenosis in patients with asymptomatic carotid bruit is only 10–20% *(12,13)*. Patients with carotid bruit and documented carotid stenosis on duplex ultrasound do have higher risk of cerebral events *(14)*. Indeed, patients with carotid bruit have been shown to have a two to fourfold higher risk of subsequent strokes when compared to controls *(12,13)*.

Carotid Intimal–Medial Thickness

There is a strong association between cerebrovascular atherosclerosis and adverse vascular events. Measurement of the intimal–medial thickness (IMT) on carotid ultrasound has evolved to be a reliable method to evaluate early carotid atherosclerosis *(15)*. Many studies have documented the link between increased IMT and future adverse vascular events. In a prospective study by O'Leary et al. involving more than 4400 elderly subjects without clinical evidence of cardiovascular disease, approx 25% of patients in the fifth IMT quintile had experienced myocardial infarction or stroke at 7 yr follow-up, compared with <5% for the first quintile (Fig. 3) *(16)*.

Concomitant Coronary Artery Disease and Peripheral Arterial Disease

Presence of severe atherosclerosis in one vascular bed may trigger screening for concomitant silent cerebrovascular disease. Among patients with severe coronary disease

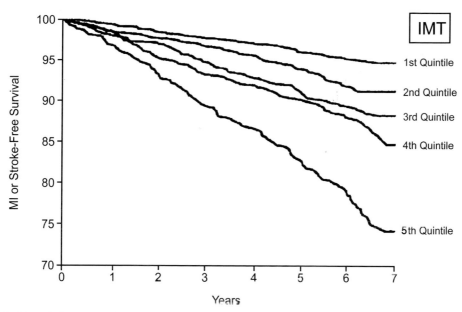

Fig. 3. Cumulative event-free (myocardial infarction or stroke) survival rates according to quintiles of combined intimal–medial thickness (IMT). (Adapted from ref. *16*.)

being considered for cardiac surgery, 17–22% have >50% carotid stenosis, and 6–12% have >80% carotid stenosis *(17)*. Among patients with peripheral arterial disease, 14–34% had carotid stenosis >50% by duplex ultrasound *(18,19)*, and 5% have carotid occlusion *(19)*.

CONSEQUENCE OF CAROTID ARTERY STENOSIS

Disease Progression

Similar to other vascular beds, atherosclerotic carotid disease is a dynamic process. In a prospective study of patients with asymptomatic carotid bruit and mild carotid stenosis, serial ultrasound studies showed that the annual rate of disease progression to >50% stenosis was 8% *(12)*. In a recent series, among patients with moderate asymptomatic carotid disease (50–79% stenosis) followed for a mean of 38 mo, 17% had evidence of disease progression documented on serial ultrasound examinations, with an estimated annual rate of progression of 4.9% *(20)*.

Risk of Stroke

The risk of stroke is highly dependent on the severity of stenosis and symptom status. Patients with known carotid artery stenosis who presented with a neurologic event within the last 6 mo are more likely to have a future stroke event. For example, in the NASCET study, the risks of ipsilateral strokes at 5 yr for patients with mild (<50%) stenosis on angiography were 18.7% and 7.8% for those with and without symptoms, respectively. For those with more severe (75–94%) stenosis, the rates were higher, 27.1% and 18.5% for symptomatic and asymptomatic patients, respectively (Fig. 4) *(21)*.

Among patients studied in the asymptomatic carotid endarterectomy trials with carotid stenosis >60%, the incidence of ipsilateral stroke at 5 yr was 11.5% in ACAS

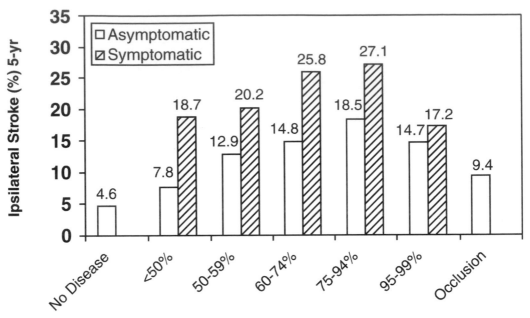

Fig. 4. Risk of ipsilateral stroke at 5 yr based on severity of carotid stenosis and symptom status. (Adapted from ref. *21*.)

Table 1
Annual Percentage Risk of Cerebrovascular Events Depending on Stenosis Severity
and Symptom Status

	Degree of stenosis			
	1–29%	*30–59%*	*60–99%*	*Occluded*
Asymptomatic patients				
Irreversible stroke	0.4	1.3	2.3	4.0
Reversible event	0.7	1.0	5.6	3.0
Symptomatic patients				
Irreversible stroke	1.3	2.0	13.0	9.1
Reversible event	—	4.0	14.5	2.0

Adapted from ref. *24*.

(Asymptomatic Carotid Endarterectomy Study) *(22)*, and 11.7% in ACST (Asymptomatic Carotid Surgery Trial) *(23)*. Table 1 provides a summary of the annual ipsilateral cerebrovascular event based on underlying stenosis severity and symptom status *(24)*.

Other Predictors of Stroke

Aside from symptom status and stenosis severity, plaque characteristics could also affect subsequent stroke risk. For example, hypoechogenic plaques as detected by high-resolution ultrasound are associated with higher stroke risk. Presumably these plaques have high lipid content and are more prone to rupture, with subsequent thrombosis and embolization *(25–27)*. Ulcerated plaques are also known to be more unstable and at higher risk for neurologic event. For example, in the medical arm of NASCET, the 2-yr stroke rate among patients without an ulcer was 21.3% irrespective of stenosis severity. However, among those with an ulcer on angiography, the 2-yr stroke event increased incrementally from 26.3% to 73.2%, as the stenosis severity increased from 75% to 95% *(28)*.

Risks of Coronary Artery Disease

It should be noted that patients with cerebrovascular disease have a high prevalence of silent coronary artery disease. Hertzer et al. performed coronary angiography on 200 asymptomatic patients (most of whom had carotid bruit). Eighty patients (40%) were found to have severe coronary artery disease (defined as >70% stenosis of ≥1 coronary artery), and 93 patients (46%) had mild or moderate disease. Only 27 patients (14%) had normal coronary arteries. In terms of extent of disease, 22% were considered to have severe but compensated coronary artery disease, 16% had severe but surgically correctable disease, and 2% had inoperable disease *(29)*.

Risk of Stroke with Coronary Artery Bypass Surgery

High-grade carotid artery stenosis (>80%) occur in roughly 8–12% of patients scheduled for coronary artery bypass grafting, and was responsible for up to 30% of hemispheric strokes that occur early after surgery. The incidence of perioperative stroke is dependent on stenosis severity, being <2% when carotid stenosis is mild (<50% severity), but increasing to 10% with moderate lesions (stenosis 50–80%), and to 11–19% with severe stenosis (>80%). Patients with bilateral high-grade stenosis (>80%) or occlusion have up to a 25% incidence of stroke perioperatively *(30)*. Therefore, screening for significant carotid stenosis is important prior to cardiac surgery, and is routinely performed in most institutions. This allows surgeons to have a better estimation of perioperative stroke risk.

CONCLUSION

Carotid artery stenosis is an important cause of stroke. Symptomatic patients with severe carotid artery stenosis are at much higher risk for future strokes than are asymptomatic patients. Patients with significant carotid artery stenosis are also at increased risk for other vascular events, as atherosclerosis is a systemic disease. Management of these patients should thus be multifaceted, and should include aggressive risk-factor modification, medical treatment to diminish global atherothrombotic risks, and carotid revascularization to lower cerebrovascular events, as appropriate.

REFERENCES

1. Fine-Edelstein JS, Wolf PA, O'Leary DH, et al. Precursors of extracranial carotid atherosclerosis in the Framingham Study. Neurology 1994;44:1046–1050.
2. Rockman CB, Jacobowitz GR, Gagne PJ, et al. Focused screening for occult carotid artery disease: patients with known heart disease are at high risk. J Vasc Surg 2004;39:44–51.
3. AHA. American Heart Association. Heart Disease and Stroke Statistics—2005 Update. Dallas, TX: American Heart Association; 2004. americanheart.org 2005.
4. Cloud GC, Markus HS. Diagnosis and management of vertebral artery stenosis. QJM 2003;96:27–54.
5. Sacco RL. Extracranial carotid stenosis. N Engl J Med 2001;345:1113–1118.
6. Petty GW, Brown RD, Jr., Whisnant JP, Sicks JD, O'Fallon WM, Wiebers DO. Ischemic stroke subtypes: a population-based study of incidence and risk factors. Stroke 1999;30:2513–2516.

7. White H, Boden-Albala B, Wang C, et al. Ischemic stroke subtype incidence among whites, blacks, and Hispanics: the Northern Manhattan Study. Circulation 2005;111:1327–1331.

8. Sacco RL, Kargman DE, Gu Q, Zamanillo MC. Race-ethnicity and determinants of intracranial atherosclerotic cerebral infarction. The Northern Manhattan Stroke Study. Stroke 1995;26:14–20.

9. Tegeler C, Shi F, Morgan T. Carotid stenosis in lacunar stroke. Stroke 1991;22:1124–1128.

10. Griffiths PD, Worthy S, Gholkar A. Incidental intracranial vascular pathology in patients investigated for carotid stenosis. Neuroradiology 1996;38:25–30.

11. Kappelle LJ, Eliasziw M, Fox AJ, Sharpe BL, Barnett HJ. Importance of intracranial atherosclerotic disease in patients with symptomatic stenosis of the internal carotid artery. Stroke 1999;30:282–286.

12. Roederer G, Langlois Y, Jager K, et al. The natural history of carotid arterial disease in asymptomatic patients with cervical bruits. Stroke 1984;15:605–613.

13. Chambers BR, Norris JW. Outcome in patients with asymptomatic neck bruits. N Engl J Med 1986;315:860–865.

14. Norris JW, Zhu CZ, Bornstein NM, Chambers BR. Vascular risks of asymptomatic carotid stenosis. Stroke 1991;22:1485–1490.

15. Mancini GB, Dahlof B, Diez J. Surrogate markers for cardiovascular disease: structural markers. Circulation 2004;109:IV22–30.

16. O'Leary DH, Polak JF, Kronmal RA, et al. Carotid-artery intima and media thickness as a risk factor for myocardial infarction and stroke in older adults. N Engl J Med 1999;340:14–22.

17. Eagle K, Guyton R, Davidoff R, et al. ACC/AHA 2004 guideline update for coronary artery bypass graft surgery: summary article. A report of the American College of Cardiology/American Heart Association Task Force on Practice Guidelines (Committee to Update the 1999 Guidelines for Coronary Artery Bypass Graft Surgery). J Am Coll Cardiol 2004;44: p1146–1154, e213–310.

18. Simons PC, Algra A, Eikelboom BC, Grobbee DE, van der Graaf Y. Carotid artery stenosis in patients with peripheral arterial disease: the SMART study. SMART study group. J Vasc Surg 1999;30: 519–525.

19. House AK, Bell R, House J, Mastaglia F, Kumar A, D'Antuono M. Asymptomatic carotid artery stenosis associated with peripheral vascular disease: a prospective study. Cardiovasc Surg 1999;7:44–49.

20. Rockman CB, Riles TS, Lamparello PJ, et al. Natural history and management of the asymptomatic, moderately stenotic internal carotid artery. J Vasc Surg 1997;25:423–431.

21. NASCET Collaborators. Beneficial effect of carotid endarterectomy in symptomatic patients with high-grade carotid stenosis. North American Symptomatic Carotid Endarterectomy Trial Collaborators. N Engl J Med 1991;325:445–453.

22. ACAS. Endarterectomy for asymptomatic carotid artery stenosis. Executive Committee for the Asymptomatic Carotid Atherosclerosis Study. JAMA 1995;273:1421–1428.

23. ACST Collaborative Group. Prevention of disabling and fatal strokes by successful carotid endarterectomy in patients without recent neurological symptoms: randomised controlled trial. Lancet 2004;363: p1491–p1502.

24. Obuchowski NA, Modic MT, Magdinec M, Masaryk TJ. Assessment of the efficacy of noninvasive screening for patients with asymptomatic neck bruits. Stroke 1997;28:1330–1339.

25. Barnett HJ, Eliasziw M, Meldrum H. Plaque morphology as a risk factor for stroke. JAMA 2000; 284:177.

26. Mathiesen EB, Bonaa KH, Joakimsen O. Echolucent plaques are associated with high risk of ischemic cerebrovascular events in carotid stenosis: the Tromso Study. Circulation 2001;103:2171–2175.

27. Polak J, Shemanski L, O'Leary D, et al. Hypoechoic plaque at US of the carotid artery: an independent risk factor for incident stroke in adults aged 65 years or older. Cardiovascular Health Study [published erratum appears in Radiology 1998 Oct;209(1):288–289]. Radiology 1998;208:649–654.

28. Eliasziw M, Streifler JY, Fox AJ, Hachinski VC, Ferguson GG, Barnett HJ. Significance of plaque ulceration in symptomatic patients with high-grade carotid stenosis. North American Symptomatic Carotid Endarterectomy Trial. Stroke 1994;25:304–308.

29. Hertzer NR, Young JR, Beven EG, et al. Coronary angiography in 506 patients with extracranial cerebrovascular disease. Arch Intern Med 1985;145:849–852.

30. Bittl JA, Hirsch AT. Concomitant peripheral arterial disease and coronary artery disease: therapeutic opportunities. Circulation 2004;109:3136–3144.

2

Medical Therapy for Carotid Artery Stenosis

David S. Lee, MD

CONTENTS

INTRODUCTION
TRADITIONAL CARDIOVASCULAR
   RISK FACTORS AND CAROTID STENOSIS
ANTIPLATELET AND ANTITHROMBOTIC THERAPY
CONCLUSION
REFERENCES

Summary

Patients with carotid atherosclerotic disease are at an increased risk for stroke. This chapter reviews the risk factors associated with carotid artery stenosis and the medical interventions that decrease the cardiovascular risk from carotid atherosclerotic disease.

Key Words: Angiotensin-converting enzyme inhibitor, antiplatelet therapy, antithrombotic therapy, cardiovascular risk factors, carotid artery stenosis, statin.

INTRODUCTION

Patients with carotid atherosclerotic disease are at an increased risk for stroke. The focus of the rest of this book is on carotid arterial revascularization, which in certain patient subsets has been shown to decrease the future risk of stroke and death *(1–4)*. This chapter focuses on medical interventions that decrease the risk from carotid atherosclerotic disease.

TRADITIONAL CARDIOVASCULAR RISK FACTORS AND CAROTID STENOSIS

Traditional cardiovascular risk factors correlate with carotid artery stenosis. In the Framingham Heart Study, the odds ratio of moderate carotid stenosis ($\geq 25\%$) in men was 2.11 (95% confidence interval [CI] 1.51–2.97) for an increase of 20 mmHg in systolic blood pressure (SBP), 1.10 (95% CI 1.03–1.16) for an increase of 10 mg/dL of total cholesterol, and 1.08 (95% CI 1.03–1.13) for an increase of 5 pack-years of smoking, with similar findings in women *(5)*. In a study of 3998 people in Osaka, Japan, the number of major coronary risk factors was associated with a higher likelihood of severe

From: *Contemporary Cardiology: Handbook of Complex Percutaneous Carotid Intervention*
Edited by: J. Saw, J. E. Exaire, D. S. Lee, and S. Yadav © Humana Press Inc., Totowa, NJ

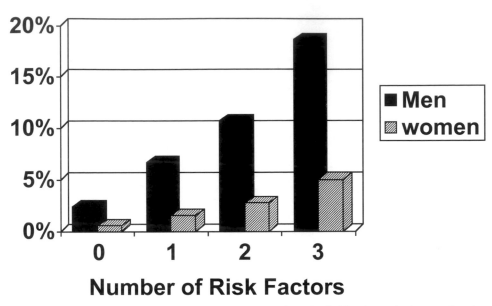

Fig. 1. Correlation between cardiac risk factors (hypertension, dyslipidemia, and tobacco abuse) and incidence of significant carotid stenosis (≥50%). A linear relationship exists between the number of risk factors and the likelihood of significant carotid stenosis. This relationship was stronger in men than in women. (Adapted from ref. *6*.)

(≥50%) carotid stenosis (Fig. 1). Major coronary risk factors in this study were hypertension (SBP ≥140, diastolic blood pressure [DBP] ≥90, or on medication), hyperlipidemia (total cholesterol >220 mg/dL or on medication), or tobacco abuse (current smoker). The mean carotid arterial intimal–medial thickness (IMT) was also increased with increasing numbers of coronary risk factors *(6)*. Another study found that patients with carotid stenosis had higher SBP and DBP, and higher plasma cholesterol and triglyceride concentrations than the control groups. They had, as well, a far greater likelihood of being cigarette smokers and a greater likelihood of having diabetes mellitus and previous evidence of coronary and peripheral arterial disease. Patients with carotid stenosis were also more likely to have two or more of these common risk factors of atherosclerosis than were the control subjects *(7)*. Other studies have suggested diabetes mellitus, family history of stroke, low high-density lipoprotein (HDL) levels, coronary artery disease (CAD), and peripheral arterial disease as associated risk factors *(7–12)*. Overall, approx 40% of the incidence of carotid stenosis can be accounted for by traditional risk factors *(10)*.

Thus, the focus of medical therapy for carotid atherosclerotic disease typically concentrates on treatment of these risk factors: hypertension, dyslipidemia, diabetes mellitus, and tobacco use. Importantly, disease in the carotid arteries suggests that atherosclerotic disease may exist elsewhere in other arterial beds. The National Cholesterol Education Program and ATP III guidelines consider the presence of carotid disease equivalent to the presence of CAD for calculating cardiovascular risk *(13)*.

What are Useful End Points or Outcomes to Measure?

The major carotid surgical revascularization studies utilized ipsilateral stroke, all-stroke, fatal stroke, and/or all-cause mortality as end points (1–4). The SAPPHIRE (Stenting and Angioplasty with Protection in Patients at High Risk for Endarterectomy) trial comparing carotid stenting to carotid endarterectomy used a composite including death, stroke, and myocardial infarction (MI) to better reflect the totality of the risk of revascularization (14).

Unfortunately, for the purposes of our discussion, nearly all clinical trials addressing medical therapies have not focused on patients with carotid stenosis. Major trials of medical therapy have focused on patients with prior cardiovascular events, known atherosclerotic disease, or with multiple cardiovascular risk factors. Trials specifically evaluating patients with carotid stenosis are lacking and generally have been under-powered and have enrolled small numbers of patients. All-cause mortality, cardiac death, MI, coronary revascularization, and/or stroke have all been used as end points in these trials. From a global perspective for the patient, these combination end points best reflect the "real world." The goal is to prevent any or all cardiovascular complications. To better determine the effect on carotid atherosclerotic disease, however, a more limited end point of ischemic ipsilateral stroke would be preferable. Unfortunately, most trials did not report the proportion of patients with carotid disease, the severity of carotid disease, or the subtype of strokes in the outcomes. Therefore, for the most part, the reduction in stroke risk specifically attributable to treated carotid disease cannot be separated from the overall reduction in stroke risk for a given therapy.

Hypertension

Hypertension is a well recognized risk factor for cardiovascular disease, and is perhaps the most important modifiable risk factor for stroke. Most evidence about the effects of blood pressure (BP) on the risk of cardiovascular complications is obtained from two types of data: prospective nonrandomized observational studies correlating the relationship between BP and the incidence of stroke and other adverse outcomes, and randomized trials of antihypertensive drug therapy.

A meta-analysis of 61 prospective observational studies including approx 1 million adults found that each 20 mmHg SBP or 10 mmHg DBP difference was associated with a more than twofold increase in the stroke or death rate. Men and women had similar findings, and hypertension was found to be associated with both fatal hemorrhagic and ischemic stroke. The risk remained elevated until the BP reached a low of 115 mmHg systolic and 75 mmHg diastolic (12). An analysis of 18 studies on Chinese and Japanese patients found a significant association between DBP and both hemorrhagic and nonhemorrhagic stroke. Each 5 mmHg reduction in DBP was associated with a reduced odds ratio (OR) of nonhemorrhagic stroke [OR = 0.61 (95% CI 0.57–0.66)] and hemorrhagic stroke [OR = 0.54 (95% CI 0.50–0.58)] (15).

In the Systolic Hypertension in the Elderly Program (SHEP) study, 4736 patients ≥60 yr of age with isolated systolic hypertension were enrolled. The average SBP was 155 mmHg in control patients compared to 143 mmHg in treated patients, resulting in a 36% relative risk reduction in total stroke ($p = 0.0003$). Nonfatal and fatal MI were reduced 27%, with a 32% reduction in cardiovascular events (16). In a meta-analysis of 37,000 patients, antihypertensive therapy resulted in a 5–6 mmHg decrease in the DBP, which was associated with a 42% reduction in stroke (95% CI 35–50%, $p < 0.0001$) and a 14% reduction in cardiovascular events (95% CI 4–22%, $p < 0.01$) with follow-up over 2–5 yr (17).

In patients with a history of stroke or transient ischemic attack (TIA), BP continues to be an important risk factor. However, concerns exist about the safety of BP reduction in this patient cohort, especially in the presence of cerebrovascular disease. The Perindopril Protection Against Recurrent Stroke Study (PROGRESS) trial studied the effect of BP reduction in 6105 patients with a history of stroke or TIA within 5 yr. Patients were treated with either perindopril or placebo. Physicians had the option of adding indapamide (a diuretic) to perindopril at their discretion. The treatment arm reduced BP (systolic/diastolic) by 9/4 mmHg. Notably, combination therapy reduced the BP by 12/5 mmHg vs 5/3 mmHg with perindopril alone. Over 4 yr of follow-up, treatment was associated with a 28% reduction in stroke (10% vs 14%, p < 0.0001) and a 26% reduction in major vascular events. Combination therapy reduced the stroke rate by 43% whereas single-agent therapy did not produce a significant reduction in stroke rate *(18)*.

COMPARATIVE TRIALS

The choice of antihypertensive agent depends on the clinical presentation and other comorbidities. While numerous trials have been performed attempting to determine which antihypertensive agent is preferable as first-line treatment, the majority of patients will likely need more than one agent, making this discussion less relevant. However, these trials (ALLHAT, HOPE, EUROPA, PEACE, VALUE, and CAMELOT) do have useful insights into which patient cohorts benefit from antihypertensive therapy, the magnitude of the treatment effect, and the utility of specific medications.

The Antihypertensive and Lipid-Lowering Treatment to Prevent Heart Attack Trial (ALLHAT) enrolled 33,357 patients ≥55 yr of age with hypertension and ≥1 cardiovascular risk factor to therapy with an angiotensin-converting enzyme inhibitor (ACE inhibitor), a calcium channel blocker, or a diuretic with mean follow-up of 4.9 yr. The α-blocker treatment arm was stopped prematurely because of an increased adverse event rate with doxazocin compared to diuretic therapy. The primary end point, combined fatal coronary heart disease or nonfatal MI, and all-cause mortality were not significantly different between treatment groups. SBP was increased in the amlodipine-treated group (0.8 mmHg, p = 0.03) and in the lisinopril-treated group (2 mmHg, p < 0.001), compared to the chlorthalidone-treated group. Treatment with amlopidine was associated with an increased rate of heart failure (10.2% vs 7.7%, RR 1.38, 95% CI 1.25–1.52), while treatment with lisinopril was associated with an increased rate of stroke (6.3% vs 5.6%, RR 1.15, 95% CI 1.02–1.30) (Fig. 2). The rate of combined cerebrovascular disease and heart failure was also higher with lisinopril *(19)*. The difference in stroke rates between lisinopril and chlorthalidone may be attributed to the BP differences achieved between the two therapies. However, thiazide-type diuretics should be preferred as first-line therapy in patients who do not have a specific indication for another agent (e.g., ACE inhibitors or β-blockers in left ventricular dysfunction, β-blockers after MI, etc.).

CARDIOPROTECTIVE EFFECT OF ACE INHIBITORS/ANGIOTENSIN RECEPTOR BLOCKER (ARBs)?

The Heart Outcomes Prevention Evaluation (HOPE) study randomized >9000 high-risk patients to treatment with ramipril or placebo. Patients were deemed high risk if they had evidence of cardiovascular disease including coronary disease, prior MI, stroke, or peripheral arterial disease, or if they had diabetes mellitus and ≥1 cardiovascular risk factor (dyslipidemia, hypertension, microalbuminuria, or tobacco abuse).

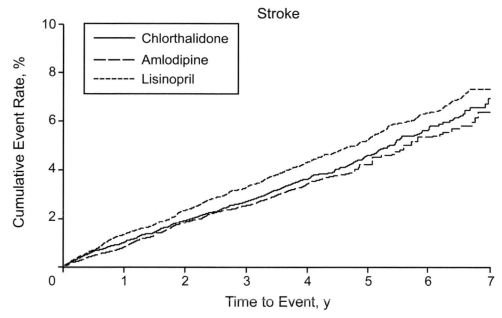

Fig. 2. Cumulative risk of stroke in patients treated with different antihypertensive medications (lisinopril, amlodipine, chlorthalidone) in the ALLHAT trial. Lisinopril therapy was associated with an increase in stroke rate compared to chlorthalidone therapy at 6 yr (6.3% vs 5.6%, RR 1.15; 95% CI 1.02–1.30). (Reproduced with permission from the ALLHAT study [19].)

The mean BP at enrollment was 139/79 mmHg. Patients treated with ramipril had a 22% reduction in MI, stroke, or cardiovascular death, a 26% reduction in cardiovascular death, a 32% reduction in stroke, a 15% reduction in revascularization, and a 23% reduction in heart failure. The benefit was seen within the first year and was consistent within all subgroups. Treatment with ramipril would prevent 18 deaths per 1000 patients treated, 16 MIs, and 9 strokes (20). The magnitude of BP lowering with ramipril was 3.3/1.4 mmHg. The benefit seen initially was thought to be much greater than what could be attributed to BP lowering alone, suggesting that ACE inhibitor may have cardiovascular benefit beyond just BP reduction. A subgroup of patients with ambulatory BP monitoring, however, had much greater BP reductions than what was recorded at office visits (21).

The EUROPA (European trial on reduction of cardiac events with perindopril in stable CAD) study also treated nearly 14,000 high-risk patients with an ACE inhibitor, perindopril, or placebo. Patients were considered high risk if they had a prior MI, known CAD, coronary revascularization, or a positive stress test. The mean BP at enrollment was 137/82 mmHg. Therapy with perindopril was associated with a 5/2 mmHg decrease in BP. Patients enrolled in EUROPA were not as high risk as patients in HOPE. The cardiovascular mortality in the placebo-treated groups was 8% for HOPE and 4% for EUROPA. Perindopril treatment, however, was still associated with a 20% reduction in the combined end point of cardiovascular death, MI, or cardiac arrest. The benefit was seen at 1 yr and was consistent among subgroups (22).

The Prevention of Events with Angiotensin Converting Enzyme Inhibition (PEACE) Trial treated patients with stable CAD [prior MI or coronary artery bypass graft (CABG) or known angiographic CAD] with either trandolapril or placebo. The mean baseline BP at enrollment was 133/78 mmHg. Treatment with trandolapril did not result in any significant reduction in adverse events. The incidence of cardiovascular death, nonfatal MI, or revascularization was 21.9% with trandolapril compared to 22.5% with placebo. Notably, the cardiovascular risk was not as high in this patient cohort as with patients enrolled in either HOPE or EUROPA, suggesting perhaps that the value of therapy may be proportional to the underlying risk (23).

The Valsartan Antihypertensive Long-Term Use Evaluation (VALUE) trial compared valsartan therapy to amlodipine therapy in hypertensive patients at high risk, defined as known coronary heart disease, dyslipidemia, diabetes mellitus type 2, cerebrovascular disease, peripheral arterial disease, left ventricular hypertrophy, reduced renal function, proteinuria, or tobacco abuse. The mean BP at enrollment was 155/88 mmHg. After mean follow-up of 4.2 yr, the primary composite end point of cardiac events, MI, stroke, and death was not significantly different between the treatment arms (24).

The Comparison of amlodipine vs enalapril to limit occurrences of thrombosis (CAMELOT) trial compared treatment with either amlodipine or enalapril to placebo in patients with known angiographic coronary disease >20% and DBP <100 mmHg. Mean baseline BP was 129/78 mmHg. The primary end point was a composite of cardiovascular death, nonfatal MI, resuscitated cardiac arrest, coronary revascularization, hospitalization for either angina or congestive heart failure, fatal or nonfatal stroke, TIA, and new diagnosis of peripheral arterial disease. The incidence of the composite end point was 23.1% in the placebo group compared to 16.6% in the amlodipine-treated group and 20.2% in the enalapril-treated group. Only the amlodipine-treated arm had a statistically significant reduction in risk (HR 0.69, 95% CI 0.54–0.88, $p = 0.003$). The enalapril-treated arm had a hazard ratio of 0.85 (95% CI 0.67–1.07, $p = 0.16$). While the BP reduction was similar with both treatment arms (4.8/2.5 mmHg with amlodipine and 4.9/2.4 mmHg with enalapril), the once daily dosing of both drugs raises the possibility that BP lowering may not have been as stable with enalapril (half-life of ~11 h) compared to amlodipine (half-life of ~50 h). Moreover, amlodipine has antianginal properties, which may have reduced the need for coronary revascularization and hospitalization for angina. The reduction in the incidence of nonfatal MI, stroke, and death was similar between amlodipine and enalapril treatments, although not statistically significant for either compared to placebo (25).

Overall, these trials suggest that high-risk patients with "normotensive" blood pressures (baseline BP of 137–139/79–82 mmHg) still benefit from therapy. Moreover, it seems likely that the magnitude of BP lowering achieved by therapy may be more important than the actual agent used, although this is controversial.

GOAL OF BLOOD PRESSURE MANAGEMENT

The Seventh Report of the Joint National Committee on Prevention, Detection, Evaluation, and Treatment of High Blood Pressure (JNC VII) issued new guidelines for the treatment of BP in 2003. The recommended target BP was <140/90 mmHg in patients with cardiovascular disease and <130/80 in patients with diabetes mellitus or chronic kidney disease with proteinuria. They concluded that most patients will require at least two BP medications to reach these goals (26). The 2003 European Society of Hypertension-European Society of Cardiology (ESH-ESC) guidelines for the management of arterial hypertension, however, recommended a goal BP <130/85 mmHg in high-risk patients with cardiovascular disease (27). Given the results of HOPE, EUROPA, PEACE, VALUE, and CAMELOT, several conclusions become evident.

Patients at higher risk derive greater benefit from BP reduction even if they are not "hypertensive." Blood pressure reduction itself may be more important than the actual agent used. Certain classes of medications are of greater benefit in certain clinical situations, such as ACE inhibitors for patients with congestive heart failure, left ventricular dysfunction, or diabetes mellitus, and β-blockers for patients with angina, prior MI, or congestive heart failure. Overall, however, the recommendations of ESH-ESC may better reflect goals of therapy in high-risk patients.

CAROTID DISEASE AND BLOOD PRESSURE REDUCTION

In patients with severe carotid atherosclerotic disease, concerns exist about decreasing the BP especially in the setting of severe bilateral carotid stenosis or carotid occlusion. Cerebral perfusion has been hypothesized to be dependent on perfusion pressure, and therefore systemic BP. Decreasing the BP in this setting may result in increasing ischemia to regions of the brain that are marginally receiving sufficient blood flow at baseline. While this hypothesis has validity in the acute stroke setting, very little clinical data exists about this possibility for long-term treatment. Rothwell et al. conducted a post hoc analysis of data from three trials, two of which were carotid revascularization trials in symptomatic patients with carotid stenosis (NASCET and ECST) and one in patients with stroke or TIA with low likelihood of carotid stenosis treated with aspirin. Increased BP correlated with higher stroke risk in patients with symptomatic carotid disease, although this relationship is blunted in comparison to other patients presenting with TIA or stroke. Carotid occlusion did not affect this, but patients with bilateral ≥70% stenosis had an increased stroke risk with decreased BP, suggesting that aggressive BP reduction may result in worse outcomes in this cohort of patients (28). However, it is important to note that this was a post hoc analysis looking at the relationship of BP at time of enrollment and subsequent stroke. This was not a trial of BP lowering, and the relatively small number of strokes in these patients with bilateral carotid disease makes the data liable to statistical variance. However, caution is still warranted in this cohort of patients.

Hyperlipidemia

EPIDEMIOLOGICAL PARADOX

Hyperlipidemia has been associated with carotid atherosclerotic disease. Elevated total cholesterol was associated with an increased likelihood of moderate carotid stenosis in the Framingham Study. Other studies have suggested a correlation between total cholesterol/HDL ratio and carotid stenosis and an inverse relationship between HDL and carotid stenosis (29,30). High HDL may be associated with reduced carotid plaque progression (31). Surprisingly, however, elevated lipid levels are not established as a risk factor for stroke (32). Our understanding of how dyslipidemia affects stroke risk comes from two types of data: observational studies looking at the association of plasma lipid levels and stroke and randomized controlled trials of lipid-lowering therapy and the effect on stroke risk. Unfortunately, unlike work on hypertension, a discordance is seen between the epidemiological studies and the therapeutic studies. Only a weak association between lipid levels and stroke is observed, but a significant benefit is seen with lipid-lowering therapy, primarily statins, in reducing stroke risk.

In a large analysis of 450,000 patients, no correlation between cholesterol levels and stroke could be found, except potentially in patients younger than 45 yr of age. This finding was not different after adjusting for gender, DBP, history of CAD, or ethnicity.

Unfortunately, three quarters of the stroke events in this analysis were from studies that recorded only fatal strokes. Moreover, the type of stroke was not recorded in any of the trials to allow for analysis by subtype *(33)*. In another analysis, Iso et al. studied more than 350,000 men to determine the relationship between total cholesterol level and risk of fatal stroke. After adjustment for age, smoking, DBP, and ethnicity, there was an association between total cholesterol level and fatal nonhemorrhagic stroke ($p = 0.007$). Interestingly, however, in men with DBP >90 mmHg, a low total cholesterol (<160 mg/dL) was associated with a threefold greater risk of fatal hemorrhagic stroke ($p = 0.05$) *(34)*. In a case control study, separating patients into quintiles based on total and HDL cholesterol values, the highest quintile of total cholesterol compared to the lowest quintile had an increased risk for nonhemorrhagic stroke (OR 1.6 [95% CI 1.3–2.0]). Atherosclerotic stroke (OR 3.2) and lacunar stroke (OR 2.4) had the strongest associations. The lowest quintile of total cholesterol had an increased risk of hemorrhagic stroke *(35)*.

Similar findings were seen in different ethnic cohorts. The Copenhagen City Heart Study found that total cholesterol only correlated with nonhemorrhagic strokes in patients with serum total cholesterol levels of >309 mg/dL (>8 mmol/L). The risk associated with lower cholesterol levels remained fairly constant. An association between plasma triglycerides and nonhemorrhagic strokes (RR 1.12 [95% CI 1.07–1.16]) and an inverse relationship between HDL levels and nonhemorrhagic strokes were found. Notably, however, the lipid studies were performed on nonfasting samples *(36)*. People in eastern Asia tend to have higher incidence of hemorrhagic stroke than Western populations. An analysis of 18 studies studying Chinese and Japanese patients found that total cholesterol levels were only weakly correlated with strokes. Each 0.6 mmol/L reduction in total cholesterol was associated with a trend to a reduced risk of nonhemorrhagic stroke (OR 0.77 [95% CI 0.57–1.06]), and an increased risk of hemorrhagic stroke (OR 1.27 [95% CI 0.84–1.91]) *(15)*.

Overall, elevated cholesterol levels correlated with ischemic stroke, albeit weakly, and an association was found between low cholesterol levels and hemorrhagic stroke.

STATIN THERAPY

Amarenco et al. performed a meta-analysis on more than 90,000 patients treated with statin therapy enrolled into randomized clinical trials published before August 2003. Statin therapy was found to reduce the stroke rate significantly (risk reduction of 21% [OR 0.79 {95% CI 0.73–0.85}]) (Fig. 3). After trials for which stroke was not a specified end point were excluded, the OR was 0.80 (95% CI 0.74–0.87). A nonsignificant reduction in fatal strokes of 9% was also found (OR 0.91 [95% CI 0.76–1.10]). Statin therapy also did not affect the likelihood of hemorrhagic stroke. The pooled OR was 0.90 (95% CI 0.65–1.22). Overall, each 10% low-density lipoprotein (LDL) reduction reduced the risk of stroke by 15.6% (95% CI 6.7–23.6%). Approximately 33–80% of the stroke reduction could be attributed to the LDL reduction. Each 10% reduction in LDL also reduced the carotid IMT by 0.73% per year (95% CI 0.27–1.19%). The correlation between LDL reduction and IMT reduction was significant ($r = 0.65$, $p = 0.004$) *(37)*.

Patients with "normal" cholesterol levels also benefit from statin therapy to reduce stroke. The Cholesterol and Recurrent Events (CARE) trial treated 4159 patients with a history of MI with average cholesterol (mean 209 mg/dL) and LDL levels (mean 139 mg/dL) with either pravastatin or placebo. The pravastatin-treated group had an

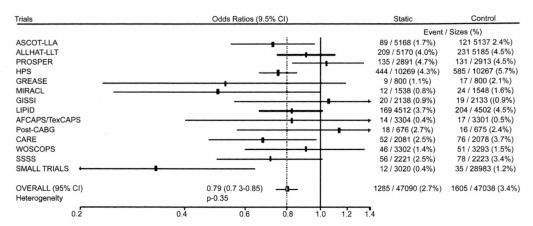

Trials	Odds Ratios (9.5% CI)	Static	Control
		Event / Sizes (%)	
ASCOT-LLA		89 / 5168 (1.7%)	121 5137 2.4%)
ALLHAT-LLT		209 / 5170 (4.0%)	231 5185 (4.5%)
PROSPER		135 / 2891 (4.7%)	131 / 2913 (4.5%)
HPS		444 / 10269 (4.3%)	585 / 10267 (5.7%)
GREASE		9 / 800 (1.1%)	17 / 800 (2.1%)
MIRACL		12 / 1538 (0.8%)	24 / 1548 (1.6%)
GISSI		20 / 2138 (0.9%)	19 / 2133 ((0.9%)
LIPID		169 4512 (3.7%)	204 / 4502 (4.5%)
AFCAPS/TexCAPS		14 / 3304 (0.4%)	17 / 3301 (0.5%)
Post-CABG		18 / 676 (2.7%)	16 / 675 (2.4%)
CARE		52 / 2081 (2.5%)	76 / 2078 (3.7%)
WOSCOPS		46 / 3302 (1.4%)	51 / 3293 (1.5%)
SSSS		56 / 2221 (2.5%)	78 / 2223 (3.4%)
SMALL TRIALS		12 / 3020 (0.4%)	35 / 28983 (1.2%)
OVERALL (95% CI)	0.79 (0.7 3-0.85)	1285 / 47090 (2.7%)	1605 / 47038 (3.4%)
Heterogeneity	p-0.35		

0.2   0.4   0.6   0.8   1.0   1.2   1.4

Fig. 3. Effects of statin therapy on fatal and nonfatal stroke risk from the study by Amarenco ct al. Odds ratios for stroke reduction with statin therapy are shown for individual trials. The small trials included in the meta-analysis were grouped together. (Reproduced with permission from ref. *37*.)

average reduction of 20% total cholesterol and 32% LDL. Patients treated with pravastatin had a 32% reduction in all-cause stroke (95% CI 4–52%, $p = 0.03$) and a 27% reduction in stroke or TIA (95% CI 4 44%, $p = 0.02$). No increase in hemorrhagic strokes was observed *(38)*. A subgroup analysis of the Anglo-Scandinavian Cardiac Outcomes Trial focused on hypertensive patients with multiple cardiac risk factors with normal total cholesterol values (<6.5 mmol/L). Patients in this cohort treated with atorvastatin had decreased nonfatal MI and cardiac death. Fatal and nonfatal stroke was also reduced by 27% (95% CI 4–44%, $p - 0.024$). The benefit of statin therapy was observed in the first year of treatment *(39)*.

Aggressive treatment with statin therapy also reduced the stroke risk. The Treating to New Targets (TNT) trial enrolled 10,0001 patients with stable coronary disease with LDL levels <130 mg/dL and treated them with either low- (10 mg daily) or high-dose (80 mg daily) atorvastatin therapy. High-dose atorvastatin therapy significantly reduced LDL more than low-dose atorvastatin (average LDL of 77 mg/dL vs 101 mg/dL) and was associated with a significant 25% reduction in fatal and nonfatal stroke (95% CI 4–41%). Cardiovascular events were also reduced *(40)*.

The Heart Protection Study (HPS) deserves special mention because it was the only large statin trial that included a significant number of patients with prior stroke and TIA. HPS studied 20,536 patients with known arterial occlusive disease or diabetes mellitus and treated them with either simvastatin 40 mg daily or placebo. The average LDL level at the time of enrollment was 131 mg/dL, of whom about one third had LDL levels of <116 mg/dL. The magnitude of reduction of LDL by simvastatin was 39 mg/dL. In all patients, there was a 25% relative risk reduction for stroke (95% CI 15–34%, $p < 0.0001$). The rate of ischemic strokes was decreased 28% (95% CI 19–37%, $p < 0.0001$) with no increase in hemorrhagic strokes. Moreover, the rate of TIA was decreased (2.0% vs 2.4%, $p = 0.02$) and the need for carotid revascularization was also reduced (0.4% vs 0.8%, $p = 0.0003$). Notably, the benefit was found by the end of the second year of therapy. The reduction in stroke was found in patients with CAD, diabetics, and patients with low LDL (<116 mg/dL) at enrollment *(41)*.

Of all the patients enrolled, 3280 had a history of cerebrovascular disease defined as prior nondisabling ischemic stroke or TIA, and/or prior carotid endarterectomy or angioplasty. In this subgroup analysis, no reduction was found in the stroke rate, although a 20% relative risk reduction was found in the rate of any vascular event (95% CI 8–29%, $p = 0.001$). Notably, patients who had a stroke within 6 mo were excluded, and on average the cerebrovascular event occurred 4.3 yr before enrollment. Stroke events were not subtyped although this was typical for most medical therapy trials. The reason for this lack of benefit in this subgroup is unclear and somewhat perplexing *(41)*.

NONSTATIN THERAPY

Nonstatin lipid-lowering therapy has not consistently shown to decrease stroke risk. A meta-analysis of lipid-lowering therapy revealed a relative risk reduction of 17% for strokes. Statin therapy had a more pronounced effect compared to other treatments (RRR of 26%). The effect was primarily seen when the total cholesterol was reduced to <232 mg/dL *(42)*. Another meta-analysis revealed only a benefit for statin therapy but not for other medication and lifestyle therapies for decreasing LDL. Some of the lack of benefit of these other therapies has been attributed to their relative lack of efficacy in reducing LDL compared to statin therapy. However, in the VA-HIT trial, patients with low HDL cholesterol (≤40 mg/dL) treated with gemfibrozil had a decreased rate of stroke compared to placebo (31% RRR [95% CI 2% to 52%, $p = 0.036$]). The rate of TIA and carotid endarterectomy were also reduced with gemfibrozil. The benefit was evident after just 6–12 mo *(43)*.

ACUTE STROKE TREATMENT WITH STATINS

Statin therapy has multiple effects beyond just lipid lowering and may provide neuroprotective effects in the setting of acute stroke. In an occlusion–reperfusion model of stroke in mice, treatment with atorvastatin for 14 d before the stroke reduced stroke volume by 40%. This protective effect was lost when the statin therapy was stopped abruptly, with complete loss of protection after 4 d. The authors concluded in this study that the neuroprotective mechanism may be due at least in part to upregulation of endothelial nitric oxide synthase *(44)*. In humans, a small retrospective study of 167 patients suggested that being on prior statin therapy at the time of acute ischemic stroke improved neurologic outcomes at 3 mo (using the modified Rankin score and the Barthel Index), although the initial stroke severity and risk of progression were not different than in patients not on statin therapy *(45)*. In a slightly larger retrospective study of 650 patients, those on lipid lowering therapy at the time of an acute ischemic stroke had a reduced risk of stroke progression and a lower 90-d mortality rate than those not on therapy. More than 90% of patients on lipid-lowering therapy were on statin therapy *(46)*. Although these findings are preliminary, they are provocative about the benefit of statins in this setting, and will hopefully lead to clinical trials assessing the value of statin therapy in acute stroke.

Diabetes Mellitus

Diabetic patients have an increased risk of cardiovascular events including ischemic stroke. The ATP III guidelines consider diabetes mellitus to be the equivalent of known coronary atherosclerotic disease for future risk, and advocates aggressive secondary prevention. Diabetic control, however, has not been as convincingly associated with reduced risk of macrovascular events including ischemic stroke. The Diabetes Control and Complications Trial (DCCT) found conclusively that aggressive diabetic control was associated with reduced microvascular events (retinopathy, nephropathy, neuropathy). However, there was only a trend to reduction of macrovascular or cardiovascular events (3.2% vs 5.4%, $p = 0.08$) *(47)*. This trial, however, focused on young type 1 diabetic patients, who likely did not have as high a likelihood of having ischemic events. However, in type 2 diabetic patients, the UK Prospective Diabetes Study (UKPDS) trial found no difference in cardiovascular events between intensive therapy and conventional therapy *(48)*. A subgroup analysis suggested that there might be a reduction in MI and stroke with improved diabetic control.

Overall, diabetic control should be advocated for reduction in microvascular complications. There may be a benefit in reducing macrovascular complications, although this has not been convincingly borne out in either type 1 or 2 diabetic patients. However, aggressive control of other risk factors especially in type 2 diabetic patients including hypertension, dyslipidemia, and smoking cessation are of great importance in reducing the cardiovascular risk, including the risk of ischemic stroke. In the UK Prospective Diabetes Study 38 Trial, intensive BP control, primarily with the use of an ACE inhibitor or β-blocker, resulted in significant BP lowering. The mean BP at baseline was 160/94 and decreased to 144/82 mmHg with intensive treatment vs 154/87 mmHg with standard treatment. Improved BP control was associated with a 32% reduction in diabetes-related death (95% CI 6–51%, $p = 0.019$), 44% reduction in strokes (95% CI 11–65%, $p = 0.013$), and 37% reduction in microvascular complications (95% CI 11–56%, $p = 0.0092$) *(49)*.

Smoking Cessation

Tobacco abuse has a known association with carotid atherosclerosis as well as adverse cardiovascular events. Smoking cessation reduces this risk eventually over time, although the risk likely does not fully normalize. One observational study in British men found that current smokers had a 3.7-fold relative risk (95% CI 2.0–6.9) for stroke compared to men who had never smoked. Men who quit had a decreased risk compared to men who were smoking, but the risk is still elevated compared to men who never smoked although not significantly (RR 1.7; 95% CI 0.9–3.3, $p = 0.11$). The reduced risk seen in men who quit smoking was seen within 5 yr. The amount of tobacco used determined the risk reduction. Light smokers (<20 cigarettes/d) had a risk similar to men who never smoked, while heavy smokers (≥20 cigarettes/d) were not able to eliminate the risk entirely (RR 2.2; 95% CI 1.1–4.3). Hypertensive men had a greater benefit from smoking cessation compared to normotensive men *(50)*. Women had similar outcomes, with a 2.6-fold risk of stroke (95% CI 2.08–3.19) compared to women who had never smoked. Women who quit smoking still had an elevated risk, although not as great as current smokers (RR 1.34, 95% CI 1.04–1.73). The risk of all stroke and ischemic stroke was reduced to similar levels as women who never smoked within 2–4 yr. Unlike the study in men, the number of cigarettes smoked did not influence the reduction in risk associated with smoking cessation *(51)*.

ANTIPLATELET AND ANTITHROMBOTIC THERAPY

Antiplatelet therapy and antithrombotic therapy continue to be important weapons in the armamentarium to decrease cardiovascular death and adverse vascular events. The value of therapy depends on both the agent and the clinical situation.

Acute Stroke

For acute treatment of ischemic events, unequivocal evidence supports the use of aspirin to treat acute ST-segment elevation MI. The value of intravenous fibrinolytic therapy has also been demonstrated in these patients, although it has been displaced by primary percutaneous coronary intervention. For acute ischemic stroke, both aspirin and fibrinolytic therapy are beneficial, but to a lesser degree and with a narrower therapeutic index than for MI.

The International Stroke Trial and the Chinese Acute Stroke Trial studied the use of aspirin in acute ischemic stroke. The International Stroke Trial was a large randomized, open-label trial of 19,435 patients comparing the use of up to 14 d of treatment with either subcutaneous unfractionated heparin (5000 or 12,500 IU bid) or aspirin 300 mg daily in a factorial design. No significant difference was seen in death at 14 d with unfractionated heparin (9.0% for heparin vs 9.3% for placebo). Notably, the recurrent ischemic stroke rate was significantly lower for the heparin group (2.9% vs 3.8%) but this was offset by an increase in the risk of hemorrhagic stroke (1.2% vs 0.4%). Therefore the rate of death or nonfatal recurrent stroke at 14 d was not significantly different (11.7% vs 12.0%). Aspirin also did not significantly reduce death at 14 d (9.0% vs 9.4%). Aspirin-treated patients, however, did have a reduced rate of recurrent ischemic strokes within 14 d (2.8% vs 3.9%) with no significant increase in the rate of hemorrhagic strokes (0.9% vs 0.8%). Aspirin therapy resulted in a significantly lower rate of death or nonfatal recurrent stroke at 14 d (11.3% vs 12.4%) *(52)*.

The Chinese Acute Stroke Trial (CAST) was a large randomized, placebo-controlled, clinical trial of 21,106 patients with acute ischemic stroke comparing aspirin 160 mg daily with placebo, started within 48 h of symptoms and continued for up to 4 wk. Aspirin-treated patients had a significant reduction in death at 4 wk (3.3% vs 3.9%, $p = 0.04$). Aspirin therapy was also associated with a decreased recurrent ischemic stroke rate (1.6% vs 2.1%, $p = 0.01$) and a nonsignificantly increased hemorrhagic stroke rate (1.1% vs 0.9%, $p > 0.1$). The composite end point of in-hospital death or nonfatal stroke at 4 wk was significantly decreased with aspirin therapy (5.3% vs 5.9%, $p = 0.03$) *(53)*.

Overall, treatment with aspirin in acute stroke was associated with an absolute reduction of death or nonfatal stroke of 9 per 1000 treated for 3 wk. Although a small increase was seen in extracranial bleeding, the benefits of therapy clearly outweighed the risks *(54)*. Although the benefit seems small compared to the magnitude of benefit seen from aspirin therapy in other clinical settings, it is important to note that the duration of therapy needed to achieve this benefit was 2–4 wk compared to the years of therapy needed to obtain benefit in secondary prevention.

Secondary Prevention

In patients presenting with TIA or minor stroke, low-dose aspirin has been shown to decrease the risk of stroke. The Swedish Aspirin Low-Dose Trial (SALT) enrolled 1360 patients presenting with TIA or minor stroke and randomized them to either therapy with low-dose aspirin (75 mg daily) or placebo. Treatment with aspirin was associated with an 18% reduction in stroke or death (RR 0.82; 95% CI 0.67–0.99, $p = 0.02$) with similar reductions for stroke, frequent TIA, and MI *(55)*. Another trial compared 30 mg of aspirin daily with 283 mg daily in patients with prior TIA or minor stroke. Low-dose aspirin was just as efficacious as the higher dose in preventing vascular death, nonfatal stroke, or nonfatal MI (14.7% in the low-dose group vs 15.2% in the high-dose group)

(56). However, the United Kingdom Transient Ischaemic Attack Aspiring Trial (UK-TIA) showed discordant results. The UK-TIA was a randomized trial of 2435 patients with presumed TIA or minor ischemic stroke treated with either 1200 mg of aspirin daily, 300 mg of aspirin daily, or placebo. Only a trend to decreased risk of major stroke, MI, or vascular death was found with aspirin (OR 0.85, 95% CI 0.71–1.03). No difference was found between low-dose and high-dose aspirin *(57)*.

In high-risk patients, a meta-analysis of six trials of low-dose aspirin (≤325 mg daily) found that aspirin therapy was associated with a 20% reduction in stroke, 18% reduction in death, 30% reduction in MI, and a 30% reduction in vascular events. However, aspirin use was associated with increased gastrointestinal bleeding *(58)*. Overall, the efficacy of aspirin for preventing strokes seems to be relatively leveled from a dose of 50 mg/dL to 1500 mg/dL daily *(59)*. The Antithrombotic Trialists' Collaboration published a meta-analysis of antiplatelet therapy in 2002. In general, in high-risk patients, antiplatelet therapy was associated with a 25% reduction in nonfatal strokes. In patients with prior TIA or stroke, antiplatelet therapy was associated with a 22% reduction in the composite end point of nonfatal stroke, nonfatal MI, or vascular death. Thirty-six events would be prevented in 2 yr for every 1000 patients treated. Aspirin was the most commonly used antiplatelet agent in this study *(60)*.

Aspirin and Treatment for Carotid Stenosis

Few studies have assessed the benefit of aspirin therapy for secondary prevention in patients with known carotid stenosis. Most have enrolled relatively few patients and have been underpowered to assess the effect of aspirin. One such study by Cote et al. evaluated 372 patients with known carotid stenosis of ≥50% treated with either aspirin 325 mg daily or placebo for 2 yr. Notably, these patients were asymptomatic from their carotid disease and did not undergo revascularization. No significant difference was found between treatment groups in the rate of death or significant ischemic event. The multivariate analysis found an adjusted hazard ratio for aspirin of 0.99 (95% CI 0.67–1.46, $p = 0.95$) *(61)*. In the Antithrombotic Trialists' Collaboration analysis, there was a trend toward improved outcomes with aspirin therapy in patients with carotid stenosis, similar in magnitude to that found with aspirin for secondary prevention *(60)*.

Patients undergoing carotid endarterectomy benefit from aspirin therapy. A small trial of 232 patients randomized to aspirin 75 mg daily or placebo starting preoperatively and continued for 6 mo after surgery found that intraoperative stroke and postoperative stroke with residual defects were lower in the aspirin-treated arm (1.7% vs 9.6%, $p = 0.01$). There was a trend toward a lower rate of any neurological event and/or death in the aspirin treated arm ($p = 0.12$). Notably, there was no significant increase in bleeding complications with aspirin therapy *(62)*. This benefit is likely the result of decreased emboli during surgery in patients treated with aspirin. When transcranial Doppler (TCD) monitoring was performed in symptomatic patients with carotid stenosis, the absence of aspirin therapy was associated with a sevenfold increase in microembolic events found via TCD *(63)*. Low-dose aspirin is preferred over high-dose aspirin in patients undergoing carotid endarterectomy. The ASA and Carotid Endarterectomy (ACE) Trial found that patients treated with aspirin 81 mg or 325 mg daily had a lower combined rate of stroke, MI, and death compared to 650 mg or 1300 mg daily at 3 mo (6.2% vs 8.4%, $p = 0.03$), and a trend toward benefit at 30 d (5.4% vs 7.0%, $p = 0.07$) *(64)*.

Primary Prevention

The Physicians' Health Study was the largest randomized clinical trial in 22,071 men evaluating the effect of low-dose aspirin on cardiovascular mortality for primary prevention. A 44% relative risk reduction was found in the risk of MI (RR 0.56; 95% CI 0.45–0.70, $p < 0.00001$). A nonsignificant but slightly increased risk of stroke was seen, primarily of hemorrhagic stroke (RR 2.14; 95% CI 0.96–4.77, $p = 0.06$). No reduction in cardiovascular mortality was found. Subgroup analysis revealed that the benefit was predominantly in patients >50 yr of age. The risk of gastrointestinal ulceration was not significantly higher (RR 1.22, 95% CI 0.98–1.53, $p = 0.08$) (65). Although the British Doctors' Trial did not show any benefit for aspirin, a meta-analysis of five major primary prevention trials including more than 55,000 patients (>11,000 women) found a 32% relative risk reduction in the risk of a first MI and overall 15% relative risk reduction in vascular events, but no significant effect on nonfatal stroke or vascular death (66).

Interestingly, the Nurses' Health Study found somewhat discordant results. In this observational study of 79,319 women, low-dose aspirin use (one to six aspirin/wk) was associated with a decreased stroke risk while higher doses of aspirin (seven or more aspirin/wk) led to a slightly increased stroke risk. Multivariate analysis revealed a relative risk of 0.50 (95% CI 0.29–0.85, $p = 0.01$) for large artery ischemic stroke in woman taking low-dose aspirin compared to women not taking aspirin. Women taking 15 or more aspirin/wk had an increased risk for subarachnoid hemorrhage (RR 2.02, 95% CI 1.04–3.91, $p = 0.02$). Subgroup analysis suggested that women who were older, hypertensive, and who smoked benefited most from low-dose aspirin therapy (67). Not surprisingly, the benefit or risk of aspirin in low-risk primary prevention cohorts will depend on their underlying risk profile.

Therefore, in patients who have a 10-yr risk of ≥10% for a coronary event, the US Preventive Services Task Force recommends the use of low-dose, long-term aspirin therapy (68). For women at increased risk of ischemic stroke, low-dose aspirin is considered beneficial.

Dipyridamole

Dipyridamole alone and in addition to aspirin has been studied extensively for secondary prevention in patients with prior stroke or TIA. Dipyridamole inhibits adenosine phosphodiesterase and adenosine deaminase, resulting in an increase and accumulation of adenosine, cyclic adenosine monophosphate (cAMP), and adenine nucleotides, with resultant platelet inhibition and vasodilation especially of the coronary circulation. The largest trial assessing the efficacy of dipyridamole was the second European Stroke Prevention Study (ESPS-2). In this study, 6602 patients with a history of stroke or TIA were randomized to 25 mg of aspirin, extended release dipyridamole 200 mg, both, or placebo, given twice daily in a factorial design. In pairwise comparisons, treatment with aspirin resulted in a 18% reduction in stroke risk ($p = 0.013$) and a 13% reduction in the risk of stroke or death ($p = 0.016$). Treatment with dipyridamole resulted in a 16% reduction in stroke risk ($p = 0.039$) and a 15% reduction in stroke or death ($p = 0.015$). More importantly, the combination of aspirin and dipyridamole was additive, leading to a 37% reduction in the stroke rate ($p < 0.001$) and a 24% reduction in stroke or death ($p < 0.001$). No significant impact on mortality was found. Similar findings were found in the rate of TIA, with a 36%

reduction for combination therapy ($p < 0.001$). Patients treated with dipyridamole had a higher incidence of headaches. All-site bleeding and gastrointestinal bleeding were significantly higher in patients treated with aspirin (69).

Prior to ESPS-2, a few studies also showed a significant reduction in stroke with the combination of aspirin and dipyridamole, compared to placebo (70). However, others comparing the addition of dipyridamole to aspirin therapy suggested no benefit, raising doubts about the value of dipyridamole (71,72). However, with the publication of ESPS-2, and a subsequent meta-analysis by Leonardi-Bee et al. (revealing a 22% reduction in recurrent stroke for the combination of dipyridamole and aspirin, compared to aspirin alone [OR 0.78, 95% CI 0.65–0.93] /73/), the combination of aspirin and dipyridamole has become accepted as first-line therapy in treating patients to prevent recurrent ischemic stroke.

Of note, dipyridamole has been used in the past as a pharmacological coronary stressor for nuclear stress tests. There has been concern about the use of dipyridamole in patients with stable angina. In fact, the American College of Cardiology has recommended against its use in this patient cohort (74). However, in the meta-analysis by Leonardi-Bee et al. combination therapy with aspirin and dipyridamole was associated with a significant reduction in the composite of nonfatal stroke, non-fatal MI, and vascular death compared to aspirin alone (OR 0.84, 95% CI 0.72–0.97) (73). In addition, a post hoc analysis of ESPS-2 did not show any increased incidence of cardiac events in patients with a history of CAD or MI treated with dipyridamole (75).

Ticlopidine

Ticlopidine has been used extensively in the past for the treatment of cardiovascular disease, after coronary stent placement, and to prevent recurrent strokes or TIA. Ticlopidine is a thienopyridine platelet antagonist that inhibits ADP-dependent platelet aggregation. Two major studies evaluated ticlopidine for secondary stroke prevention. The Canadian American Ticlopidine Study (CATS) randomized 1072 patients with recent ischemic stroke to either ticlopidine 250 mg twice daily or placebo between 1 wk and 4 mo after their index event. Treatment with ticlopidine resulted in a 30.2% relative risk reduction in stroke, MI, or vascular death (15.3% vs 10.8%, 95% CI 7.5–48.3%, $p = 0.006$). Intention-to-treat analysis found a 23.3% relative risk reduction of the combined end point ($p = 0.02$) (76). The magnitude of benefit compares favorably to aspirin therapy. The Ticlopidine Aspirin Stroke Study compared ticlopidine therapy (500 mg daily) to aspirin (1300 mg daily) in 3069 patients with recent TIA, amaurosis fugax, or stroke. The risk of nonfatal stroke or death was 17% for the ticlopidine arm and 19% for the aspirin arm at 3 yr (RRR 12%, $p = $ NS). The rate of all strokes (fatal and nonfatal) at 3 yr was 10% for ticlopidine and 13% for aspirin (RRR 21%, 95% CI 4–38%, $p = 0.024$) (77). Overall, ticlopidine seems to have slightly greater efficacy compared to aspirin therapy.

Ticlopidine, however, has a significant risk profile of side effects. Patients in CATS had a 1% incidence of severe neutropenia, and 2% incidence of skin rash and diarrhea, all of which were found to be reversible after discontinuation of ticlopidine (76). In the Ticlopidine Aspirin Stroke Study, patients treated with ticlopidine had a 20% incidence of diarrhea, a 14% incidence of skin rash, and a <1% incidence of severe neutropenia (77). Given its side-effect profile in addition to its cost, ticlopidine has not been used as a first-line agent.

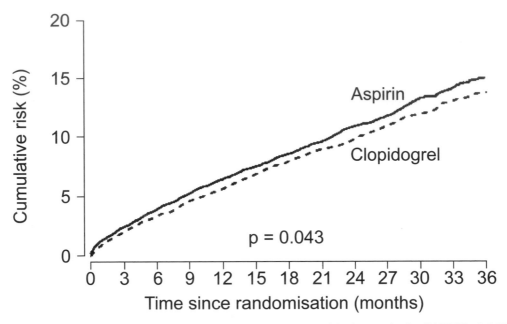

Fig. 4. Risk of adverse vascular events with clopidogrel and aspirin therapy in the CAPRIE trial. The annual rate of ischemic stroke, MI, or vascular death was reduced with clopidogrel therapy compared to aspirin therapy (5.32% vs 5.83%, RRR of 8.7%; 95% CI 0.3–16.5%, $p = 0.043$). (Reproduced with permission from ref. *78*.)

Clopidogrel

Clopidogrel is also a thienopyridine platelet antagonist that inhibits ADP-mediated platelet inhibition. It has a better side-effect profile than ticlopidine, without the incidence of neutropenia. Clopidogrel has a once daily dosing, and has supplanted ticlopidine in most settings. The largest trial of clopidogrel for secondary prevention was the Clopidogrel versus Aspirin in Patients at Risk of Ischaemic Events (CAPRIE) trial, which randomized 19,185 patients to either clopidogrel 75 mg daily or aspirin 325 mg daily. These patients had a recent ischemic stroke, recent MI, or symptomatic peripheral arterial disease. The annual rate of ischemic stroke, MI, or vascular death was 5.32% in patients treated with clopidogrel compared to 5.83% with aspirin, with a relative risk reduction of 8.7% for clopidogrel (95% CI 0.3–16.5%, $p = 0.043$) (Fig. 4). Actual treatment analysis revealed a relative reduction of 9.4% *(78)*.

In the CURE (Clopidogrel in Unstable angina to prevent Recurrent Events) study of patients presenting with acute coronary syndromes, combination therapy with aspirin and clopidogrel was shown to be more beneficial than aspirin therapy alone for reducing the number of cardiovascular events. For secondary stroke prevention, however, the benefit of combination therapy is less clear. The MATCH trial treated 7599 patients with recent ischemic stroke or TIA already on clopidogrel 75 mg daily with aspirin 75 mg daily or placebo. The primary end point was a combination of ischemic stroke, MI, vascular death, or hospitalization for acute ischemia at 18 mo. Patients treated with the combination of aspirin and clopidogrel had a nonsignificant reduction in the primary end point (6.4%, 95% CI −4.6 to 16.3%) compared to treatment with clopidogrel alone. Major and life-threatening bleeding was significantly higher in the combination therapy group, however *(79)*. The MATCH trial has been criticized for numerous reasons, including its entry criteria and its use of a composite end point. However, for stroke prevention, the combination of aspirin and clopidogrel has not been proven to be better than clopidogrel monotherapy. More recently, a study involving 100 patients undergoing CEA who were treated with aspirin and clopidogrel showed a 10-fold reduction in the number of patients having more than 20 emboli detected by TCD within 3 h of surgery (OR 10.23; 95% CI 1.3–83.3, $p = 0.01$) *(80)*.

Warfarin

Antithrombotic therapy with warfarin has not been shown to be effective in preventing recurrent stroke. In the Warfarin-Aspirin Recurrent Stroke Study (WARSS), 2206 patients presenting with ischemic stroke within 30 d were randomized to either aspirin (325 mg daily) or warfarin (INR 1.4–2.8) for >2 yr. The risk of recurrent ischemic stroke or death was 17.8% in the warfarin-treated group and 16.0% in the aspirin-treated group (hazard ratio 1.13, 95% CI 0.92–1.38, $p = 0.25$). No significant differences were found in the rates of TIA, MI, or hemorrhage (2.22 major hemorrhage/100 patient-years in the warfarin group and 1.49/100 patient-years in the aspirin group). Importantly, patients with operable carotid stenosis were excluded from this trial *(81)*. Overall, aspirin is generally preferred to warfarin for secondary prevention in patients with carotid disease. Possible exceptions are patients with thrombus in the carotid artery, critical carotid stenosis awaiting surgery, and carotid dissection in whom anticoagulation may be beneficial.

CONCLUSION

Patients with carotid artery stenosis likely have atherosclerotic disease elsewhere. Overall, the goal of therapy in these patients is not only to reduce the stroke risk attributable to the carotid stenosis, but also to decrease their global risk of cardiovascular death, MI, and stroke. To achieve this goal, therapy should focus on aggressive treatment of an individual patient's cardiovascular risk factors including hypertension, dyslipidemia, and tobacco abuse. Blood pressure reduction, even in "normotensive" patients, has a substantial impact in reducing the likelihood of stroke as well as cardiovascular death and MI. Reaching target blood pressure is likely more important than the agent used to achieve it, with notable exceptions in patients who have other indications for particular agents (e.g., ACE inhibitors in patients with congestive heart failure or diabetes mellitus). Caution should be exercised in aggressively lowering blood pressure in patients with bilateral carotid stenoses. Lipid lowering therapy, specifically statin therapy, has significant value in reducing cardiovascular risk including stroke reduction. However, the value of statin therapy in patients who have a history of cerebrovascular disease is uncertain for stroke reduction. Statin therapy should still be utilized because of its impact on overall vascular risk. Patients at high risk for vascular events will also benefit from aspirin therapy. Patients with prior stroke or TIA definitely benefit. Depending on other comorbidities, these patients may also benefit from either dipyridamole–aspirin combination therapy (patients with isolated TIAs without other significant vascular disease) or clopidogrel therapy (patients with other established vascular disease). Smoking cessation should also be advocated strongly. The value of aggressive glucose control in diabetic patients is not entirely clear for the reduction of macrovascular events. Aggressive control should still be encouraged for its favorable effect on microvascular events. In summary, although carotid revascularization is indicated for only a minority of patients with carotid atherosclerotic disease, aggressive medical therapy is indicated for all patients with carotid atherosclerotic disease.

REFERENCES

1. Beneficial effect of carotid endarterectomy in symptomatic patients with high-grade carotid stenosis. North American Symptomatic Carotid Endarterectomy Trial Collaborators. N Engl J Med 1991;325: 445–453.
2. Endarterectomy for asymptomatic carotid artery stenosis. Executive Committee for the Asymptomatic Carotid Atherosclerosis Study. JAMA 1995;273:1421–1428.
3. Barnett HJ, Taylor DW, Eliasziw M, et al. Benefit of carotid endarterectomy in patients with symptomatic moderate or severe stenosis. North American Symptomatic Carotid Endarterectomy Trial Collaborators. N Engl J Med 1998;339:1415–1425.
4. Halliday A, Mansfield A, Marro J, et al. Prevention of disabling and fatal strokes by successful carotid endarterectomy in patients without recent neurological symptoms: randomised controlled trial. Lancet 2004;363:1491–1502.
5. Wilson PW, Hoeg JM, D'Agostino RB, et al. Cumulative effects of high cholesterol levels, high blood pressure, and cigarette smoking on carotid stenosis. N Engl J Med 1997;337:516–522.
6. Mannami T, Baba S, Ogata J. Strong and significant relationships between aggregation of major coronary risk factors and the acceleration of carotid atherosclerosis in the general population of a Japanese city: the Suita Study. Arch Intern Med 2000;160:2297–2303.
7. Duncan GW, Lees RS, Ojemann RG, David SS. Concomitants of atherosclerotic carotid artery stenosis. Stroke 1977;8:665–669.
8. Bogousslavsky J, Regli F, Van Melle G. Risk factors and concomitants of internal carotid artery occlusion or stenosis. A controlled study of 159 cases. Arch Neurol 1985;42:864–867.
9. Candelise L, Bianchi F, Galligoni F, et al. Italian multicenter study on reversible cerebral ischemic attacks: III—Influence of age and risk factors on cerebrovascular atherosclerosis. Stroke 1984;15: 379–382.
10. Crouse JR, Toole JF, McKinney WM, et al. Risk factors for extracranial carotid artery atherosclerosis. Stroke 1987;18:990–996.
11. Crouse JR, 3rd, Tang R, Espeland MA, Terry JG, Morgan T, Mercuri M. Associations of extracranial carotid atherosclerosis progression with coronary status and risk factors in patients with and without coronary artery disease. Circulation 2002;106:2061–2066.
12. Lewington S, Clarke R, Qizilbash N, Peto R, Collins R. Age-specific relevance of usual blood pressure to vascular mortality: a meta-analysis of individual data for one million adults in 61 prospective studies. Lancet 2002;360:1903–1913.
13. Executive Summary of The Third Report of The National Cholesterol Education Program (NCEP) Expert Panel on Detection, Evaluation, and Treatment of High Blood Cholesterol in Adults (Adult Treatment Panel III). JAMA 2001;285:2486–2497.
14. Yadav JS, Wholey MH, Kuntz RE, et al. Protected carotid-artery stenting versus endarterectomy in high-risk patients. N Engl J Med 2004;351:1493–1501.
15. Blood pressure, cholesterol, and stroke in eastern Asia. Eastern Stroke and Coronary Heart Disease Collaborative Research Group. Lancet 1998;352:1801–1807.
16. Prevention of stroke by antihypertensive drug treatment in older persons with isolated systolic hypertension. Final results of the Systolic Hypertension in the Elderly Program (SHEP). SHEP Cooperative Research Group. JAMA 1991;265:3255–3264.
17. Collins R, Peto R, MacMahon S, et al. Blood pressure, stroke, and coronary heart disease. Part 2, Short-term reductions in blood pressure: overview of randomised drug trials in their epidemiological context. Lancet 1990;335:827–838.
18. Randomised trial of a perindopril-based blood-pressure-lowering regimen among 6,105 individuals with previous stroke or transient ischaemic attack. Lancet 2001;358:1033–1041.
19. Major outcomes in high-risk hypertensive patients randomized to angiotensin-converting enzyme inhibitor or calcium channel blocker vs diuretic: the Antihypertensive and Lipid-Lowering Treatment to Prevent Heart Attack Trial (ALLHAT). JAMA 2002;288:2981–2997.
20. Yusuf S, Sleight P, Pogue J, Bosch J, Davies R, Dagenais G. Effects of an angiotensin-converting-enzyme inhibitor, ramipril, on cardiovascular events in high-risk patients. The Heart Outcomes Prevention Evaluation Study Investigators. N Engl J Med 2000;342:145–153.
21. Svensson P, de Faire U, Sleight P, Yusuf S, Ostergren J. Comparative effects of ramipril on ambulatory and office blood pressures: a HOPE Substudy. Hypertension 2001;38:E28–E32.
22. Fox KM. Efficacy of perindopril in reduction of cardiovascular events among patients with stable coronary artery disease: randomised, double-blind, placebo-controlled, multicentre trial (the EUROPA study). Lancet 2003;362:782–788.

23. Braunwald E, Domanski MJ, Fowler SE, et al. Angiotensin-converting-enzyme inhibition in stable coronary artery disease. N Engl J Med 2004;351:2058–2068.
24. Julius S, Kjeldsen SE, Weber M, et al. Outcomes in hypertensive patients at high cardiovascular risk treated with regimens based on valsartan or amlodipine: the VALUE randomised trial. Lancet 2004; 363:2022–2031.
25. Nissen SE, Tuzcu EM, Libby P, et al. Effect of antihypertensive agents on cardiovascular events in patients with coronary disease and normal blood pressure: the CAMELOT study: a randomized controlled trial. JAMA 2004;292:2217–2225.
26. Chobanian AV, Bakris GL, Black HR, et al. The Seventh Report of the Joint National Committee on Prevention, Detection, Evaluation, and Treatment of High Blood Pressure: the JNC 7 report. JAMA 2003;289:2560–2572.
27. 2003 European Society of Hypertension-European Society of Cardiology guidelines for the management of arterial hypertension. J Hypertens 2003;21:1011–1053.
28. Rothwell PM, Howard SC, Spence JD. Relationship between blood pressure and stroke risk in patients with symptomatic carotid occlusive disease. Stroke 2003;34:2583–2590.
29. Ford CS, Crouse JR, 3rd, Howard G, Toole JF, Ball MR, Frye J. The role of plasma lipids in carotid bifurcation atherosclerosis. Ann Neurol 1985;17:301–303.
30. van Merode T, Hick P, Hoeks PG, Reneman RS. Serum HDL/total cholesterol ratio and blood pressure in asymptomatic atherosclerotic lesions of the cervical carotid arteries in men. Stroke 1985;16:34–38.
31. Johnsen SH, Mathiesen EB, Fosse E, et al. Elevated high-density lipoprotein cholesterol levels are protective against plaque progression: a follow up study of 1952 persons with carotid atherosclerosis the Tromso study. Circulation 2005;112:498–504.
32. Gorellck PB, Mazzone T. Plasma lipids and stroke. J Cardiovasc Risk 1999;6:217–221.
33. Cholesterol, diastolic blood pressure, and stroke: 13,000 strokes in 450,000 people in 45 prospective cohorts. Prospective studies collaboration. Lancet 1995;346:1647–1653.
34. Iso H, Jacobs DR, Jr., Wentworth D, Neaton JD, Cohen JD. Serum cholesterol levels and six-year mortality from stroke in 350,977 men screened for the multiple risk factor intervention trial. N Engl J Med 1989;320:904–910.
35. Tirschwell DL, Smith NL, Heckbert SR. Association of cholesterol with stroke risk varies in stroke subtypes and patient subgroups. Neurology 2004;63:1868–1875.
36. Lindenstrom E, Boysen G, Nyboe J. Influence of total cholesterol, high density lipoprotein cholesterol, and triglycerides on risk of cerebrovascular disease: the Copenhagen City Heart Study. BMJ 1994;309:11–15.
37. Amarenco P, Labreuche J, Lavallee P, Touboul PJ. Statins in stroke prevention and carotid atherosclerosis: systematic review and up-to-date meta-analysis. Stroke 2004;35:2902–2909.
38. Plehn JF, Davis BR, Sacks FM, et al. Reduction of stroke incidence after myocardial infarction with pravastatin: the Cholesterol and Recurrent Events (CARE) study. The Care Investigators. Circulation 1999;99:216–223.
39. Sever PS, Dahlof B, Poulter NR, et al. Prevention of coronary and stroke events with atorvastatin in hypertensive patients who have average or lower-than-average cholesterol concentrations, in the Anglo-Scandinavian Cardiac Outcomes Trial–Lipid Lowering Arm (ASCOT-LLA): a multicentre randomised controlled trial. Lancet 2003;361:1149–1158.
40. LaRosa JC, Grundy SM, Waters DD, et al. Intensive lipid lowering with atorvastatin in patients with stable coronary disease. N Engl J Med 2005;352:1425–1435.
41. Collins R, Armitage J, Parish S, Sleight P, Peto R. Effects of cholesterol-lowering with simvastatin on stroke and other major vascular events in 20536 people with cerebrovascular disease or other high-risk conditions. Lancet 2004;363:757–767.
42. Corvol JC, Bouzamondo A, Sirol M, Hulot JS, Sanchez P, Lechat P. Differential effects of lipid-lowering therapies on stroke prevention: a meta-analysis of randomized trials. Arch Intern Med 2003;163: 669–676.
43. Bloomfield Rubins H, Davenport J, Babikian V, et al. Reduction in stroke with gemfibrozil in men with coronary heart disease and low HDL cholesterol: the Veterans Affairs HDL Intervention Trial (VA-HIT). Circulation 2001;103:2828–2833.
44. Gertz K, Laufs U, Lindauer U, et al. Withdrawal of statin treatment abrogates stroke protection in mice. Stroke 2003;34:551–557.
45. Marti-Fabregas J, Gomis M, Arboix A, et al. Favorable outcome of ischemic stroke in patients pretreated with statins. Stroke 2004;35:1117–1121.

46. Elkind MS, Flint AC, Sciacca RR, Sacco RL. Lipid-lowering agent use at ischemic stroke onset is associated with decreased mortality. Neurology 2005;65:253–258.
47. Effect of intensive diabetes management on macrovascular events and risk factors in the Diabetes Control and Complications Trial. Am J Cardiol 1995;75:894–903.
48. Intensive blood-glucose control with sulphonylureas or insulin compared with conventional treatment and risk of complications in patients with type 2 diabetes (UKPDS 33). UK Prospective Diabetes Study (UKPDS) Group. Lancet 1998;352:837–853.
49. Tight blood pressure control and risk of macrovascular and microvascular complications in type 2 diabetes: UKPDS 38. UK Prospective Diabetes Study Group. Bmj 1998;317:703–713.
50. Wannamethee SG, Shaper AG, Whincup PH, Walker M. Smoking cessation and the risk of stroke in middle-aged men. JAMA 1995;274:155–160.
51. Kawachi I, Colditz GA, Stampfer MJ, et al. Smoking cessation and decreased risk of stroke in women. JAMA 1993;269:232–236.
52. The International Stroke Trial (IST): a randomised trial of aspirin, subcutaneous heparin, both, or neither among 19435 patients with acute ischaemic stroke. International Stroke Trial Collaborative Group. Lancet 1997;349:1569–1581.
53. CAST: randomised placebo-controlled trial of early aspirin use in 20,000 patients with acute ischaemic stroke. CAST (Chinese Acute Stroke Trial) Collaborative Group. Lancet 1997;349:1641–1649.
54. Eknoyan G, Levin N. K/DOQI Clinical Practice Guidelines for Chronic Kidney Disease: Evaluation, Classification, and Stratification. Am J Kidney Dis 2002;39:S1–246.
55. Swedish Aspirin Low-Dose Trial (SALT) of 75 mg aspirin as secondary prophylaxis after cerebrovascular ischaemic events. The SALT Collaborative Group. Lancet 1991;338:1345–1349.
56. A comparison of two doses of aspirin (30 mg vs. 283 mg a day) in patients after a transient ischemic attack or minor ischemic stroke. The Dutch TIA Trial Study Group. N Engl J Med 1991;325:1261–1266.
57. Farrell B, Godwin J, Richards S, Warlow C. The United Kingdom transient ischaemic attack (UK-TIA) aspirin trial: final results. J Neurol Neurosurg Psychiatry 1991;54:1044–1054.
58. Weisman SM, Graham DY. Evaluation of the benefits and risks of low-dose aspirin in the secondary prevention of cardiovascular and cerebrovascular events. Arch Intern Med 2002;162:2197–2202.
59. Johnson ES, Lanes SF, Wentworth CE, 3rd, Satterfield MH, Abebe BL, Dicker LW. A metaregression analysis of the dose-response effect of aspirin on stroke. Arch Intern Med 1999;159:1248–1253.
60. Hennekens CH. Update on aspirin in the treatment and prevention of cardiovascular disease. Am J Manag Care 2002;8:S691–S700.
61. Cote R, Battista RN, Abrahamowicz M, Langlois Y, Bourque F, Mackey A. Lack of effect of aspirin in asymptomatic patients with carotid bruits and substantial carotid narrowing. The Asymptomatic Cervical Bruit Study Group. Ann Intern Med 1995;123:649–655.
62. Lindblad B, Persson NH, Takolander R, Bergqvist D. Does low-dose acetylsalicylic acid prevent stroke after carotid surgery? A double-blind, placebo-controlled randomized trial. Stroke 1993;24:1125–1128.
63. Goertler M, Blaser T, Krueger S, Lutze G, Wallesch CW. Acetylsalicylic acid and microembolic events detected by transcranial Doppler in symptomatic arterial stenoses. Cerebrovasc Dis 2001;11:324–329.
64. Taylor DW, Barnett HJ, Haynes RB, et al. Low-dose and high-dose acetylsalicylic acid for patients undergoing carotid endarterectomy: a randomised controlled trial. ASA and Carotid Endarterectomy (ACE) Trial Collaborators. Lancet 1999;353:2179–2184.
65. Final report on the aspirin component of the ongoing Physicians' Health Study. Steering Committee of the Physicians' Health Study Research Group. N Engl J Med 1989;321:129–135.
66. Eidelman RS, Hebert PR, Weisman SM, Hennekens CH. An update on aspirin in the primary prevention of cardiovascular disease. Arch Intern Med 2003;163:2006–2010.
67. Iso H, Hennekens CH, Stampfer MJ, et al. Prospective study of aspirin use and risk of stroke in women. Stroke 1999;30:1764–1771.
68. Summaries for patients. Aspirin for the prevention of heart attacks in people without previous cardiovascular events: recommendations from the United States Preventive Services Task Force. Ann Intern Med 2002;136:I55.
69. Diener HC, Cunha L, Forbes C, Sivenius J, Smets P, Lowenthal A. European Stroke Prevention Study. 2. Dipyridamole and acetylsalicylic acid in the secondary prevention of stroke. J Neurol Sci 1996;143:1–13.
70. The European Stroke Prevention Study (ESPS). Principal end-points. The ESPS Group. Lancet 1987;2:1351–1354.

71. Bousser MG, Eschwege E, Haguenau M, et al. "AICLA" controlled trial of aspirin and dipyridamole in the secondary prevention of athero-thrombotic cerebral ischemia. Stroke 1983;14:5–14.
72. Persantine Aspirin Trial in cerebral ischemia. Part II: Endpoint results. The American-Canadian Co-Operative Study group. Stroke 1985;16:406–415.
73. Leonardi-Bee J, Bath PM, Bousser MG, et al. Dipyridamole for preventing recurrent ischemic stroke and other vascular events: a meta-analysis of individual patient data from randomized controlled trials. Stroke 2005;36:162–168.
74. Gibbons RJ, Abrams J, Chatterjee K, et al. ACC/AHA 2002 guideline update for the management of patients with chronic stable angina—summary article: a report of the American College of Cardiology/American Heart Association Task Force on practice guidelines (Committee on the Management of Patients With Chronic Stable Angina). J Am Coll Cardiol 2003;41:159–168.
75. Diener HC, Darius H, Bertrand-Hardy JM, Humphreys M. Cardiac safety in the European Stroke Prevention Study 2 (ESPS2). Int J Clin Pract 2001;55:162–163.
76. Gent M, Blakely JA, Easton JD, et al. The Canadian American Ticlopidine Study (CATS) in thromboembolic stroke. Lancet 1989;1:1215–1220.
77. Hass WK, Easton JD, Adams HP, Jr., et al. A randomized trial comparing ticlopidine hydrochloride with aspirin for the prevention of stroke in high-risk patients. Ticlopidine Aspirin Stroke Study Group. N Engl J Med 1989;321:501–507.
78. A randomised, blinded, trial of clopidogrel versus aspirin in patients at risk of ischaemic events (CAPRIE). CAPRIE Steering Committee. Lancet 1996;348:1329–1339.
79. Diener HC, Bogousslavsky J, Brass LM, et al. Aspirin and clopidogrel compared with clopidogrel alone after recent ischaemic stroke or transient ischaemic attack in high risk patients (MATCH): randomised, double-blind, placebo-controlled trial. Lancet 2004;364:331–337.
80. Payne DA, Jones CI, Hayes PD, et al. Beneficial effects of clopidogrel combined with aspirin in reducing cerebral emboli in patients undergoing carotid endarterectomy. Circulation 2004;109:1476–1481.
81. Mohr JP, Thompson JL, Lazar RM, et al. A comparison of warfarin and aspirin for the prevention of recurrent ischemic stroke. N Engl J Med 2001;345:1444–1451.

3

Carotid Endarterectomy

Techniques and Evidence-Based Medicine

Joël Gagnon, MD *and*
York N. Hsiang, MB ChB, MHSc, FRCSC

CONTENTS

Summary

Internal carotid artery stenosis is responsible for approx 30% of ischemic strokes. Since the beginning of the 20th century, various surgical procedures were used for the prevention of stroke. The first successful case of carotid endarterectomy (CEA) was reported by DeBakey in 1953. Since then, CEA has been continually refined and is now the gold standard procedure to prevent large-artery stroke. In this chapter we describe the procedure, and discuss the benefits and risks of CEA as compared with medical treatment.

Key Words: Carotid artery stenosis, carotid endarterectomy, ischemic stroke.

HISTORICAL BACKGROUND

Death from stroke is the third leading cause of mortality in the United States *(1)*. For survivors, stroke is an important cause of disability for patients, their families, and society. Stroke may be caused by ischemia or hemorrhage. Ischemia, from thromboembolic causes, accounts for stroke in 75% of patients and hemorrhage in 25% of stroke patients. Internal carotid artery stenosis is responsible for approx 30% of ischemic strokes *(2,3)*.

Since the beginning of the 20th century, various procedures such as the stellate ganglion block, cervical sympathectomy, thrombectomy of occluded carotid arteries, and carotid bifurcation ligation were used for the prevention of stroke. The first successful case of carotid endarterectomy (CEA) was reported by DeBakey in 1953. Since then, CEA has been continually refined and is now the gold standard procedure to prevent large-artery stroke.

From: *Contemporary Cardiology: Handbook of Complex Percutaneous Carotid Intervention*
Edited by: J. Saw, J. E. Exaire, D. S. Lee, and S. Yadav © Humana Press Inc., Totowa, NJ

Over the course of the last two decades, CEA has become the most studied surgical procedure ever *(4–16)*. The result of this intense scrutiny have provided irrefutable evidence of its safety, performance, and durability. Indications, risks, and expectations for this procedure have also been determined. As newer procedures become available, in particular carotid angioplasty and stenting, they will be compared to this gold standard. In this chapter we describe the procedure, and discuss the benefits and risks of CEA as compared with medical treatment.

TECHNIQUE

CEA is a meticulous procedure that minimizes trauma to the carotid arteries, avoids injury to the surrounding structures, and removes the offending plaque to leave a smooth interior vessel wall free of particulate debris. There are two well accepted techniques for CEA: the classical procedure and eversion endarterectomy. The results of both techniques are largely comparable in terms of stroke prevention. In this chapter, only the classical technique is described.

Anesthesia

CEA can be performed safely under local, regional, or general anesthesia. The choice of anesthesia depends on the experience of the surgeon and anesthetist, as well as patient factors. Known patient factors influencing this decision include comorbidities such as poor cardiac and pulmonary reserve, as well as local factors such as a short wide neck. In approx 10% of patients, surgery cannot be performed under local anesthesia *(17)*. This issue of anesthetic type and outcome is discussed further below.

Incision and Dissection

A thorough understanding of the anatomy of the neck, in particular, the relationship of the carotid arteries to important nerves and other organs, is essential. A 10- to 15-cm skin incision is made along the anterior border of the sternocleidomastoid muscle. The skin incision is then deepened through the subcutaneous fat and platysma muscle to expose the carotid sheath. Once the sheath is entered, the internal jugular vein is dissected and retracted to expose the carotid vessels. The common facial vein is a landmark for the carotid bifurcation where it obliquely crosses the carotid arteries to the internal jugular vein. The surgeon will then divide this vein, to allow for dissection of the carotid vessels. If necessary, the posterior belly of the digastric muscle may also be divided to allow adequate exposure of the distal internal carotid artery.

Care is taken to avoid injury to the important nerves in this area. These include the hypoglossal, vagus, and recurrent laryngeal nerves. Damage to the recurrent laryngeal nerve, a branch of the vagus nerve, may cause hoarseness from vocal cord paralysis. The hypoglossal nerve passes across the internal and external carotid arteries. Injury to this nerve causes lateral deviation of the tongue toward the ipsilateral side during protrusion and can cause difficulty with chewing and swallowing. During dissection of the carotid bifurcation, stimulation of the sinus nerve may cause a reflex vagal response resulting in bradycardia and subsequent hypotension. This reflex can be abolished by injecting the carotid sinus area with a local anesthetic. In addition, care must be taken when dissecting the carotid vessels to avoid disturbing

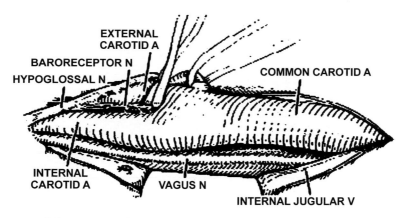

Fig. 1. Anatomy of the common, internal, and external carotid arteries. (From Brewster DC, ed: Common Problems in Vascular Surgery. Chicago: Year Book Medical, 1989.)

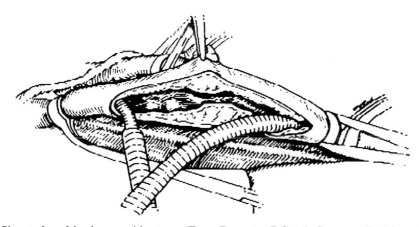

Fig. 2. Shunt placed in the carotid artery. (From Brewster DC, ed: Common Problems in Vascular Surgery. Chicago: Year Book Medical, 1989.)

the atheromatous lesions causing fragmentation and subsequent embolization and strokc.

Once the common, internal, and external carotid arteries have been dissected, isolated, and controlled with vascular loop tapes, the patient is heparinized in preparation for endarterectomy (Fig. 1).

Clamping and Shunting

Once the patient has been adequately heparinized, clamps are applied to the common, external, and internal carotid arteries. A longitudinal arteriotomy is made in the distal common carotid and extended distally into the internal carotid artery, beyond the stenosis. At this point, a decision to use a shunt is made, based on the results of intraoperative EEG monitoring, cerebral oximetry, or carotid stump back pressures. Some surgeons routinely shunt. A shunt is a hollow silicone tube that is secured to the common and internal carotid arteries to allow continuous flow to the ipsilateral cerebral hemisphere during the procedure. Total cerebral clamp time is usually monitored (Fig. 2).

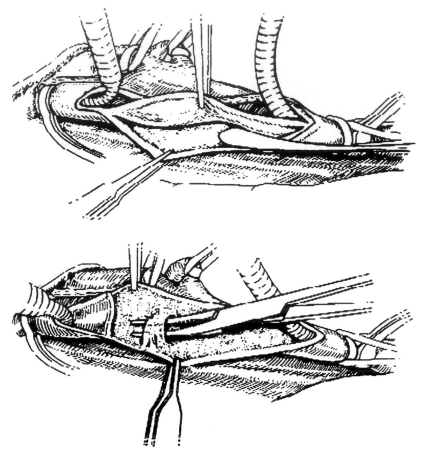

Fig. 3. Endarterectomy of the atherosclerotic plaque. (From Brewster DC, ed: Common Problems in Vascular Surgery. Chicago: Year Book Medical, 1989.)

Endarterectomy

To remove the atheromatous plaque (the endarterectomy), the optimal plane between the diseased intima is identified and separated from the deep media layer. At the distal extent of this plane, the plaque is progressively thinned out or divided (Fig. 3a and 3b).

Sutures to tack down the divided plaque may be required to prevent dissection (Fig. 4). Plaque from the external carotid artery is removed using an eversion technique. When the endarterectomy has been completed, the remaining vessel wall is irrigated with heparin saline, and any loose debris removed to yield a smooth surface.

Closure

A fine polypropylene suture is used to close the arteriotomy. Commonly, a vein or prosthetic patch may be used for arteriotomy closure to increase the diameter of the vessel, thereby decreasing the risk of early vessel thrombosis and late restenosis (Fig. 5a and 5b). If a shunt has been used, it is removed before completion of the anastomosis. Once flow has been restored, completeness of the procedure is assessed by Doppler ultrasound or completion angiography. Drains are commonly used to prevent hematoma formation.

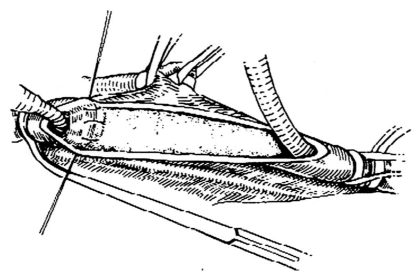

Fig. 4. Tacking stitches. (From Brewster DC, ed: Common Problems in Vascular Surgery. Chicago: Year Book Medical, 1989.)

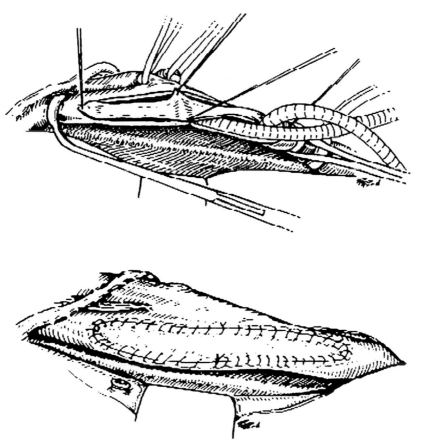

Fig. 5. Patch graft closure. (From Brewster DC, ed: Common Problems in Vascular Surgery. Chicago: Year Book Medical, 1989.)

Factors Affecting Surgical Outcome

ANESTHESIA

The issue of anesthesia affecting surgical outcome was addressed using a meta-analysis by the Cochrane database in 2004 *(17)*. Seven randomized trials with 554 operations and 41 nonrandomized trials with 25,622 operations were reviewed. The results from the randomized trials showed that there was no significant difference between local anesthesia (LA) or general anesthesia (GA) use in terms of perioperative death from all cause, any stroke, any stroke or death, or cranial nerve injury. Fewer local hemorrhages (odds ratio [OR] 0.31 [0.12–0.79]) and fewer shunts (OR 0.68 [0.40–1.14]) were needed in the LA group compared to the GA group.

The results of the nonrandomized trials showed less death (OR 0.67 [0.46–0.97]), perioperative stroke (OR 0.56 [0.44–0.70]), any stroke or death (OR 0.61 [0.48–0.77]), and fewer shunts needed (OR 0.11 [0.10–0.12]), in favor of LA. There was no difference in the frequency of local hemorrhage or cranial nerve palsies.

These results must be analyzed with caution because of the heterogeneity of the studies and the small number of patients in the randomized trials. In addition, the majority of nonrandomized trials were retrospective (29/41), and the procedures were performed with different closure techniques (patch or no patch), as well as different prognostic factors (symptomatic or asymptomatic). Based on this, the authors concluded that there was no reliable evidence to guide the choice of whether to use local or general anesthesia for CEA *(17)*.

CLOSURE/PATCH

The goal of CEA is to prevent stroke by removing the atherosclerotic plaque causing arterial stenosis. During primary closure of the arteriotomy, a stenosis may be involuntarily caused from direct suture of the vessel wall. Interposing a piece of tissue (patch) within the arteriotomy avoids this issue. Patch grafting, however, has its own minor problems such as increasing the length of the operative procedure, rupture (for vein patches), and infection (prosthetic patches). Bond et al. *(18)* reviewed the results of primary closure and patch graft closure. Their meta-analysis included 7 controlled trials, which enrolled a total of 1127 patients. The results showed that carotid patch angioplasty was associated with a reduction in the risk of stroke of any type (OR = 0.33 [0.15–0.70]), ipsilateral stroke (OR = 0.31 [0.15–0.63]), and stroke or death not only during the perioperative period (OR = 0.39 [0.20–0.78]) but also in the long term (OR = 0.59 [0.42–0.84]). It was also associated with a reduced risk of perioperative arterial occlusion (OR = 0.15 [0.06–0.37]) and decreased restenosis during long-term follow-up in five trials (OR = 0.20 [0.13–0.29]). Overall, these results support a recommendation in favor of routine patching.

SHUNT

To lower perioperative stroke, blood flow is often "shunted" from the common carotid to the distal internal carotid artery while CEA is performed. This procedure allows ipsilateral cerebral blood flow during the CEA. Shunting, however, may also be responsible for causing stroke by introducing air or plaque embolism, or cause intimal wall damage leading to dissection or acute occlusion of the internal carotid artery. In addition, intimal injury may cause premature postoperative stenosis by initiating neointimal hyperplasia.

Selective shunting has been advocated to minimize these complications. However, the important clinical question to decide which patients to shunt remains unresolved.

Many indirect methods of assessing intraoperative cerebral blood flow have been used, for example, monitoring electroencephalographic activity, somatosensory evoked potentials, measuring carotid stump back pressure, or a combination of these. Equally, direct assessments of cerebral blood flow during the operation have also been used, for example, intraarterial radiolabeled xenon, transcranial Doppler, or clinical assessment for the development of new neurological signs in awake patients who undergo the procedure under local anesthesia. None of these assessments can predict late postoperative stroke with complete certainty.

A meta-analysis by the Cochrane group (19) to analyze this issue of routine shunting included only two randomized trials. A total of 273 patients were randomized to the shunt group and 286 to the nonshunt group. The results of this meta-analysis showed a trend favoring a reduction in both deaths and strokes within 30 d of surgery when routine shunting was used, although the overall result was not significant. However, both studies were flawed. In one, the study was not truly randomized and in the other, more patching occurred in the shunt group, introducing a major bias. The conclusion of this meta-analysis was a lack of sufficient evidence to support the use of routine or selective shunting in CEA.

Our group reported on a retrospective study of 305 patients, 92 of whom were routinely shunted and 213 who were selectively shunted based on EEG monitoring. The incidence of major strokes in the routine shunt group was significantly higher than in the selective shunt group, 4.4% vs 0.5%, $p < 0.05$ (20).

Complications

Stroke and acute coronary events are the most feared complications after CEA. The risk of perioperative stroke varies with the indication for surgery, age of the patient, and skill of the surgeon. The best reported series of perioperative stroke ranges from 1% for an asymptomatic stenosis to 9.6% for a completed stroke. Community-based surveys show that the risk of stroke is higher than in tertiary care institutions, with rates ranging from 5.6% for an asymptomatic stenosis to 21% for a completed stroke (21).

Cardiac complications (myocardial infarction [MI], arrhythmia, and congestive heart failure) occurred in 3.9% of patients in the NASCET study (5). For older or higher-risk patients, the incidence of cardiac complications may be even higher.

Other important complications are wound infection, hematoma, and cranial nerve injury. The rates of these are shown in Table 1. Usually, cranial nerve injuries are transient and improve over time. In our own experience, we reported a lower incidence of acute MI (0.7%), wound hematoma (2.3%), wound infection (0.3%), and cranial nerve injury (6%) (20).

Recurrent (>50%) stenosis following CEA is relatively frequent based on regular carotid duplex ultrasound follow-up. At 3 years post-CEA, the incidence is approx 10% and increases to 13% by 5 yr (22,23). However, the clinical significance of recurrent stenosis demonstrated by ultrasound is much less. In fact, the 5-yr ipsilateral stroke-free rate was the same in patients with or without internal carotid restenosis, 94.4% and 94.2%, respectively (23).

CEA is a durable procedure. The prognosis of future ipsilateral stroke varies according to the age of the patient and the original indication for surgery. The annual risk of stroke after an uncomplicated CEA for patients presenting with asymptomatic carotid stenosis, transient ischemic attacks (TIAs), and for completed stroke is 1.0%, 2.3%, and 4.5%, respectively (21).

Table 1
Perioperative Complications Within 30 d
of Carotid Endarterectomy

Complication	Percentage
Cardiac	
Myocardial infarction	0.9
Congestive heart failure	0.6
Arrhythmia	1.2
Other	1.2
Wound	
Hematoma	5.5
Infection	3.4
Cranial nerve injury	7.6

RESULTS OF RANDOMIZED CLINICAL TRIALS

As CEA became refined, many authors demonstrated its safety, effectiveness, and durability. The popularity of this procedure continued to grow as an important method of stroke prevention, despite reports of poor results, especially when reported in larger databases such as statewide surveys. Because of the concern that widespread application of this technique would lead to greater harm than good, randomized controlled clinical trials were recommended as the definitive method of addressing the value of CEA.

The trials comparing CEA to medical treatment have focused on a patient's original *symptoms* and the *degree of stenosis*. Using this convention, the trials can be categorized as symptomatic or asymptomatic. Regarding the degree of stenosis, there has been no uniform method of measuring stenosis between trials. Initially, all studies required the gold standard diagnostic test, carotid angiography. Because of the demonstrated accuracy of ultrasound in high-quality departments, and the lack of morbidity, more contemporary studies have occasionally used the results of ultrasound instead of angiography. Despite these differences, trials have concentrated on the effect of CEA on carotid stenosis, usually >50% stenosis.

Trials of Symptomatic Carotid Stenosis

The indication for CEA in symptomatic stenosis is based on the results of three prospective randomized trials.

The first published study, the VA symptomatic trial, randomized 189 men over 5 yr who had symptomatic internal carotid stenosis >50% to either medical treatment or medical treatment plus CEA *(4)*. After a median follow-up of 11.9 mo, this study showed that the risk of stroke or further TIAs was 7.7% in the surgical and 19.4% in the medical group ($p = 0.011$). Further, the benefit of CEA for patients with >70% stenosis was even greater: Patients randomized to CEA had a combined stroke and TIA risk of 7.9% compared with 25.6% in the medical group ($p = 0.004$). This study was criticized because of the small number of patients enrolled; it excluded female patients; and the composite end point of death, stroke, and TIA deviated from the more traditional end point of stroke and death.

The North American Symptomatic Carotid Endarterectomy Trial (NASCET) was a landmark study, randomizing 659 patients to either medical treatment (aspirin ≤1300 mg daily) or medical treatment plus CEA for symptomatic carotid artery stenosis (5). All eligible patients needed to have had a symptomatic event (TIA, stroke, or amaurosis) within 90 d prior to randomization. After only 18 mo, the study was prematurely stopped because of the clear evidence that surgery was superior to medical treatment in symptomatic patients who had an angiographically proven stenosis of 70–99%. The 2-yr risk of ipsilateral stroke was 9% in the surgical group and 26% in the medical group ($p < 0.001$). Moreover, the number of patients needed to be treated (NNT) to prevent another stroke was 6.

Lesser degrees of stenosis were addressed in a later study published by the NASCET investigators in 1998 (6). In a subset of 2267 patients, they showed that for stenosis between 50% and 69%, the 5-yr risk of ipsilateral stroke was 15.7% for CEA plus medical therapy, and 22.2% for medical therapy alone ($p = 0.045$). The NNT was 15. Conversely, for stenosis <50%, the 5-yr risk of ipsilateral stroke was 14.9% for surgery and 18.7% for medical therapy ($p = 0.16$, NS).

The reported results by European surgeons supported the findings described by NASCET. In the European Carotid Stenosis Trial (ECST), 778 patients with severe (70–99%) internal carotid artery stenosis were randomized over 10 yr to either best medical therapy or medical therapy plus CEA. For severe stenosis (80–100%), the 3-yr risk of ipsilateral stroke was 6.8% for CEA and 20.6% for best medical therapy ($p < 0.0001$). For lesser degrees of stenosis, there was no benefit of CEA over medical treatment for mild (0–29%) and moderate (30–69%) stenosis.

Although the results were similar to NASCET, there was a difference in the way carotid stenosis was measured angiographically (7–9). In the ECST study, the estimated degree of stenosis was more conservative than the method of determining carotid artery stenosis used by NASCET. Accordingly, a 70–99% stenosis according to the ECST method corresponded to a NASCET measurement of 50–69%.

In summary, the results of these three trials delineated the indications for CEA in symptomatic patients. In patients with 70–99% stenosis, CEA was highly beneficial. For patients with 50–69% stenosis, the procedure was moderately beneficial. However, for patients with <50% carotid stenosis, the procedure was no better than medical therapy alone. Table 2 summarizes the findings from these three trials.

Trials of Asymptomatic Carotid Stenosis

The recommendation of CEA in asymptomatic stenosis is based on the results of five randomized trials.

The carotid surgery vs medical therapy in asymptomatic carotid stenosis (CASANOVA) trial was the first to address this problem (10). Four hundred and ten patients with an internal carotid artery stenosis between 50% and 90% were randomized to either group A or group B. In group A, patients were operated on unilaterally if they had a unilateral stenosis and bilaterally if they had bilateral stenosis. Patients enrolled in group B with bilateral stenosis were operated on the more stenotic side. All patients received acetylsalicylic acid and dipyridamole. After 3 yr, the risk of stroke and death was 10.7% in group A and 11.3% in group B ($p = $ NS). This trial was criticized for many methodologic faults. For example, patients with a known carotid stenosis >90% were excluded and were referred for surgical treatment. During the trial, surgical treatment was offered to the medical group if the degree of carotid stenosis progressed to >90%, if patients developed bilateral carotid stenosis >50%, or if they developed hemispheric TIAs. In total, 118 of a total of 204 medical patients crossed over to the surgical group.

The Mayo Clinic asymptomatic carotid endarterectomy trial was a small study and randomized only 71 patients to either CEA without aspirin or medical therapy (aspirin) *(11)*. Notably, this study was terminated prematurely because of a significantly higher MI rate in the surgical group. MI occurred in 8 of 36 (22.2%) patients in the surgical arm compared with none in the medical arm ($p = 0.0037$). This study demonstrated the importance of antiplatelet therapy in surgical patients.

The VA asymptomatic trial was a prospective randomized study of men with an asymptomatic carotid stenosis of at least 50% or more, as shown by angiography *(12)*. Four hundred and forty-four men were assigned to either medical treatment, aspirin 650 mg twice daily, or surgical treatment plus the same medical treatment. The rate of stroke was 4.7% in the surgical group and 9.4% in the medical group ($p = 0.056$). However, the combined incidence of ipsilateral neurologic events was 8% in the surgical arm and 20.6% in the medical arm ($p < 0.001$). In summary, the VA asymptomatic trial demonstrated that men with asymptomatic internal carotid stenosis >50% benefited by having CEA to reduce ipsilateral neurologic events (TIAs plus stroke).

The Asymptomatic Carotid Endarterectomy Study (ACAS) was the largest North America trial comparing CEA with medical treatment for stroke prevention in patients with asymptomatic carotid artery stenosis *(13)*. A total of 1662 patients with angiographically determined (using the NASCET method) asymptomatic internal carotid stenosis >60% were randomized to either medical treatment or medical treatment plus CEA. The stenosis was confirmed by angiography, primarily in the surgical arm. Both arms received aspirin 325 mg daily. After a mean follow-up of 2.5 yr, the 5-yr risk of ipsilateral stroke by the Kaplan–Meier projection was 5.1% in the surgery arm and 11% in the medical arm ($p = 0.004$). This represented a relative risk and absolute risk reduction of 53% and 5.9%, respectively. The NNT was 19. Although both men and women were entered into the study, the relative risk reduction was 66% in men and 17% in women. This suggested that CEA was more beneficial for men than women who had asymptomatic carotid stenosis. These results were based on a very low perioperative complication rate of only 2.3% and perioperative death rate of 0.1%. In summary, ACAS showed that patients with asymptomatic internal carotid stenosis >60% benefited from CEA by reducing stroke risk. The benefit was more evident in men than in women.

Finally, the United Kingdom Medical Research Council sponsored Asymptomatic Carotid Surgery Trial (ACST) conclusively defined the role of surgery for patients with asymptomatic carotid stenosis *(14)*. This was the largest carotid surgery trial. A total of 3120 patients with asymptomatic internal carotid stenosis >60% by ultrasonography (angiography during first few years of the study, but later angiography was not an ACST requirement) were randomized to either medical therapy or medical therapy plus CEA. After a follow-up of 10 yr, the 5-yr stroke risk was 6.4% in the surgical arm and 11.8% in the medical arm ($p < 0.001$). These significant benefits applied equally to men and women, for those younger than 65 yr and for those 65–74 yr of age. The risk of stroke or death within 30 d of surgery was 3.1%. In summary, this study showed that patients younger than 75 yr old with an internal carotid artery stenosis >70% benefited with surgical treatment by lowering the relative risk of stroke by 50%. The results of these trials are summarized in Table 3.

Table 2
Summary of Symptomatic Controlled, Randomized Trials

Trial	No. of pts.	% Women	Method of assessment	Length F/U	Stroke		RRR (%)	ARR (%)	NNT	Year of risk	p
					Surgical	Medical					
VA	189	0	Angio	11.9	7.7[c]	19.4[a]	60.3	11.7	9	0.99	0.011
NASCET I	659	32	Angio	18	15.8[b]	32.3[b]	51.1	16.5	6	2	<0.001
NASCET II	2226	29	Angio	5 y	33.2[b]	43.3[b]	23.3	10.1	10	5	0.005
ECST	3024	28	Angio	6.1	14.9[c]	26.5[c]	43.8	11.6	9	3	0.001

[a]Ipsilateral stroke or crescendo TIAs.
[b]Any stroke/death.
[c]Major stroke/death.
ARR, Absolute risk reduction; NNT, number needed to treat; RRR, relative risk reduction.

Table 3
Summary of Asymptomatic Controlled, Randomized Trials

Trial	No. of pts.	% Women	Method of assessment	Length F/U	Stroke/Death		RRR (%)	ARR (%)	NNT	Year of risk	p
					Surgical	Medical					
VA	444	0	Angio	47.9 m	41.2[b]	44.2[b]	6.8	3.0	33	4	NS
ACAS	1662	34	Angio	2.7 y	5.1[b]	11.0[b]	53.6	5.9	17	5	0.004
ACST	3120	34	Angio & U.S	3.4 y	6.4[b]	11.8[b]	45.8	5.4	19	5	<0.0001

[a]Ipsilateral stroke or crescendo TIAs.
[b]Any stroke/death.
[c]Major stroke/death.
ARR, absolute risk reduction; NNT, number needed to treat; RRR, relative risk reduction.

SURGICAL INDICATIONS AND CONTRAINDICATIONS

The indications and contraindications of CEA are based on the results of the randomized controlled studies conducted over the last two decades. In essence, they are the summary of the natural history of carotid stenosis, the skill of the surgical team, and specific patient factors. By carefully observing patients, the natural history of both symptomatic and asymptomatic carotid stenosis has now been well determined. In the presence of a high-grade (>70%) stenosis, a symptomatic lesion is associated with a 13% annual stroke risk. Moderate carotid stenosis is associated with a lower annual stroke risk of 5%. Asymptomatic lesions carry the lowest annual stroke risk, 2%. Thus, an effective procedure requires surgical skill that is much better than the natural history of untreated carotid stenosis. Based on the very good results achieved by the trialist surgeons, the recommended surgical performance should be a perioperative stroke and death rate of <6% for symptomatic and <3% for asymptomatic lesions, in order to achieve the same efficacious results. Surgical results outside of these requirements negates the benefit of CEA for these patients.

In addition to the degree of carotid stenosis, other risk factors that favor intervention include male gender, hemispheric as opposed to retinal presentation, a stroke as opposed to TIA, plaque ulceration, contralateral carotid occlusion, intraluminal thrombus, the presence of intracranial atherosclerosis, the absence of collateral pathways to the distal internal carotid artery, and the presence of white-matter changes on brain CT scanning *(24)*.

Despite the positive findings from the asymptomatic trials, in practice, the role of CEA for asymptomatic stenosis is more controversial than for symptomatic stenosis. The reasons for the controversy are the low natural history of stroke in asymptomatic patients and whether the results achieved by the trialist surgeons can be reproduced in standard clinical practice. Nonetheless, some factors increase the risk of stroke, which may require consideration on an individual basis. These include male sex, higher degrees of stenosis, ipsilateral brain infarction on CT or MRI, plaque ulceration, presence of an occluded contralateral carotid artery, stenosis that progresses over time, an echolucent or heterogeneous plaque, or evidence of intraplaque hemorrhage on ultrasound *(25)*.

Contraindications for CEA include patients with unstable medical (e.g., unstable angina, recent MI, and uncontrolled congestive heart failure) or unstable neurologic (e.g., recent large cerebral infarction, hemorrhagic brain infarction, progressive stroke, decreased level of consciousness) status, and surgically inaccessible lesions. Unstable medical patients and those with inaccessible lesions may be the optimal patients for new lower risk technologies, for example, angioplasty and stenting.

CONCLUSION

Carotid endarterectomy is the most studied surgical procedure ever. Originally described in 1954, this procedure has been carefully scrutinized over the past two decades. Eight prospective randomized clinical trials (three for symptomatic patients and five for asymptomatic patients) have been done. The results of these studies have conclusively shown the benefit of this procedure in the hands of skilled surgeons for patients with symptoms and a carotid stenosis of >50%, or in asymptomatic carotid stenosis >60%. Although it is currently recognized as the gold standard treatment, the emergence of new techniques to treat carotid artery disease, namely carotid angioplasty and stenting, may well alter the role of carotid endarterectomy in the future. There are presently several ongoing randomized clinical trials examining this issue.

REFERENCES

1. CDC database (2003), http://www.cdc.gov/nchs/products/pubs/pubd/hus/trendtables.htm.
2. Barnett HJ, Gunton RW, Eliaszim M, Fleming L, Sharpe B, Gates P, Meldrum H. Causes and severity of ischemic stroke in patients with internal carotid artery stenosis. JAMA 2000;283:1429–1436.
3. Dodick DW, Meissner I, Meyer FB, Cloft HJ. Evaluation and management of asymptomatic carotid artery stenosis. Mayo Clin Proc 2004;79:937–944.
4. Mayberg MR, Wilson SE, Yatsu F, et al. Carotid endarterectomy and prevention of cerebral ischemia from symptomatic carotid stenosis. JAMA 1991;266:3289–3294.
5. North American Symptomatic Carotid Endarterectomy Trial Collaborators. Beneficial effect of carotid endarterectomy in symptomatic patients with high-grade stenosis. N Engl J Med 1991;325:445–453.
6. Barnett HJ, Taylor DW, Eliasziw M, et al. Benefit of carotid endarterectomy in patients with symptomatic moderate to severe stenosis: North American Symptomatic Carotid Endarterectomy Trial Collaborators. N Engl J Med 1998;339:1415–1425.
7. European Carotid Surgery Trialist's Collaborative Group. European Carotid Surgery Trial: interim results for symptomatic patients with severe (70%–99%) or with mild (0%–29%) carotid stenosis. Lancet 1991;337:1235–1243.
8. European Carotid Surgery Trialists's Collaborative Group. Endarterectomy for moderate symptomatic carotid stenosis: interim results from the MRC European Carotid surgery Trial. Lancet 1996;347. 1591–1593.
9. Randomised trial of endarterectomy for recently symptomatic carotid stenosis: final results of the MRC European Carotid Surgery Trial (ECST). Lancet 1998;351:1379–1387.
10. CASANOVA Study Group. Carotid surgery versus medical therapy in asymptomatic carotid stenosis. Stroke 1991;22:1229–1235.
11. Mayo Asymptomatic Carotid Endarterectomy Study group. Results of a randomised controlled trial of carotid endarterectomy for asymptomatic carotid stenosis. Mayo Clin Proc 1992;67:513–518.
12. Hobson R, Weiss D, Fields W, et al. Efficacy of carotid endarterectomy for asymptomatic carotid stenosis. N Engl J Med 1993;328:221–227.
13. Executive Committee for Asymptomatic Carotid Atherosclerosis Study. Endarterectomy for asymptomatic carotid artery stenosis. JAMA 1995;273:1421–1428.
14. MRC Asymptomatic Carotid Surgery Trial (ACST) Collaborative Group. Prevention of disabling and fatal strokes by successful carotid endarterectomy in patients without recent neurological symptoms: randomised controlled trial. Lancet 2004;363:1491–1502.
15. Rothwell PM, Eliasziw M, Gutnikov SA, et al. Analysis of pooled data from the randomised controlled trials of endarterectomy for symptomatic stenosis. Lancet 2003;361:107–116.
16. Mayberg MR. Carotid artery disease: from knife to stent. Cleve Clin J Med 2004;71 (Suppl 1):S42–S44.
17. Rerkasem K, Bond R, Rothwell PM. Local versus general anaesthesia for carotid endarterectomy [Review] Cochrane Database of Systematic Reviews 2004;2:CD000126.
18. Bond R, Rerkasem K, AbuRahma AF, Naylor AR, Rothwell PM. Patch angioplasty versus primary closure for carotid endarterectomy [Review] Cochrane Database of Systematic Reviews 2004; 2:CD000160.
19. Bond R, Rerkasem K, Rothwell PM. Routine or selective carotid artery shunting for carotid endarterectomy (and different methods of monitoring in selective shunting) Cochrane Database of Systematic Reviews 2004;2:CD000190.
20. Salvian AJ, Taylor DC, Hsiang YN, et al. Selective shunting with EEG monitoring is safer than routine shunting for carotid endarterectomy. Cardiovasc Surg 1997;5:481–485.
21. Taylor LM, Porter JM. Basic data related to carotid endarterectomy. Ann Vasc Surg 1986;1:264–266.
22. Ricotta JJ, O'Brien-Irr MS. Conservative management of residual and recurrent lesions after carotid endarterectomy: long-term results. J Vasc Surg 1997;26:963–970.
23. Mattos MA, Van Bemmelen PS, Barkmeier ID, et al. Routine surveillance after carotid endarterectomy: does it affect clinical management? J Vasc Surg 1993;17:819–830.
24. Findlay JM, Marchak BE, Pelz DM, Feasby TE. Carotid endarterectomy: a review. Can J Neurol Sci 2004;31:22–36.
25. Barnett HJM, Meldrum HE, Eliasziw M. The appropriate use of carotid endarterectomy. Can Med Assoc J 2002;166:1169–1179.

4 Carotid Angioplasty and Stenting Trials

A Historical Perspective and Evidence-Based Medicine

David S. Lee, MD *and Jay S. Yadav,* MD

CONTENTS

Summary

The goal of treatment of carotid artery stenosis is to prevent stroke and death. Stroke is the third leading cause of death in the United States. This chapter focuses on the evidence supporting the use of carotid artery stenting for treatment of carotid artery stenosis. The data supporting carotid angioplasty and stenting have been primarily observational registries and a few randomized controlled trials comparing carotid angioplasty and stenting to carotid endarterectomy. No trial has compared carotid angioplasty and stenting to medical therapy.

Key Words: Carotid artery stenosis, carotid artery stenting, carotid endarterectomy.

INTRODUCTION

This chapter focuses on the evidence supporting the use of carotid artery stenting (CAS) to treat carotid artery stenosis. The goal of any treatment for carotid stenosis is to prevent stroke and death. Stroke is the third leading cause of death in the United States *(1,2)*. One quarter of stroke survivors eventually will have another event. Half of the survivors will be deceased by 5 yr after the index event, and a substantial proportion of those alive will be disabled *(3)*. Because the treatment of acute stroke is currently limited with few options and a narrow temporal window, the primary focus continues to be on stroke prevention. The most effective means to achieve this goal have been aggressive treatment of hypertension, antithrombotic therapy for atrial fibrillation, and carotid revascularization. Currently, the standard of care for carotid revascularization is surgical carotid endarterectomy (CEA).

From: *Contemporary Cardiology: Handbook of Complex Percutaneous Carotid Intervention*
Edited by: J. Saw, J. E. Exaire, D. S. Lee, and S. Yadav © Humana Press Inc., Totowa, NJ

For any carotid revascularization treatment to be evaluated, the risk of the procedure and the procedure's impact on long-term risk must be compared to the long-term risk from best alternative therapy. For almost any intervention, an up-front risk is taken for the long-term benefit that accrues. The data supporting carotid angioplasty and stenting have been primarily observational registries and a few randomized controlled trials comparing carotid angioplasty and stenting to CEA. No trial has compared carotid angioplasty and stenting to medical therapy. The historical context is important to understand how carotid intervention has evolved and the types of trials that have been performed.

Chiari and later Hunt described the association of carotid occlusion and disease to stroke in the early 20th century. Eastcott performed the first successful surgical removal of an area of carotid stenosis and reconstruction of the carotid artery in 1954 *(4,5)*. Following this, anecdotal case reports and series continued to be reported about the potential benefit of carotid revascularization, and in the mid-1970s to early 1980s, CEA became the standard of care with hundreds of thousands of cases performed *(6)*. Data in the mid-1980s suggested that the complication rates for CEA were much higher than previously thought. For example, Brott et al. analyzed all CEA performed in the Cincinnati area in 1980, half of which were done in asymptomatic patients. The perioperative mortality was 2.8% and the perioperative stroke was 8.6%. The stroke rate was significantly higher in symptomatic vs asymptomatic patients (11.6% vs 5.6%, $p < 0.05$) *(7)*. This report and others like it dampened the enthusiasm for CEA and the number of procedures performed dropped in the late 1980s *(8)*. Finally, in 1991, more than 37 yr after the procedure was first performed, the first major randomized trial results comparing CEA to medical therapy (the NASCET trial) were reported.

REVIEW OF CAROTID ENDARTERECTOMY TRIALS

NASCET

The North American Symptomatic Carotid Endarterectomy Trial (NASCET) enrolled 659 patients with a symptomatic carotid stenosis of 70–99% and a nondisabling stroke, transient ischemic attack (TIA), or amaurosis fugax within 120 d and randomized them to either CEA or medical therapy. This trial was stopped prematurely because of the significant benefit seen in the surgical arm. At 30 d, patients treated with CEA had higher event rates than those treated medically as a result of the perioperative risk of the procedure. The 30-d risk of stroke and/or death was 5.8% in CEA-treated patients vs 3.3% in medically treated patients. Patients undergoing CEA also had a 0.9% risk of myocardial infarction (MI). At 2 yr, however, the risk of ipsilateral stroke was significantly decreased in CEA-treated patients (9% vs 26%, $p < 0.001$) with an absolute risk reduction of 17% (Fig. 1). The reduction in the risk of major or fatal ipsilateral strokes was even more striking (2.5% vs 13.1%, $p < 0.001$). The benefit was stratified by the degree of stenosis, with patients with 90–99% stenosis having the greatest absolute risk reduction and patients with 70–79% stenosis having the least (26% vs 12%) *(9)*.

The NASCET trial also recruited 2226 patients with less severe stenosis (30–69%) and a nondisabling stroke, TIA, or amaurosis fugax within 120 d and randomized them to either CEA or medical therapy. At 5 yr, for patients with 50–69% stenosis, the risk of any ipsilateral stroke was 15.7% for CEA and 22.2% for medical therapy ($p < 0.045$) (Fig. 1). This benefit was much less compelling with an absolute risk reduction of 6.5% over 5 yr or 1.3% per year compared to an absolute risk reduction of 17% over 2 yr or 8.5% per year for patients with 70–99% stenosis. No statistically significant improvement in the

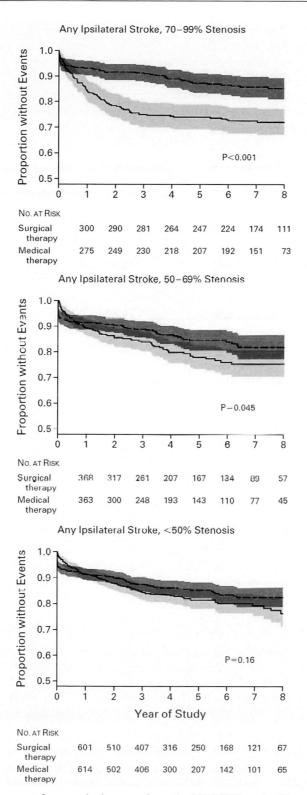

Fig. 1. Kaplan-Meier event-free survival curves from the NASCET study. (Reproduced with permission from ref. 9.)

ipsilateral stroke risk was seen in patients with <50% stenosis. At 5 yr, the risk of any ipsilateral stroke was 14.9% for CEA and 18.7% for medical therapy *(10)*.

While NASCET and several other trials including ECST provided compelling evidence for the use of CEA to treat symptomatic patients with severe stenosis, the value of treating asymptomatic patients was uncertain until the publication of ACAS in 1995. Other trials were published before ACAS but were limited by methodological flaws and a lack of acceptance. At the time of its publication, ACAS was the largest, best-designed trial to address the utility of CEA in asymptomatic patients.

ACAS

The Asymptomatic Carotid Atherosclerosis Study (ACAS) trial enrolled 1662 patients with asymptomatic carotid stenosis ≥60% and randomized them to CEA or medical therapy. The perioperative mortality rate was 0.1% while the perioperative stroke or death rate was 2.3%. The reported outcome was an actuarial estimate of 5-yr risk with median 2.7-yr follow-up. The risk of any ipsilateral stroke or perioperative stroke/death was reduced in the CEA cohort (5.1% vs 11%, $p = 0.004$) with an absolute risk reduction of 5.9% at 5 yr *(11)*. The risk of major ipsilateral stroke or perioperative stroke/death was not significantly reduced with CEA (3.4% vs 6%). ACAS also found that the benefit of CEA was not as great in women compared to men (absolute risk reduction of 1.4% vs 8%). The benefit of CEA in women was not statistically significant. The reasons for this were not clear. Further, unlike in symptomatic stenosis, no gradation between severity of stenosis and magnitude of benefit with CEA was clearly demonstrated *(11)*. Regardless of any criticisms, the ACAS trial was the basis for the treatment of asymptomatic patients, and its results were confirmed with the publication of ACST in 2004.

ACST

The Asymptomatic Carotid Surgery Trial (ACST) was the most contemporary and largest trial of CEA in asymptomatic patients. In this study, 3120 patients with carotid stenosis ≥60% by duplex ultrasound evaluation were randomized to either immediate CEA or deferral of endarterectomy until a specific indication for it arose. Half of the patients in the immediate CEA arm had surgery within 1 mo and nearly 90% by 1 yr. The rate of surgery in the deferred arm was approx 4% annually. The primary end point was perioperative death, stroke, or MI and long-term stroke. The CEA treated cohort had a perioperative stroke or death rate of 3.1% at 30 d. The 5-yr risk for all strokes and perioperative death was reduced with immediate CEA (6.4% vs 11.8%) (Fig. 2). The rate of major stroke or fatal stroke was also decreased (3.5% vs 6.1%). Subgroup analysis revealed a benefit for immediate CEA for both men and women, although the benefit was not as significant for women as for men. Insufficient numbers of patients older than 75 yr of age were enrolled, so conclusions about its benefit in this cohort are unclear *(12)*.

Recommendations for Carotid Revascularization

Overall, the data suggested that the greatest benefit of surgical carotid revascularization occurred in symptomatic patients with 70–99% stenosis, with some benefit in symptomatic patients with 50–69% stenosis and in asymptomatic patients with 60–99% stenosis. The effect on overall outcomes is impacted heavily by perioperative risk. In ACST, for example, even with a 3.1% rate of perioperative stroke or death, it still took 2 yr for a net benefit in stroke reduction to emerge with CEA. Therefore, the American Heart Association (AHA) recommended that symptomatic patients meeting criteria

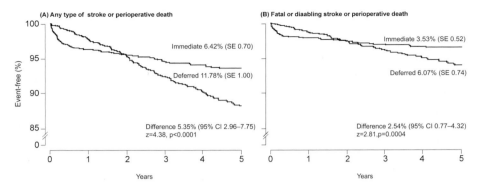

Fig. 2. Kaplan-Meier event-free survival curves from the ACST study. (Reproduced with permission from ref. *12.*)

Table 1
Exclusion Criteria for NASCET and ACAS

Medical exclusion criteria	Anatomic exclusion criteria
Age >79 yr	Prior ipsilateral endarterectomy
Unstable angina	Tandem lesions
Recent myocardial infarction (within	Contralateral occlusion
6 mo)	Total occlusion
Cardiac valvular or rhythm abnormality	Prior contralateral endarterectomy
likely to cause embolic cerebrovascular	within 4 mo
events	
Uncontrolled hypertension	
Uncontrolled diabetes mellitus	
Renal failure	
Liver failure	
Severe lung condition	
Major surgery within the past month	
Prior severe stroke	
Progressing neurological symptoms	

should undergo CEA if their perioperative stroke or death risk was <6% *(13)*. For asymptomatic patients, the AHA recommended that the perioperative risk should be <3% *(13)*. While these benchmarks were based on clinical trials, it is notable that many patients were excluded from these studies.

Patient Exclusion from CEA Trials

The exclusion criteria of NASCET and ACAS can be divided into high-risk clinical criteria and high-risk anatomic criteria (Table 1). Medical criteria included age >79 yr, unstable angina, recent MI (within past 6 mo), cardiac valvular or rhythm abnormality likely to cause embolic cerebrovascular events, uncontrolled hypertension, uncontrolled diabetes mellitus, renal failure, liver failure, severe lung condition, major surgery within the past month, prior severe stroke, or progressing neurologic symptoms. Anatomic criteria included prior ipsilateral endarterectomy, tandem lesions, contralateral occlusion, total occlusion, or prior contralateral endarterectomy within 4 mo.

The 30-d mortality in the most frequently quoted clinical trials were very low, 0.1% in ACAS and 0.6% in NASCET. Wennberg et al. studied 113,000 Medicare patients in 1992–93 who underwent CEA. Perioperative mortality was 1.4% at trial hospitals (institutions participating in NASCET and ACAS). At nontrial hospitals (all other hospitals performing CEA), mortality correlated with the number of CEA performed: high volume 1.7%, average volume 1.9%, and low volume 2.5% (*p* for trend <0.001). In multivariate modeling, patients who had their procedures at trial hospitals had a 25% reduction in mortality compared with average volume hospitals, and there was a 43% reduction in mortality compared with low-volume hospitals *(14)*. This suggests that the institution at which the surgery is performed and the experience of the surgeon were important factors in determining outcome. Even at hospitals that participated in ACAS and NASCET, however, the perioperative mortality was still strikingly higher than what was reported in these trials. This finding is likely due to the stringent exclusion criteria in these trials, and that "real world" experience likely reflected a more diverse and higher-risk population of patients who underwent this procedure.

Patients at High Risk for CEA

These higher-risk cohort of patients were never studied in randomized clinical trials (with the exception of SAPPHIRE; see below) but several registries and observational series have evaluated outcomes in these patients. In one retrospective analysis of >1100 patients undergoing CEA at 12 academic centers in the United States, the rates of death/stroke/MI were 6.9% in all patients, 9.5% in patients with symptomatic disease, 9.9% in patients with a history of angina, and 11.8% in patients older than 75 yr of age. In fact, having at least two high-risk criteria was associated with a nearly twofold increase in risk *(15)*. Ouriel et al. reported the 10-yr experience in >3100 CEA from the Cleveland Clinic. Patients were considered high risk if they had significant medical comorbidities—coronary disease with revascularization within 6 mo prior to CEA, history of congestive heart failure (CHF), severe obstructive lung disease, or renal insufficiency. High-risk patients had a greater than 2.5-fold higher risk of in-hospital death or stroke than low risk patients (2.9% vs 7.4%, *p* < 0.0005) *(16)*. In multiple series, several high-risk factors have become evident including age >75 yr, concomitant coronary disease requiring bypass surgery, CHF, and renal insufficiency. The risk in patients with contralateral occlusion and with prior CEA and restenosis was also higher *(17,18)*.

More recently, some of these high-risk criteria have been criticized, and several series have reported acceptable surgical risk in elderly patients as well as patients with coronary artery disease and other high-risk features *(19,20)*. As these discordant studies are being evaluated, several important considerations must be kept in mind. Rothwell et al. performed a systematic review of CEA in >16,000 symptomatic patients between 1980 and 1995. Overall, the risk of death was 1.62%, and the risk of stroke and/or death was 5.6%. However, there was significant study variability in the risk of stroke and death depending on the methodology of the study. Studies in which a neurologist assessed patients after surgery had the highest risk of stroke and/or death (7.7%; 95% CI, 5.0–10.2) while studies with a single surgeon author had the lowest risk (2.3%; 95% CI, 1.8–2.7) *(21)*. These results speak to the need for uniform, independent follow-up to ensure no bias in the reporting of events. Notably, nearly all major carotid stenting trials and registries in the United States have had independent neurologist adjudication of stroke events.

Complications Associated with CEA

Carotid endarterectomy was also associated with other complications beyond stroke or death. In NASCET, nearly 9% of patients suffered cranial nerve palsy. In addition, hemorrhage and infection at the surgical site complicated the hospital course in nearly 9% of patients *(22)*. An analysis of NASCET also revealed a 8.1% medical complication rate of various cardiac, pulmonary, infectious, and other complications, which usually resolved but did prolong hospitalization *(23)*. In ACAS, restenosis also complicated up to 10% of cases *(11)*. Surgical series have suggested up to a fivefold increase in risk with reoperation for restenosis after CEA *(24)*.

Given these concerns, carotid angioplasty and/or stenting provide a less invasive alternative to CEA that might be better tolerated, especially in patients at high risk. While concern was raised about the likelihood of embolization and stroke during the procedure, hope was raised that carotid angioplasty and stenting would evolve similarly to coronary angioplasty and stenting. CEA, however, is still the accepted standard of care for treatment of severe carotid stenosis, especially in symptomatic patients. Any new treatment modality must be compared to this "gold standard"; therefore, it is not surprising that no clinical trial comparing CAS to medical therapy has thus far been performed. Clinical trials and registries have either compared CAS to CEA or to historical controls. Moreover, with the availability of a treatment with a proven track record especially in low-risk patients, clinical trials evaluating CAS have focused on the high-risk cohort of patients at increased risk from CEA.

CAROTID ANGIOPLASTY AND STENTING STUDIES

The first extracranial carotid angioplasty to treat carotid artery stenosis was reported by Kerber et al. in 1980 *(25)*. Over the next several years, a number of pioneers, including Mathias and Theron, reported their experience with percutaneous carotid intervention, primarily as observational series *(26)*. Percutaneous carotid intervention has evolved during the past 25 years; Operators have become more experienced, especially in the last decade. Equipment has become more sophisticated, with the development of specific carotid stent platforms. Wire diameters have been reduced from 0.035 in. to 0.014 in. Over-the-wire stent platforms are increasingly being replaced by monorail systems. Multiple embolic protection devices (EPD) have been devised, including distal balloon occlusion, distal filter systems, and proximal flow reversal systems.

Over the past decade, multiple carotid angioplasty and stenting trials have been published or reported. By and large, these trials were either single-center or multi-center, prospective, single-arm registries of carotid angioplasty and/or stenting or were randomized or nonrandomized trials comparing carotid angioplasty and/or stenting to CEA. A summary of published trials of patients undergoing carotid angioplasty/stenting using EPD is shown in Table 2. Only four major trials that compared CEA to carotid angioplasty and/or stenting have been performed with results that have been presented or published: the WallStent Trial, CAVATAS, SAPPHIRE, and CARESS. Of these, only SAPPHIRE and CARESS utilized EPD, and only SAPPHIRE enrolled exclusively high-risk patients. The CREST trial CAS to CEA in low-risk patients is ongoing, although the lead-in results have been released.

WallStent Trial (The "Stopped" Trial)

The first randomized trial of CAS vs surgery was the WallStent Trial reported in 1999. Importantly, no EPD were used during the intervention. The trial end points were

Table 2
Carotid Registries Using Embolic Protection Devices—30-d Events

	Year	EPD	N	Stroke (%)	Death (%)	Composite (%)
Theron et al. (41)	1996	Coaxial cath	69	3	0	3
Jaeger et al. (42)	2001	AngioGuard	20	0	0	0
Tubler et al. (43)	2001	GuardWire	58	3.4	0	3.4
Al-Mubarak et al. (44)	2002	Multiple	164	1	1	2
Guimaraens et al. (45)	2002	Multiple	194	1	1.9	2.9
Angelini et al. (46)	2002	AngioGuard	38	0	2.8	2.8
Schluter et al. (47)	2002	GuardWire	99	3.1	0	3.1
Macdonald et al. (48)	2002	Neuroshield	75	—	—	4.0
Cremonesi et al. (49)	2004	Multiple	442	2.0	0	2.0
Reimers et al. (50)	2004	Multiple	815	2.9	0.5	3.3
Cremonesi et al. (51)	2005	Spider	73	6.8	0	6.8
Reimers et al. (52)	2005	MO.MA	157	5.1	0.6	5.7
Coppi et al. (53)	2005	MO.MA	416	4.1	0.5	4.6

a safety end point of 30-d death/stroke/MI and an efficacy end point of ipsilateral stroke from d 30 to 365. The risk of any ipsilateral stroke or study-related death at 30 d was higher in patients treated with CAS vs CEA although not significant (9% vs 4%, $p = 0.105$). This difference was maintained at 1 yr, although still not significant (13% vs 5%, $p = 0.113$). This trial has been widely criticized. Surprisingly no phase I trial using this system had been performed prior to the initiation of the randomized trial. Training of the operators on the carotid stent system was thought to be suboptimal. Moreover, no principal investigator or executive committee was ever established, and the trial design was criticized. This study was stopped prematurely after it was concluded that the end points were unlikely to be reached (27).

CAVATAS

CAVATAS was one of the first randomized trials of carotid angioplasty vs CEA. Patients did not have to be high-risk to participate in this study. Five hundred and four patients were enrolled, 253 treated with CEA and 251 treated with carotid angioplasty. Stents were used in only 26% of cases. No EPD was utilized in the angioplasty arm. Medical therapy was identical in both arms, and patients were followed for 3 yr. The risk of disabling stroke or death at 30 d was similar between treatment groups and not statistically significant (6.4% for angioplasty vs 5.9% for CEA). Similar findings were reported for any stroke or death (10.0% for angioplasty and 9.9% for CEA). Notably, the risks of cranial nerve palsy and of hematoma were significantly reduced with carotid angioplasty vs surgery. During 3 yr of follow-up, the risk of death or major stroke was nearly identical between treatment groups (14.3% for carotid intervention and 14.2% for CEA) (28).

SAPPHIRE

Aside from the flawed WallStent trial, the Stenting and Angioplasty with Protection in Patients at High Risk for Endarterectomy (SAPPHIRE) trial was the first randomized trial truly comparing CAS to CEA. Importantly, this trial focused on high-risk patients for CEA. In addition, EPD was utilized in this trial, unlike the WallStent study.

CAS was performed using the Angioguard XP device and the PRECISE nitinol self-expanding stent. Patients had to have ≥50% stenosis if symptomatic and ≥80% stenosis if asymptomatic. A consensus agreement needed to be reached by a multi-disciplinary team including a vascular surgeon, an interventionalist, and a neurologist. Patients thought too high-risk for CEA could be entered into a high-risk CAS registry, and patients thought too high-risk for CAS could be entered into a high-risk CEA registry. Patients need to be considered high-risk either from clinical comorbidities or from anatomic criteria. A total of 307 patients (156 patients treated with stent and 151 patients treated with surgery) were randomized while 409 were entered into the stent registry and 7 patients were entered into the surgery registry. Successful delivery and retrieval of the Angioguard was achieved in 98.6% of cases. Successful stent delivery with residual stenosis of <30% was achieved in 91.2% of cases. The 30-d risk of death/stroke/MI was 4.4% in the stent arm vs 9.9% in the surgery arm ($p = 0.06$). Notably, the risk of cranial nerve injury was 0.0% in the stent arm vs 5.3% in the surgery arm ($p < 0.01$). At 1 yr, the risk of death/stroke/MI was 12.0% in the stent arm vs 20.1% in the surgery arm ($p = 0.048$) (Fig. 3). In addition, target lesion revascularization was lower with CAS compared with CEA (0.7% CAS, 4.6% CEA, $p = 0.04$) (29).

The SAPPHIRE stent registry, which included only high-risk CAS patients who were rejected for CEA, likely represents a higher risk cohort than the other high-risk registries (reported below). In the 409 patients enrolled, the 30-d risk of death was 2.5%, stroke 5.6%, and MI 1.7%, for a composite event rate of 7.8%. Target lesion revascularization in the stent registry was 0.8%. The SAPPHIRE CEA registry included only seven patients, one of whom had a perioperative MI, for a 30-d composite event rate of 14.3% (29).

Overall, the SAPPHIRE results reveal a trend for reduced adverse events with CAS compared to CEA with significant reductions in the likelihood of MI, cranial nerve damage, and need for repeat revascularization. Thus, CAS with EPD is at least equivalent to CEA in high-risk patients.

Embolic Protection Device

No CAS trial has been performed that has specifically evaluated the utility of embolic protection in reducing periprocedural adverse events. No significant difference was found in the stroke and/or death rates in ARCHeR 1 (no EPD) vs ARCHeR 2 (EPD), although the number of patients in each arm were small, and the trials were underpowered to detect any difference.

The Endarterectomy vs Angioplasty of Patients with Severe Symptomatic Carotid Stenosis (EVA-3S) Trial is an ongoing, prospective, randomized trial comparing CEA to CAS. Initially operators were allowed to use an EPD at their discretion. The Safety Committee stopped the arm of CAS without EPD because interim analysis suggested that the 30-d risk of stroke was substantially higher without EPD (26.7% vs 8.6%). While this trial was not designed as a randomized comparison of CAS with and without EPD, the findings suggest that EPD reduced periprocedural stroke risk (30).

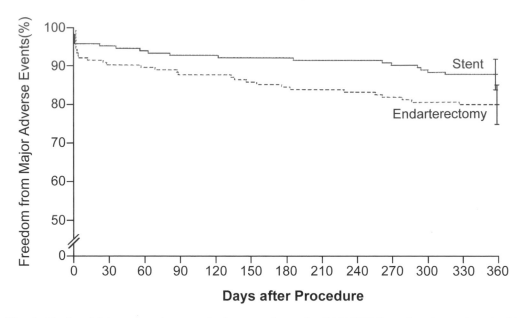

Fig. 3. Kaplan-Meier event-free survival curves from the SAPPHIRE study. (Reproduced with permission from ref. *36.*)

The Wholey global carotid artery stent registry also recorded data on embolic protection. Of 4221 procedures performed with EPD, the stroke/procedural death rate was 2.23%. Of 6753 procedures performed without EPD, the stroke/procedural death rate was 5.29% (Fig. 4) *(31)*. While this was not a randomized comparison, and other factors including operator experience, temporal bias, and availability of improved equipment also may have played significant roles, these results were concordant with the likely benefit of EPD for CAS.

High-Risk Carotid Stenting Registries

The majority of data supporting CAS in the United States have come from industry sponsored, prospective, single-arm registries evaluating specific carotid stent platforms and EPD including ARCHeR, BEACH, SECURITY, MAVeRIC, CABERNET, and the registry arm of SAPPHIRE. The results of these registries have been reported in major cardiology meetings, although few if any have yet been published (Table 3). Most required as inclusion criteria, a ≥50% stenosis in symptomatic patients or ≥80% stenosis in asymptomatic patients, with ≥1 clinical or anatomical high-risk criteria (Table 4).

ARCHeR

The Acculink for Revascularization of Carotids in High Risk Patients (ARCHeR) trials were three separate prospective, nonrandomized, multicenter registries of high-risk patients undergoing CAS. The equipment used were the Accunet filter and the Acculink nitinol self-expanding stent, both straight and tapered versions. ARCHeR 1 enrolled 158 patients including 51 lead-in patients. No EPD was used, and the stent system was over-the-wire. ARCHeR 2 enrolled 278 patients with 25 lead-in patients. Over-the-wire Accunet EPD and over-the-wire Acculink stent system were used. ARCHeR 3 enrolled 145 patients and used the Rx (monorail) versions of the Accunet EPD and Acculink stent system. Outcomes were compared to a weighted historical control for CEA derived

Carotid Stenting With & Without Emboli Protection

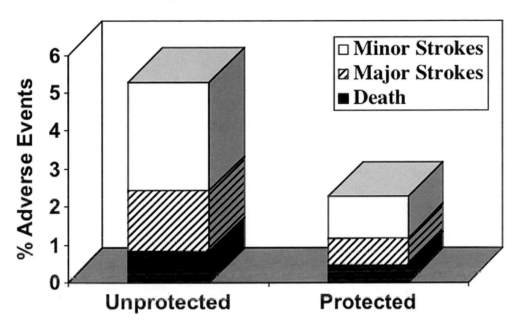

Fig. 4. Stroke/procedural death rate in procedures performed with and without embolic protection from the Wholey global carotid artery registry. In procedures with EPD, the adverse event rate was 2.23% vs 5.29% in procedures without EPD. (Adapted from ref. *30*.)

from published data for CEA in high-risk patients. Using the patient demographic data from ARCHER 1 and 2, a calculated risk was obtained adjusting for medical high-risk features and anatomical high-risk features. The adjusted 1-yr risk for the weighted historical control was 14.5%. Successful filter delivery, placement, and retrieval were seen in >95% of cases. Successful placement of the stent with <50% residual stenosis was seen in >98–99% of cases. The risk of death or any stroke at 30 d were 6.3% for ARCHeR 1, 6.8% for ARCHeR 2, and 7.6% for ARCHeR 3. The risk of death/stroke/MI at 30 d was 7.6% for ARCHeR 1, 8.6% for ARCHeR 2, and 8.3% for ARCHeR 3. The risk of major stroke or fatal stroke was 1.9% for ARCHeR 1 and 1.4% in both ARCHeR 2 and 3. From days 31 to 365, three additional minor strokes were observed in ARCHeR 1 and 3 in ARCHeR 2. In long-term follow-up (2.5 yr), freedom from death/major stroke up to 30 d and major ipsilateral stroke from 1 mo to 2.5 yr in asymptomatic patients was 95.7% and in symptomatic patients it was 93.1%. Target lesion revascularization at 12 mo due to recurrent stenosis of ≥80% in asymptomatic patients and ≥50% in symptomatic patients was 2.2% in ARCHeR 1 and 2.8% in ARCHeR 2. Overall, the risk of adverse outcome was 91.7% in ARCHeR 1 and 2 compared to 85.5% in the weighted historical control *(32)*.

BEACH

The Boston Scientific EPI: A Carotid Stent Trial for High Risk Surgical Patients Trial enrolled 747 patients. One hundred and eighty-nine patients were in the roll-in group, with an additional 78 patients in the bilateral group. Overall, 480 patients were in the pivotal group. The equipment used were the EPI Filterwire EX or EZ filter, and

Table 3
High-Risk Criteria for Carotid Artery Stenting Trials

Medical/surgical comorbidities	Anatomic comorbities
Age >80 yr	Post-radical neck surgery
LVEF <30%	Post-radiation therapy to neck
NYHA functional class ≥III	Surgically inaccessible lesions (high
FEV1 <30% predicted	cervical ICA lesions or low CCA lesions
Renal failure on hemodialysis	below clavicle)
Uncontrolled diabetes mellitus	Severe tandem lesions
Need for open heart surgery (CABG or	Spinal immobility
valve surgery) within 4–6 wk	Tracheostomy stoma
Known coronary artery disease (≥2	Contralateral laryngeal nerve paralysis
vessels with ≥70% stenosis)	Restenosis after prior CEA
Recent MI (within 30 d)	
Unstable angina	
Contralateral carotid occlusion	

CABG, Coronary artery bypass surgery; CCA, common carotid artery; CEA, carotid endarterectomy; FEV, forced expiratory volume; ICA, internal carotid artery; LVEF, left ventricular ejection fraction; MI, myocardial infarction; NYHA, New York Heart Association.

Table 4
US Carotid Registries Using Embolic Protection Devices EPD—30-d Events

	Year	EPD	N	Stroke (%)	Death (%)	MI (%)	Composite (%)
ARCHeR I	2003	AccuNet	158	4.4	2.5	2.9	8.6
ARCHeR II	2003	AccuNet	278	5.8	2.9	2.5	7.6
SECURITY	2003	Emboshield	305	6.9	0.7	0.3	7.2
BEACH	2004	FilterWire	480	4.2	1.5	0.8	5.4
MAVeRIC I, II	2004	GuardWire	498	3.6	1.0	1.8	5.2
CABERNET	2004	FilterWire	488	3.4	0.5	0.2	3.8
SAPPHIRE Registry	2002	AngioGuard	408	5.6	2.5	1.7	7.8

the Wallstent. The 30-d risk of ipsilateral major stroke, minor stroke, or hemorrhage was 3.1%. The risk of contralateral major stroke, minor stroke, or hemorrhage was 1.0%. The risk of all stroke at 30 d was 4.2%, death 1.5%, and MI 0.8%, with a composite end point of 5.4%. At 1 year, the risk of all stroke was 7.0%, death 3.2%, and MI 1.1% for a 1-yr composite end point of 9.1% *(33)*.

SECURITY

The Registry Study to Evaluate the Neuroshield Bare Wire Cerebral Protection System and X-Act Stent in Patients at High Risk for Carotid Endarterectomy (SECURITY) trial was a multicenter, prospective, carotid stent registry in high-risk patients treated with the MedNova Bare Wire Filter and the Xact stent. Of 305 patients were enrolled, filter deployment was successful in 97.3% of cases, and stent deployment successful in 96% of cases. The 30-d risk of major stroke was 2.3%, minor stroke 4.6%, all stroke 6.9%, death 0.7%, and MI 0.3% for a 30-d composite end point of 7.2% *(34)*.

MAVeRIC

The Evaluation of the Medtronic AVE Self-expanding Carotid Stent System in the Treatment of Carotid Stenosis (MAVeRIC) trials were registries in high-risk patients treated with the GuardWire EPD and the Exponent stent. Procedural success was 85.9% in MAVeRIC 1 (feasibility trial) and 90.1% in MAVeRIC 2. The 30-d risk of stroke was 3.6%, death 1.0%, and MI 1.8% for a 30-d composite of 5.2% *(35)*.

CABERNET

The Carotid Artery Revascularization Using the Boston Scientific EPI Filterwire EX/EZ and the EndoTex NexStent trial was a registry of 454 high-risk patients treated using the Filterwire EPD and the EndoTex NexStent. Patients were on average 72.5 yr of age, 65% male, and 76% asymptomatic. Twenty-one percent of CAS was performed for restenosis after CEA. System success was achieved in 96% of patients with a reduction in stenosis from 84% to 6.5%. At 30 d, the rate of death was 0.5%, stroke 3.4% (major 1.3%, minor 2.1%), and MI 0.2%, for a composite of 3.9%. The primary end point of the study, death/stroke/MI within 30 d and ipsilateral stroke or death from days 31 to 365, was 4.5%, primarily owing to additional minor strokes during a time interval from 1 mo to 1 yr. No additional major strokes were seen during this interval. The end point of all death/stroke/MI at 1 yr was 11.5% *(36)*.

Systematic Reviews of Randomized CAS Trials

Coward et al. performed a systematic review of randomized trials comparing carotid angioplasty and/or stenting to CEA. Only five randomized trials were included in the analysis involving 1269 patients. The majority of patients came from CAVATAS (*n* = 504), followed by SAPPHIRE (*n* – 334) and the WallStent trial (*n* – 219). No significant difference was found between carotid angioplasty/stenting vs CEA with respect to treatment-related death or any stroke (odds ratio [OR] 1.33, 95% confidence interval [CI], 0.86–2.04), death or disabling stroke (OR 1.22, 95% CI 0.61–2.41), or death, any stroke, or MI (OR 1.04, 95% CI, 0.69–1.57). At 1 yr, the risk of any stroke or death was similar (OR 1.01, 95% CI, 0.71–1.44). Notably, the risk of cranial nerve injury was reduced with carotid angioplasty/stenting (OR 0.13, 95% CI, 0.06–0.25) *(37)*. Unfortunately, this analysis included heterogeneous patients treated with angioplasty with selective stenting and no EPD (CAVATAS), patients treated with CAS without EPD (WallStent), and high-risk patients treated with CAS with EPD (SAPPHIRE). Given the disparate trials included in this analysis, clear conclusions about the utility of carotid intervention were difficult. In this instance, more can perhaps be learned by evaluating the trials individually.

Since the publication of that meta-analysis, several more trials were published. The Carotid Revascularization Using Endarterectomy or Stenting Systems (CaRESS) trial was a Phase I multicenter, nonrandomized study comparing CAS with EPD to CEA in patients "reflective of broad clinical practice," not isolated to patients at high risk for CEA. Patients with >50% symptomatic stenosis and >75% asymptomatic stenosis were enrolled in a 2:1 ratio of CEA to CAS. The Guardwire Plus was the distal EDP utilized in this study. The primary end points were death or stroke at 30 d and a composite of death, stroke, or MI within 30 d, and death or stroke at 31–365 d. A total of 397 patients were treated with either CEA (*n* = 254) or CAS (*n* = 143). Sixty-eight percent of patients were asymptomatic. The risk of death or stroke was similar between the treatments at 30 d (3.6% for CEA vs 2.1% for CAS) and at 1 yr (13.6% for CEA vs 10.0%

for CAS). The rate of death, stroke, or MI at 30 d was also not significantly different (4.4% for CEA vs 2.1% for CAS), and the composite end point at 1 yr also showed no significant difference (14.3% for CEA vs 10.9% for CAS). The rates of repeat carotid revascularization were similar between groups (1.0% for CEA vs 1.8% for CAS). The results of this phase I study suggested that CAS with EPD was equivalent to CEA *(38)*.

The Global Carotid Artery Stent Registry

The largest series on CAS was summarized by Wholey et al. They collected data from 53 centers worldwide from surveys to determine the current status of CAS. As of 2003, 12,392 procedures were performed in 11,243 patients. The technical success rate was 98.9%. At 30 d, the procedure-related death rate was 0.64%, major stroke rate 1.20%, minor stroke rate 2.14%, and TIA rate 3.07%. Combined stroke and procedure related deaths complicated 3.98% of procedures. The nonprocedure death rate was 0.77%, for a total death or stroke rate of 4.75%. Restenosis occurred in 2.7% at 1 yr, 2.6% at 2 yr, and 2.4% at 3 yr. Subsequent neurologic events beyond the periprocedural period occurred in 1.2% at 1 yr, 1.3% at 2 yr, and 1.7% at 3 yr. These data are limited as they are self-reported through surveys without independent adjudication of events. However, they do demonstrate a wide breadth of experience with this procedure and suggest that it can be performed with an acceptable risk *(31)*.

Summary of CAS Studies

In summary, the data on CAS are most robust in high-risk patients, suggesting that CAS with EPD is at least equivalent to CEA. Trials focusing on low-risk patients (International Carotid Stenting Study [ICSS], Stent-supported Percutaneous Angioplasty of the Carotid Artery vs Endarterectomy [SPACE] trial, Carotid Revascularization Endarterectomy vs Stent Trial [CREST], and Endarterectomy vs Angioplasty in patients with Symptomatic Severe Carotid Stenosis [EVA-3S]) are currently enrolling patients, and results are expected from both US and European sites within the next 3–5 yr. Trials focusing on low-risk asymptomatic patients are also either enrolling or in the planning stages (e.g., Carotid Angioplasty and Stenting vs Endarterectomy in Asymptomatic Patients with Significant Extracranial Carotid Occlusive Disease Trial [ACT I]). The results in low-risk patients have thus far been encouraging (e.g., CARESS).

CURRENT STATUS OF CAS IN THE UNITED STATES

In April 2004, the Circulatory Device Panel of the FDA recommended approval of CAS using the Angioguard XP and the Precise stent. On August 31, 2004, the FDA approved the Accunet and Acculink carotid stent system for the treatment of patients at high risk from CEA who require carotid revascularization, and are symptomatic with ≥50% stenosis or are asymptomatic with ≥80% stenosis. On September 15, 2005, the FDA approved the Xact Carotid Stent and the Emboshield Embolic Protection System for the treatment of patients requiring carotid revascularization who are not favorable candidates for surgery.

Unfortunately, the Centers for Medicare & Medicaid Services (CMS) on March 17, 2005 announced limited coverage for CAS to high-risk patients with ≥70% symptomatic stenosis. CMS will cover patients meeting the FDA-labeled criteria for CAS in Category B IDE clinical trials or in post-approval studies. Asymptomatic patients with severe stenoses will not be covered by CMS outside of clinical trials. Notably, the rate of asymptomatic patients undergoing CEA has been increasing. An analysis of CEA performed in 1993–94 in Ohio found only 25% of patients treated were asymptomatic *(39)*. More recent data from 1997–98 found that nearly 73% of patients treated were asymptomatic *(40)*. CAS registry data also suggest that the majority of patients undergoing this procedure are asymptomatic. Although clinical trials are continuing to enroll patients who are asymptomatic and patients who are low-risk, this limitation in coverage substantially reduces the pool of patients who are eligible for CAS.

REFERENCES

1. Council TNANDaS. Stroke and Cerebrovascular Disease: National Institutes of Health Report, 1992.
2. Bonita R, Beaglehole R. Stroke: populations, cohorts, and clinical trials. In: Whisnant JP, ed. Stroke Mortality. Oxford, England: Butterworth-Heinemann, 1993:59–79.
3. 1999 Heart and Stroke Statistical Update. Dallas: American Heart Association, 1998:13–15.
4. Eastcott HH, Pickering GW, Rob CG. Reconstruction of internal carotid artery in a patient with intermittent attacks of hemiplegia. Lancet 1954;267:994–996.
5. Eastcott HH. Late thoughts and reflections on carotid reconstruction for the prevention of ischemic stroke. J Endovasc Surg 1996;3:5–6.
6. Barnett HJ. Symptomatic carotid endarterectomy trials. Stroke 1990;21:III2–III5.
7. Brott T, Thalinger K. The practice of carotid endarterectomy in a large metropolitan area. Stroke 1984;15:950–955.
8. Tu JV, Hannan EL, Anderson GM, et al. The fall and rise of carotid endarterectomy in the United States and Canada. N Engl J Med 1998;339:1441–1447.
9. Beneficial effect of carotid endarterectomy in symptomatic patients with high-grade carotid stenosis. North American Symptomatic Carotid Endarterectomy Trial Collaborators. N Engl J Med 1991;325: 445–453.
10. Barnett HJ, Taylor DW, Eliasziw M, et al. Benefit of carotid endarterectomy in patients with symptomatic moderate or severe stenosis. North American Symptomatic Carotid Endarterectomy Trial Collaborators. N Engl J Med 1998;339:1415–1425.
11. Endarterectomy for asymptomatic carotid artery stenosis. Executive Committee for the Asymptomatic Carotid Atherosclerosis Study. JAMA 1995;273:1421–1428.
12. Halliday A, Mansfield A, Marro J, et al. Prevention of disabling and fatal strokes by successful carotid endarterectomy in patients without recent neurological symptoms: randomised controlled trial. Lancet 2004;363:1491–1502.
13. Biller J, Feinberg WM, Castaldo JE, et al. Guidelines for carotid endarterectomy: a statement for healthcare professionals from a Special Writing Group of the Stroke Council, American Heart Association. Circulation 1998;97:501–509.
14. Wennberg DE, Lucas FL, Birkmeyer JD, Bredenberg CE, Fisher ES. Variation in carotid endarterectomy mortality in the Medicare population: trial hospitals, volume, and patient characteristics. JAMA 1998;279:1278–1281.
15. McCrory DC, Goldstein LB, Samsa GP, et al. Predicting complications of carotid endarterectomy. Stroke 1993;24:1285–1291.
16. Ouriel K, Hertzer NR, Beven EG, et al. Preprocedural risk stratification: identifying an appropriate population for carotid stenting. J Vasc Surg 2001;33:728–732.
17. Goldstein LB, Samsa GP, Matchar DB, Oddone EZ. Multicenter review of preoperative risk factors for endarterectomy for asymptomatic carotid artery stenosis. Stroke 1998;29:750–753.
18. Wong JH, Findlay JM, Suarez-Almazor ME. Regional performance of carotid endarterectomy. Appropriateness, outcomes, and risk factors for complications. Stroke 1997;28:891–898.
19. Lepore MR, Jr., Sternbergh WC, 3rd, Salartash K, Tonnessen B, Money SR. Influence of NASCET/ACAS trial eligibility on outcome after carotid endarterectomy. J Vasc Surg 2001;34: 581–586.
20. Gasparis AP, Ricotta L, Cuadra SA, et al. High-risk carotid endarterectomy: fact or fiction. J Vasc Surg 2003;37:40–46.
21. Rothwell PM, Slattery J, Warlow CP. A systematic review of the risks of stroke and death due to endarterectomy for symptomatic carotid stenosis. Stroke 1996;27:260–265.
22. Ferguson GG, Eliasziw M, Barr HW, et al. The North American Symptomatic Carotid Endarterectomy Trial: surgical results in 1415 patients. Stroke 1999;30:1751–1758.

23. Paciaroni M, Eliasziw M, Kappelle LJ, Finan JW, Ferguson GG, Barnett HJ. Medical complications associated with carotid endarterectomy. North American Symptomatic Carotid Endarterectomy Trial (NASCET). Stroke 1999;30:1759–1763.

24. Meyer FB, Piepgras DG, Fode NC. Surgical treatment of recurrent carotid artery stenosis. J Neurosurg 1994;80:781–787.

25. Kerber CW, Cromwell LD, Loehden OL. Catheter dilatation of proximal carotid stenosis during distal bifurcation endarterectomy. AJNR Am J Neuroradiol 1980;1:348–349.

26. Bockenheimer SA, Mathias K. Percutaneous transluminal angioplasty in arteriosclerotic internal carotid artery stenosis. AJNR Am J Neuroradiol 1983;4:791–792.

27. Alberts MJ. Results of a multicenter prospective randomized trial of carotid artery stenting vs. carotid endarterectomy. (abstract). Stroke 2001;32:325.

28. Endovascular versus surgical treatment in patients with carotid stenosis in the Carotid and Vertebral Artery Transluminal Angioplasty Study (CAVATAS): a randomised trial. Lancet 2001;357:1729–1737.

29. Yadav JS, Wholey MH, Kuntz RE, et al. Protected carotid-artery stenting versus endarterectomy in high-risk patients. N Engl J Med 2004;351:1493–1501.

30. Mas JL, Chatellier G, Beyssen B. Carotid angioplasty and stenting with and without cerebral protection: clinical alert from the Endarterectomy Versus Angioplasty in Patients With Symptomatic Severe Carotid Stenosis (EVA-3S) trial. Stroke 2004;35:e18–e20.

31. Wholey MH, Al-Mubarek N. Updated review of the global carotid artery stent registry. Catheter Cardiovasc Interv 2003;60:259–266.

32. Gray W. The Acculink for Revascularization of Carotids in High Risk Patients (ARCHeR) Trial results. (Presentation). American College of Cardiology Scientific Sessions. New Orleans, LA, 2004.

33. White C. The Boston Scientific EPI: A Carotid Stent Trial for High Risk Surgical Patients Trial Results. (Presentation). Peripheral Angioplasty and All That Jazz. New Orleans, LA, 2005.

34. Whitlow P. The SECURITY Trial results. (Presentation). Transcatheter Therapeutics. Washington, DC, 2003.

35. Ramee S. Evaluation of the Medtronic AVE Self-expanding Carotid Stent System in the Treatment of Carotid Stenosis Results. (Presentation). Transcatheter Therapeutics. Washington, DC, 2004.

36. Hopkins LN. The Carotid Artery Revascularization Using the Boston Scientific EPI Filterwire EX/EZ and the EndoTex NexStent trial results. (Presentation). Transcatheter Therapeutics. Washington, DC, 2005.

37. Coward LJ, Featherstone RL, Brown MM. Safety and efficacy of endovascular treatment of carotid artery stenosis compared with carotid endarterectomy: a Cochrane systematic review of the randomized evidence. Stroke 2005;36:905–911.

38. Carotid Revascularization Using Endarterectomy or Stenting Systems (CaRESS) phase I clinical trial: 1-year results. J Vasc Surg 2005;42:213–219.

39. Cebul RD, Snow RJ, Pine R, Hertzer NR, Norris DG. Indications, outcomes, and provider volumes for carotid endarterectomy. JAMA 1998;279:1282–1287.

40. Halm EA, Chassin MR, Tuhrim S, et al. Revisiting the appropriateness of carotid endarterectomy. Stroke 2003;34:1464–1471.

41. Theron JG, Payelle GG, Coskun O, Huet HF, Guimaraens L. Carotid artery stenosis: treatment with protected balloon angioplasty and stent placement. Radiology 1996;201:627–636.

42. Jaeger H, Mathias K, Drescher R, et al. Clinical results of cerebral protection with a filter device during stent implantation of the carotid artery. Cardiovasc Intervent Radiol 2001;24:249–256.

43. Tubler T, Schluter M, Dirsch O, et al. Balloon-protected carotid artery stenting: relationship of periprocedural neurological complications with the size of particulate debris. Circulation 2001;104:2791–2796.

44. Al-Mubarak N, Colombo A, Gaines PA, et al. Multicenter evaluation of carotid artery stenting with a filter protection system. J Am Coll Cardiol 2002;39:841–846.

45. Guimaraens L, Sola MT, Matali A, et al. Carotid angioplasty with cerebral protection and stenting: report of 164 patients (194 carotid percutaneous transluminal angioplasties). Cerebrovasc Dis 2002;13:114–119.

46. Angelini A, Reimers B, Della Barbera M, et al. Cerebral protection during carotid artery stenting: collection and histopathologic analysis of embolized debris. Stroke 2002;33:456–461.

47. Schluter M, Tubler T, Mathey DG, Schofer J. Feasibility and efficacy of balloon-based neuroprotection during carotid artery stenting in a single-center setting. J Am Coll Cardiol 2002;40:890–895.

48. Macdonald S, McKevitt F, Venables GS, Cleveland TJ, Gaines PA. Neurological outcomes after carotid stenting protected with the NeuroShield filter compared to unprotected stenting. J Endovasc Ther 2002;9:777–785.

49. Cremonesi A, Manetti R, Setacci F, Setacci C, Castriota F. Protected carotid stenting: clinical advantages and complications of embolic protection devices in 442 consecutive patients. Stroke 2003;34:1936–1941.
50. Reimers B, Schluter M, Castriota F, et al. Routine use of cerebral protection during carotid artery stenting: results of a multicenter registry of 753 patients. Am J Med 2004;116:217–222.
51. Cremonesi A. The SPIDER Embolic Protection Device performance evaluation in the carotid artery during percutaneous transluminal angioplasty and or stenting. J Invasive Cardiol 2005;17:463–467.
52. Reimers B, Sievert H, Schuler GC, et al. Proximal endovascular flow blockage for cerebral protection during carotid artery stenting: results from a prospective multicenter registry. J Endovasc Ther 2005;12:156–165.
53. Coppi G, Moratto R, Silingardi R, et al. PRIAMUS — Proximal flow blockage cerebral protection during carotid stenting: Results from a Multicenter Italian registry. J Cardiovasc Surg (Torino) 2005;46:219–227.

5

Cerebrovascular Anatomy

Ravish Sachar, MD and Samir Kapadia, MD

CONTENTS

    INTRODUCTION
    GREAT VESSELS
    ANTERIOR CIRCULATION
    POSTERIOR CIRCULATION
    REFERENCES

Summary

Defining and understanding cerebrovascular anatomy is the cornerstone of a safe and successful carotid stenting procedure. A thorough pre-procedural angiogram with detailed documentation of cerebral anatomy and collateral flow is essential for procedural success. This chapter details supra-aortic anatomy, including the aortic arch, subclavian arteries, common and internal carotid arteries, vertebral arteries, and intracranial vessels. In each section, commonly found anatomic variations are discussed. The chapter has been divided into three main sections, the great vessels, the anterior circulation, and the posterior circulation.

Key Words: Cerebrovascular anatomy, anterior circulation, posterior circulation, internal carotid arteries, middle cerebral artery, anterior cerebral artery, posterior cerebral artery.

INTRODUCTION

Defining and understanding cerebrovascular anatomy is the cornerstone of a safe and successful carotid stenting procedure. A thorough pre-procedural angiogram with detailed documentation of cerebral anatomy and collateral flow is essential for procedural success. This chapter details supra-aortic anatomy, including the aortic arch, subclavian arteries, common and internal carotid arteries, vertebral arteries, and intracranial vessels. In each section, commonly found anatomic variations are discussed. The chapter has been divided into three main sections, the great vessels, the anterior circulation, and the posterior circulation.

GREAT VESSELS

Aortic Arch

The embryologic origin of the aortic arch is the truncus arteriosus, which descends along with the bulbus cordis and forms the aortic sac from which the six aortic arches

From: *Contemporary Cardiology: Handbook of Complex Percutaneous Carotid Intervention*
Edited by: J. Saw, J. E. Exaire, D. S. Lee, and S. Yadav © Humana Press Inc., Totowa, NJ

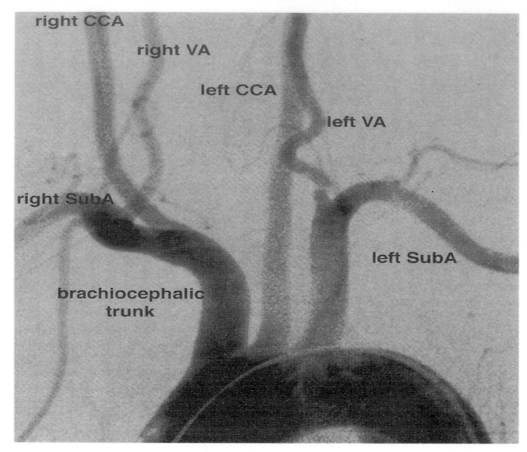

Fig. 1. The aortic arch in the LAO projection: VA, vertebral artery; CCA, common carotid artery; SubA, subclavian artery.

arise. These eventually give rise to the ascending aorta and the pulmonary trunk. The adult ascending aorta gives rise to the innominate (brachiocephalic) artery, the left common carotid artery, and the subclavian artery, although variations are common.

Aortic arch angiography should be the first step of a cerebral angiogram, and is best performed in the left anterior oblique (LAO 30–50°) projection (Fig. 1). Valuable information can be obtained on atherosclerotic burden, calcification, aneurysmal disease, arch type, and anatomic variations. Determining arch type is an essential first step in planning a percutaneous carotid intervention. Anatomically, the aortic arch can be divided into three categories: Types I, II, and III (Fig. 2). The nomenclature is based on the angle of curvature through which the great vessels arise. In general, the steeper the angle of the aorta between the origins of the left subclavian and innominate arteries, the higher the grade of the arch. The exact criteria for determining the type of arch is based on using the diameter of the proximal left common carotid artery as the reference diameter. If all the great vessels arise from within one reference diameter of the apex of the aortic arch, then the arch is termed Type I. Similarly, if the great vessels all arise from within two or three reference diameters from the apex of the aortic arch, then the arches are termed Type II and Type III, respectively.

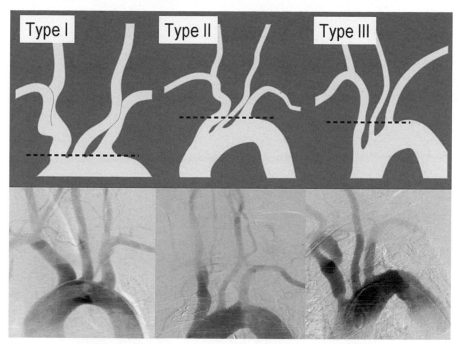

Fig. 2. Classification of the aortic arch. See text for details.

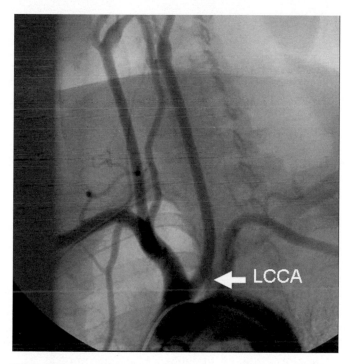

Fig. 3. Bovine origin of the left common carotid artery (LCCA).

Anatomic variations of the aortic arch are quite common. The most common is a bovine aortic arch (Fig. 3), where the left common carotid artery arises from the innominate artery. For an arch to be truly bovine, the entire ostium of the left common carotid artery must originate from the innominate artery.

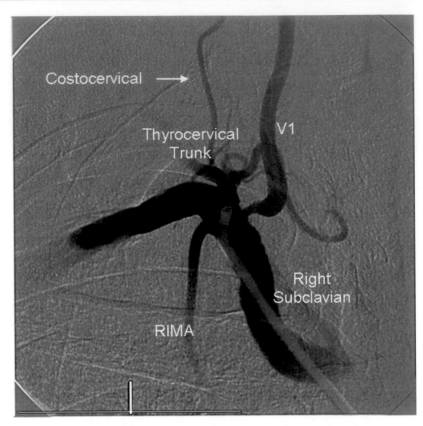

Fig. 4. The right subclavian artery and its branches in the LAO projection. V1, the first segment of the vertebral artery from its origin from the subclavian to transverse foramen of the C6 vertebral body. RIMA, right internal mammary artery.

Subclavian Arteries

Typically, the right subclavian artery arises from the innominate artery and the left subclavian artery arises from the aortic arch. Each subclavian artery can be divided into three sections. The first section of each artery extends from its origin to the medial border of the respective anterior scalene muscle. The second part lies behind the muscle, and the third part extends from the lateral border of the anterior scalene muscle to the lateral border of the first rib, after which it is termed the axillary artery. Hypertrophy of the anterior scalene muscle can result in thoracic outlet syndrome due to compression of the subclavian artery in the second section.

The second and third parts of the left and right subclavian arteries are anatomically similar. The first sections on each side are more unique. The first section of the right subclavian artery (Fig. 4) arises from the innominate artery behind the upper part of the right sternoclavicular joint. It courses laterally and superiorly above the level of the clavicle until the medial border of the anterior scalene muscle. The left subclavian artery is normally the third of the great vessels to arise from the aortic arch. Its origin is posterior to the origin of the left common carotid artery at the level of the fourth thoracic vertebra (T4), after which it courses superiorly and laterally until the medial border of the left anterior scalene muscle. The structures medial to it are the esophagus, trachea, thoracic duct, and the left recurrent nerve, while the structures lateral to it are

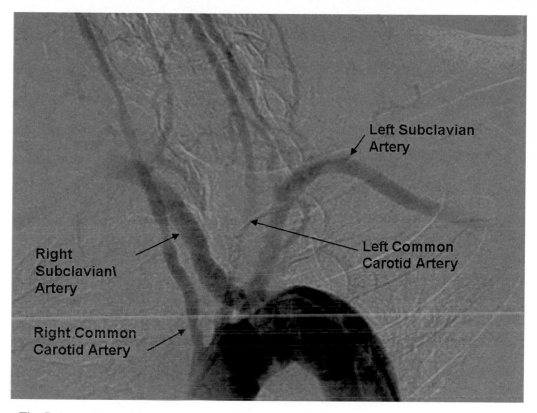

Fig. 5. Anomalous origin of the right subclavian artery from the distal portion of the aortic arch.

the left pleura and lung. These are important to keep in mind as aggressive percuta-neous interventions of heavily calcified ostial or proximal left subclavian arteries can result in perforations and compromise of these structures.

There are several anatomic variations commonly seen with both subclavian arteries. The right subclavian artery can arise independently from the aortic arch, and in such cases it is usually the first or last branch arising from the aortic arch. If it is the first branch, it takes the place of the innominate artery, and if it is the last branch, it arises obliquely from the far left of the aortic arch and courses rightward behind the trachea, esophagus, and the right carotid (Fig. 5). The left subclavian artery can occasionally share a common origin with the left common carotid artery, although variations of the left subclavian are less frequent than those of the right subclavian.

There are four main branches of each subclavian artery: the vertebral, internal mam-mary, thyrocervical, and costocervical (Fig. 4). On the left, all four originate from the first section of the subclavian artery, and on the right three of the four originate from the first section whereas the costocervical originates from the second section behind the anterior scalene muscle. The first 1–2 cm of both subclavian arteries usually do not have any branches, and the vertebral arteries are typically the first branches. The verte-bral arteries are discussed in a separate section below.

The thyrocervical trunk is usually a short trunk that arises from the superior portion of the subclavian artery after the vertebral artery. Soon after its origin it divides into three branches, the inferior thyroid, the transverse scapular, and the transverse cervical. The internal mammary artery arises inferiorly from the subclavian artery opposite the thyrocervical trunk. Finally, the costocervical artery is typically the last branch of the subclavian artery and arises from the first section of the left subclavian artery, medial to the anterior scalene muscle, and from the second section of the right subclavian artery behind the anterior scalene muscle.

ANTERIOR CIRCULATION

Common Carotid Arteries

The right common carotid artery arises at the bifurcation of the innominate artery behind the sternoclavicular joint. Anatomic variations are not common, although the vessel can originate from the aortic arch. The left common carotid artery typically originates from the aortic arch between the innominate and subclavian arteries, and is situated anteriorly compared to the origin of the subclavian and innominate arteries. Anatomic variations of the left common carotid occur more frequently than those of the right common carotid, and it is not uncommon for it to originate from the innominate artery, in which case it is known as a bovine origin of the left common carotid. Rarely, both vessels can originate from a common trunk, and in these cases the right subclavian tends to arise directly from the aortic arch. The right and left carotid can have separate origins when the right subclavian is the last branch of the aortic arch (Fig. 5).

The common carotid arteries usually do not give off any branches proximal to the bifurcation, but occasionally can give rise to the superior thyroid, the ascending pharyngeal, the inferior thyroid, or, more rarely, the vertebral artery. The common carotid arteries divide into the internal and external carotids at the C4–C5 level in approx 50% of patients. In 40% of patients the bifurcation is higher, and in the remaining 10% it is lower.

External Carotid Artery

The external carotid artery originates at the distal bifurcation of the common carotid artery and supplies blood flow to structures in the neck, face, scalp, maxilla, and tongue. At its origin, the external carotid is usually the same size as the internal carotid artery, but diminishes in size as it courses through the neck due to the large number of branches that originate from it. After its origin, the vessel courses superiorly and anteriorly before coursing posteriorly behind the mandible. It then divides into the internal maxillary artery and the superficial temporal artery. The branches of the external carotid artery are highly variable in location and size and are, in order of origination, the superior thyroid artery, lingual artery, facial artery, ascending pharyngeal artery, occipital artery, posterior auricular artery, maxillary artery, and the superficial temporal artery (Fig. 6). The external carotid arteries are often compromised during percutaneous and surgical carotid revascularization procedures. However, owing to an extensive and complex system of collaterals between the distal portions of the right and left external carotid arteries, closure of one of the arteries rarely results in symptoms. If the origins of both vessels are compromised, patients may rarely develop jaw claudication, but this usually resolves within 3–4 wk in most patients.

Internal Carotid Artery

The internal carotid artery supplies blood to the anterior part of the brain and the ipsilateral eye, along with parts of the forehead and nose. It originates as one of the two terminal branches of the common carotid artery, and at its origin is lateral and posterior to the external carotid. It can be divided into five main segments: cervical, petrous, cavernous, clinoid, and supra-clinoid (Fig. 7).

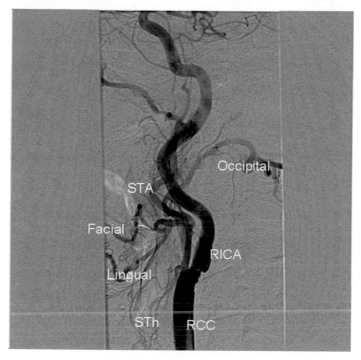

Fig. 6. Branches of the external carotid artery. RCC, right common carotid artery; STh, superior thyroidal artery; RICA, right internal carotid artery; STA, superficial temporal artery.

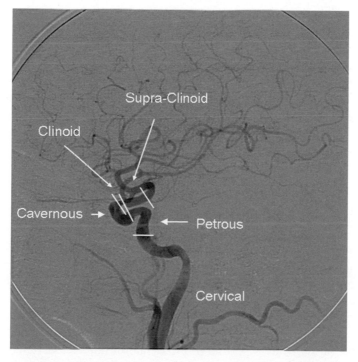

Fig. 7. The five segments of the internal carotid artery: cervical, petrous, cavernous, clinoid, and supra-clinoid. See text for details.

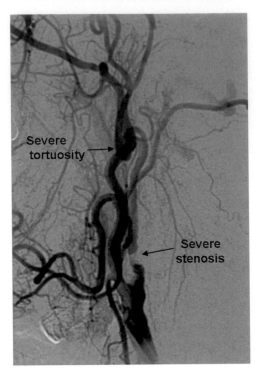

Fig. 8. Severe tortuosity in the distal cervical portion of the internal carotid artery.

The cervical portion of the internal carotid extends from the origin to the skull base, and does not give rise to any branches. Anatomically it lies anterior of the transverse processes of the first three cervical vertebrae (C1–C3). The very proximal portion is known as the carotid bulb due to its shape. There are usually one or two gentle curves in the cervical segment before reaching the petrous portion. However, considerable tortuosity can exist within the cervical portion, including cases of complete 360° loops (Fig. 8). Such tortuosity can be challenging to negotiate while deploying emboli protection devices for percutaneous carotid interventions. Tortuosity immediately after a stenosis in the proximal cervical carotid can also be a challenge during the placement of carotid stents, as curves will tend to be displaced superiorly, increasing the risk of kinking in the distal portion of the cervical portion proximal to the skull base (Fig. 9). Atherosclerotic disease of the internal carotid artery is most commonly located at its origin at the common carotid bifurcation or in the very proximal cervical portion. Lesions often encompass the distal common carotid artery and the proximal internal carotid artery, and can involve the ostium of the external carotid. Considerable calcification, sometimes circumferential, can exist with these atherosclerotic lesions. This is an important angiographic finding to note during carotid interventions as calcification can result in an inability to completely expand carotid stents and may also result in a pronounced hemodynamic response during carotid stent post dilation due to increased pressure on the carotid body.

The petrous segment extends from the base of the skull where the carotid artery enters the carotid canal of the petrous portion of the temporal bone and extends to the apex of the petrous bone. Angiographically, the petrous portion can be distinguished by a sharp perpendicular turn, which corresponds to its anatomic course medially and anteriorly as it

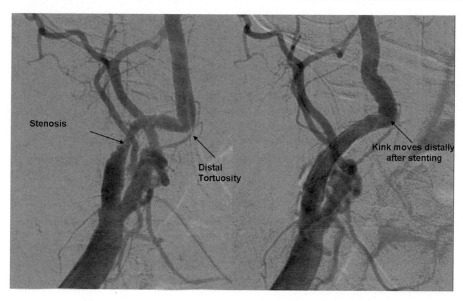

Fig. 9. Superior transmission of tortuosity with resultant kinking of the internal carotid artery as a result of stent development.

enters the foramen lacerum. Atherosclerotic disease in the petrous internal carotid artery is relatively common, but hemodynamically significant stenoses accour less frequently than in the proximal internal carotid artery. Percutaneous interventions within this segment are generally reserved for patients with symptomatic disease or for dissections, and delivery of stents as well as positioning of the emboli protection devices distal to the lesion can be challenging. The petrous portion gives rise to two branches, the tympanic artery and the artery of the pterygoid canal. These are usually not visible angiographically but may increase in size with occlusions of the distal portions of the vessel.

The cavernous segment, also known as the carotid siphon, is the most tortuous portion of the internal carotid artery, and is readily distinguished in the lateral projection as the area with the sharpest curve. This portion of the artery lies between the two layers of the dura mater that form the cavernous sinus. It extends from the foramen lacerum to the anterior clinoid and gives rise to the meningohypophyseal and inferolateral trunk branches. As this portion is restricted by the dura of the sinus (the dura is in fact the wall of the cavernous sinus), it lacks flexibility, and can limit the passage of equipment during percutaneous treatment of intracranial vascular disease. The cavernous segment gives rise to the ophthalmic artery and the hypophyseal branches. The clinoid is a very short segment during which the vessel pierces the dura mater and becomes intracranial. There are no branches from this segment. The supra-clinoid portion is the final segment and gives rise to the posterior communicating artery and the anterior choroidal artery. However, the hypophyseal branches and the ophthalmic artery can sometimes arise from this segment. The supra-clinoid segment ends as the carotid terminus by bifurcating into the middle cerebral and anterior cerebral arteries.

The ophthalmic artery can be most readily identified angiographically in the lateral projection as the vessel that originates from the very distal portion of the cavernous segment or just beyond the cavernous segment and courses anteriorly. Anatomically, its origin is normally intradural and is located on the medial side of the anterior clinoid process, and enters the orbital cavity through the optic foramen. Its branches anastomose

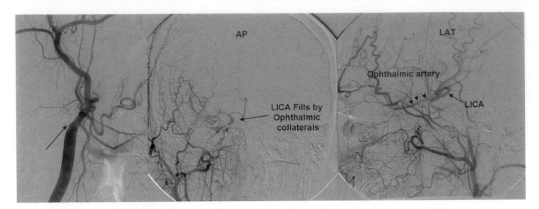

Fig. 10. The ophthalmic artery can be a source of collateral flow to the distal internal carotid in patients with proximal internal carotid occlusion. This is best viewed in the lateral projection. AP, anteroposterior projection; LAT, lateral projection; ICA, internal carotid artery.

with branches of the maxillary artery and can be an important source of external–internal carotid collaterals in patients with internal carotid occlusions (Fig. 10).

The posterior communicating artery is also identified most readily in the lateral projection angiographically (Fig. 16C). If it is present, it connects the anterior circulation with the posterior circulation, and can be an important source of collateral flow to the ipsilateral anterior circulation in cases of internal carotid occlusion. It anastomoses with the posterior cerebral artery at the junction between the P1 and P2 segments. (The P1 segment is the distance between the basilar artery and the origin of the posterior communicating artery.) It supplies the thalamus, hypothalamus, optic chiasm, and mamillary bodies, and is a common site for aneurysms.

The anterior choroidal artery is an intradural structure and is the last branch from the internal carotid artery before the carotid terminus. It provides flow to the optic tract, posterior limb of the internal capsule, the lateral geniculate nucleus, and the choroid plexus.

Anatomic variations of the internal carotid are rare, and the most common source of variability is the length or the cervical segment, which corresponds to the length of the patient's neck. Rarely, the vessel can originate directly from the aortic arch, and even more rarely, there can be a congenital absence of one or both internal carotid arteries. In such cases, anterior brain flow is normally provided by branches of the external carotid artery.

Middle Cerebral Artery

The middle cerebral artery (Fig. 11) is the largest branch of the circle of Willis and supplies most of the temporal lobe, anterolateral frontal lobe, insula, and parietal lobe. Anatomically, it begins at the inner aspect of the sylvian fissure, and runs laterally within the fissure and then courses posteriorly and superiorly on the surface of the insula. Strokes of the middle cerebral artery are usually embolic in nature and result in contralateral hemiplegia, with the arm and face being more affected than the leg. It also results in homonymous hemianopia, which is homolateral to the hemiplegia but contralateral to the MCA occlusion.

Angiographically, the middle cerebral artery can be divided into four segments, M1–M4. It is important to note that in this classification system the segments of the MCA are not defined by branches, but rather by anatomical location. The M1 segment is the horizontal portion in the AP cranial projection and starts at the carotid terminus.

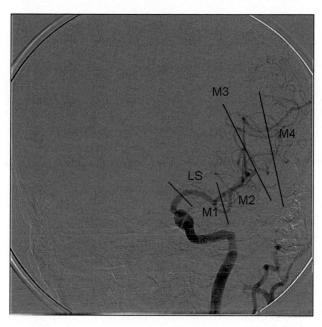

Fig. 11. The left middle cerebral artery in the AP cranial projection. The four segments, M1–M4, are defined by anatomical location and not by branches. LS, lenticulostriate perforators.

It gives rise to the lenticulostriate perforators, which are small arteries that originate from the superior aspect of the M1 segment when viewed in the AP cranial projection. These perforators supply the posterior limb of the internal capsule, and part of the head and body of the caudate and globus pallidus. Angioplasty and stenting of lesions in the M1 segment can result in plaque shift and closure of these perforators with resultant ischemia of the internal capsule. The M1 segment normally divides into a superior and inferior subdivision. Emboli often lodge at this bifurcation. The M2 segment usually begins after the M1 bifurcation and is anatomically defined as the segment extending from the superior turn of the MCA into the insula to the circular sulcus of the insula. It is also known as the insular segment. Distally, as it turns horizontally in the AP cranial projection, it is known as the M3, or opercular segment. The M3 segment extends to the lateral convexity, after which it is termed M4, or the cortical segment. Embolic strokes involving only the M3 and M4 segments result in more specific neurological deficits, and are highly variable depending on the location of the infarct.

Anterior Cerebral Artery

The anterior cerebral artery (Figs. 12A, B) supplies most of the medial surface of the cerebral cortex, the frontal pole, and the anterior portions of the corpus callosum. It originates at the carotid bifurcation and in the AP cranial projection, courses medially briefly, gives rise to the anterior communicating artery, and then runs superiorly. In the lateral projection, it curves around the corpus callosum. Strokes involving the anterior cerebral artery result in contralateral motor deficits, which are most profound in the lower extremities. Occlusions of bilateral anterior cerebral territories can result in frontal lobe symptoms. The most severe of these is akinetic mutism, a condition in which the patient recognizably has sleep–waking cycles, but is unresponsive, mute, and paralyzed.

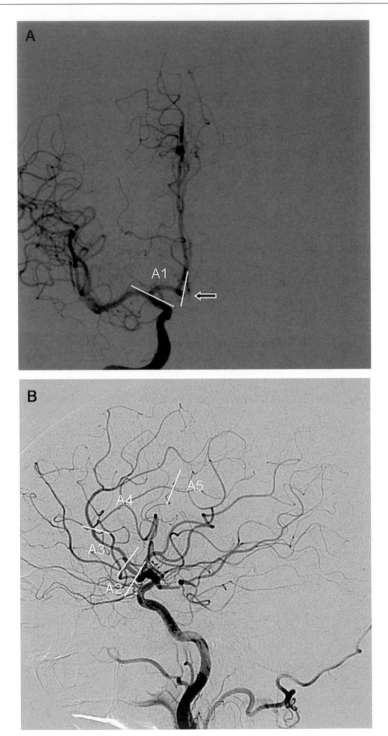

Fig. 12. The anterior cerebral artery (ACA) in the AP cranial (**A**) and lateral (**B**) projections. Segments A2–A5 are best visualized in the lateral projection and are defined by branches arising from anterior cerebral artery as it courses around the corpus callosum. The A1 segment is best seen in the AP cranial projection.

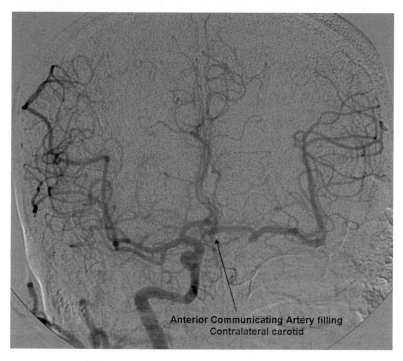

Fig. 13. The anterior communicating artery allows blood flow between the right and left hemispheres by forming a short connection between the distal A1 segments of the bilateral anterior cerebral arteries.

The anterior cerebral artery can be divided into five segments, A1–A5. The A1 segment originates at the carotid bifurcation and extends to the origin of the anterior communicating artery, which allows blood flow between the right and left hemispheres by forming a short connection between the distal A1 segments of the bilateral anterior cerebral artery (Fig. 13). The anterior communicating artery can often be atretic, resulting in no cross-filling between the two cerebral hemispheres. The A2 segment starts after the anterior communicating artery and from this point the bilateral anterior cerebral arteries course adjacently as they arch superiorly and posteriorly around the genu of the corpus callosum. The remaining segments are defined by branches arising from the anterior cerebral. The distal branches of the anterior cerebral artery anastomose with the distal branches of the posterior cerebral artery.

POSTERIOR CIRCULATION

Vertebral Arteries

The vertebral arteries arise superiorly and posteriorly from the proximal portions of the respective subclavian arteries (Fig. 14A, B). The ostia of both vertebral arteries are normally located just proximal to the origin of the thyrocervical trunk and opposite the origin of the internal mammary artery. It is common for the left vertebral artery to arise directly from the aortic arch, typically between the origins of the left subclavian artery and the left common carotid artery. Other variations include the left vertebral artery originating from the proximal portions of the left common carotid artery or the left subclavian artery. Variations of the right vertebral artery are relatively uncommon, but can include origins from the right common carotid, innominate, or directly from the arch. It

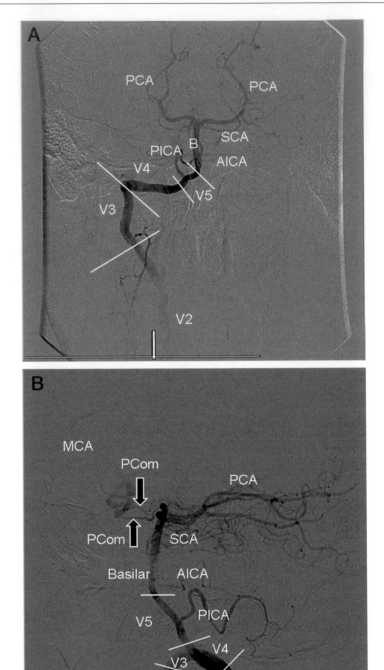

Fig. 14. The right vertebral artery and posterior circulation in the AP cranial (**A**) and lateral (**B**) projections. The V2 and V4 segments of the right vertebral artery are depicted. The posterior inferior cerebellar artery (PICA) normally originates from the V4 segment. The anterior inferior cerebellar artery (AICA) normally originates from the proximal basilar artery. The posterior communicating artery is best seen in the lateral projection (PCom). SCA, superior cerebellar artery; PCA, posterior cerebral artery; MCA, middle cerebral artery.

is extremely rare for the left vertebral artery to arise from the right subclavian. In 3% of cases, either vertebral artery may arise from the thyrocervical trunk or from the costo-cervical trunk. In the majority of patients, the two vertebrals are unequal in size, with one of the two vertebral arteries being dominant. In such cases, the non-dominant vertebral artery may be functional and small in caliber, but can often be atretic or non-existent. Angiographically, the ostia of the vertebral arteries are best visualized in the contralateral oblique view in about 60–70% of patients, and in the ipsilateral oblique view in the remainder.

Proximally, the vertebral arteries usually do not have any branches, but rarely can give rise to the inferior thyroid, the superior intercostal, deep cervical, or occipital artery. The vertebral artery can be divided into five segments, V1–V5. The first segment, V1, begins at the ostium and courses superiorly and posteriorly in front of the transverse process of the C7. It then enters the foramen of the C6 transverse process after which it is termed V2. It then courses superiorly through the foramina of C6 to C2. As it exits the transverse foramen of C2, it is termed V3, and extends superiorly to the atlanto-occipital membrane. At the atlanto-occipital membrane, the artery becomes V4 and courses medially to the foramen magnum. At this point it pierces through the dura mater, enters the foramen magnum, and extends to the basilar artery as V5.

The posterior inferior cerebellar artery (PICA) is the largest branch of the vertebral arteries and originates from the V5 segment just proximal to basilar artery. It supplies lower medulla, inferior fourth ventricle, tonsils, vermis, as well as the inferior and lateral cerebellum. The anterior inferior cerebellar artery (AICA) arises from the proximal to mid basilar artery (see below) and perfuses the pons, cranial nerves VI–VIII, and the middle cerebellar peduncle. The distal AICA and PICA anastomose at the lateral border of cerebellum and can form a large AICA–PICA complex (Fig. 15). As a result, if the anterior inferior cerebellar artery is dominant, the PICA may be absent, or vice versa. A stroke of the PICA territory is known as Wallenberg's syndrome, resulting in an *ipsilateral* nystagmus, Horner's syndrome, reduced corneal reflex, and loss of pain and temperature sensation on the face; and *contralateral* loss of pain and temperature sensation in the body and extremities.

Other branches of the vertebral artery include the posterolateral spinal artery, which can arise from the PICA in 73% of individuals, and the anterior spinal artery, which arises from two small branches that leave the vertebral arteries just before the vertebrals unite to form the basilar artery.

Basilar Artery

The basilar artery is formed by the convergence of the two vertebral arteries at the pontomedullary junction, except in cases where one of the vertebral arteries is atretic. It lies in the median groove of the pons where it courses from the lower to the upper border of the pons. It is a short artery and ends by bifurcating into the two posterior cerebral arteries. It gives rise to several pontine perforators, which originate at right angles to the basilar artery and, as the name suggests, supply the pons. Percutaneous interventions of the basilar artery are high risk partially because inadvertent closure of these branches can result in pontine infarcts and sudden death. The internal auditory artery arises from the mid portion of the basilar artery and supplies the inner ear. Distally, the basilar artery gives rise to the bilateral superior cerebellar arteries just proximal to bifurcating into the bilateral posterior cerebral arteries, and these vessels perfuse the lower mid-brain, upper pons, upper vermis, and superior cerebellum. Branches of the

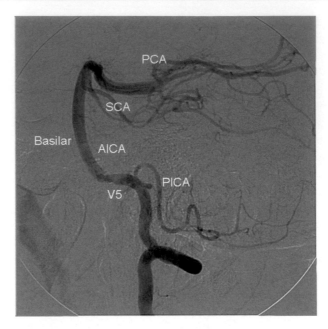

Fig. 15. The anterior inferior cerebellar artery (AICA) and the posterior inferior cerebellar artery (PICA) in the lateral projecion. One of the two arteries may be dominant, and the distal portions of the vessels can form an anastomotic network creating an AICA–PICA complex. SCA, superior cerebellar artery; PCA, posterior cerebral artery.

superior cerebellar arteries form an anastomosis with branches of the inferior cerebellar arteries (PICA and AICA) in the pia mater.

Posterior Cerebral Artery

The posterior cerebral artery can be divided into three sections, P1, P2, and P3 (Figs. 16A, B, C). The P1 segment courses laterally parallel to the superior cerebellar artery and receives the posterior communicating artery from the ipsilateral internal carotid artery. The P1 segment gives rise to the thalamic perforators, which supply the thalamus and subthalamic nuclei. If the P1 segment is atretic, or a majority of the flow to posterior cerebral artery is via the anterior circulation from the posterior communicating artery, the posterior cerebral artery is termed as being of fetal origin. Approximately 20–30% of people have fetal origins of this vessel, and this is an important angiographic finding as it may result in a posterior circulation stroke from occlusive disease of the anterior circulation. The P2 segment begins after the posterior communicating artery and provides perfusion to lateral thalamus, posterior limb of internal capsule, and part of the optic tract. The P3 segment is variable and typically perfuses the posterior temporal, parietal, and occipital lobes.

Circle of Willis

The circle of Willis is named after Thomas Willis, who is credited with being one of the first people to describe and illustrate the structure. It consists of the basilar artery, the anterior communicating artery, and the bilateral internal carotid arteries, middle cerebral arteries, posterior cerebral arteries, anterior cerebral arteries, and posterior communicating arteries. It is the major collateral pathway of the brain and connects the anterior and

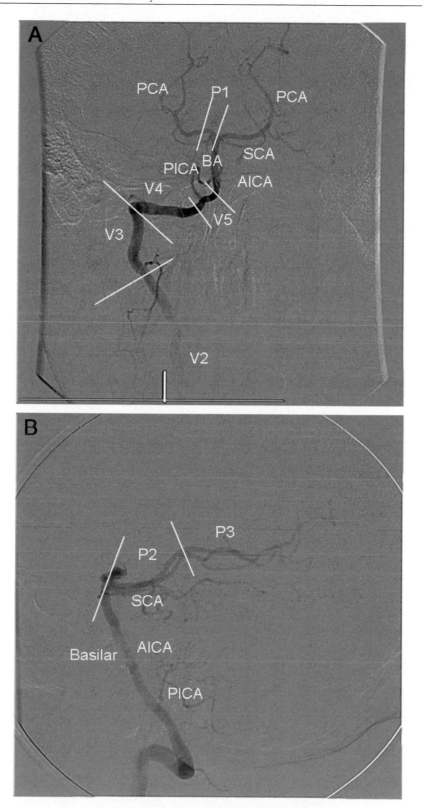

Fig. 16. (*Continued*)

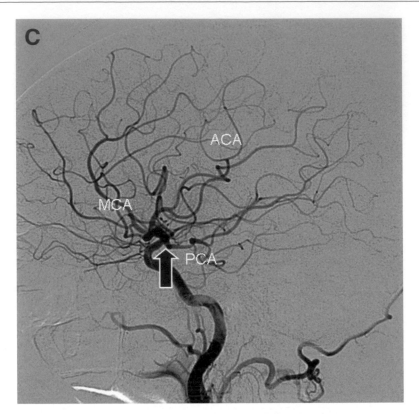

Fig. 16. The posterior cerebral artery (PCA) in the AP cranial projection (**A**) and lateral projection (**B**). The P1 segment extends from the basilar artery (BA) bifurcation to origin of the posterior communicating artery, and provides perfusion to thalamus and subthalamic nuclei, upper midbrain, and posterior portion of the internal capsule. The P2 segment extends from its origin at the posterior communicating artery to back of the mid-brain. The posterior cerebral artery is termed fetal if the P1 segment is atretic and the majority of its flow is derived from the anterior circulation via the posterior communicating artery (**C**). PICA, posterior inferior cerebellar artery; AICA, anterior inferior cerebellar artery; ACA, anterior cerebral artery; MCA, middle cerebral artery; SCA, superior cerebellar artery.

posterior circulations bilaterally via the posterior communicating arteries, as well as the left and the right anterior hemispheric circulation via the anterior communicating artery. Theoretically, if all the vessels are patent, the circle will allow continuous perfusion of all parts of the brain in the event of an occlusion of one of the source vessels. In reality, however, the anterior communicating artery or one or both of the posterior communicating arteries may not be patent, thereby resulting in incomplete collateralization.

REFERENCES

1. Netter FH. Atlas of Human Anatomy. Ciba-Geigy Corporation, Summit, NJ, 1989.
2. Standring S. (ed.) Gray's Anatomy: The Anatomical Basis of Clinical Practice, 39th ed. Elsevier/Churchill Livingstone, London, UK, 2004.
3. Morris P. Interventional and Endovascular Therapy of the Nervous System—A Practical Guide. Springer-Verlag, New York, NY, 2002.

6

Noninvasive Imaging of the Carotid Artery

J. Emilio Exaire, MD, Mikhael Mazighi, MD, Jacqueline Saw, MD, and Alex Abou-Chebl, MD

CONTENTS

Summary

Noninvasive carotid artery evaluation is an essential tool to assess patients who are at risk of atherosclerotic carotid artery disease because digital subtraction angiography is invasive and carries a 0.3 1% risk of periprocedural transient ischemic attack or stroke. Currently, duplex ultrasound, computed tomography angiography, magnetic resonance angiography, and transcranial Doppler are available to noninvasively evaluate the severity of carotid artery disease. The relative merits and limitations of each technique are reviewed in this chapter.

Key Words: Computed tomography angiography, duplex ultrasound, magnetic resonance angiography, transcranial doppler.

INTRODUCTION

The carotid artery is frequently affected by atherosclerosis, and as a consequence is a common cause of cerebral ischemia. The demonstrated efficacy of carotid endarterectomy (CEA) to prevent recurrent cerebral ischemic events in symptomatic high-grade internal carotid artery (ICA) stenosis *(1,2)*, and the potential benefit in asymptomatic high-grade ICA stenosis *(3)*, underscores the importance of grading the stenosis. Noninvasive carotid artery evaluation is an essential tool to assess patients who are at risk of atherosclerotic carotid artery disease because digital subtraction angiography (DSA), the gold-standard imaging modality for the detection and assessment of carotid

From: *Contemporary Cardiology: Handbook of Complex Percutaneous Carotid Intervention*
Edited by: J. Saw, J. E. Exaire, D. S. Lee, and S. Yadav © Humana Press Inc., Totowa, NJ

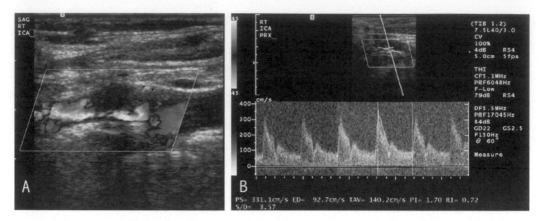

Fig. 1. (A) B-Mode and **(B)** color Doppler ultrasound of a calcified carotid artery bifurcation stenosis.

artery stenosis, is invasive and carries a 0.3–1% risk of periprocedural transient ischemic attack (TIA) or stroke *(4)*.

Currently, duplex ultrasound (DUS), computed tomography angiography (CTA), magnetic resonance angiography (MRA), and transcranial Doppler (TCD) are available to noninvasively evaluate the severity of carotid artery disease. The relative merits and limitations of each technique will be reviewed in this chapter. Because of the scope of this book and the complexity of the imaging techniques discussed in this chapter, only a cursory introduction is presented. Those seeking detailed information on the various radiographic techniques are referred to the numerous radiological texts available.

DUPLEX ULTRASOUND

Duplex ultrasonography is the standard first-line noninvasive method for the evaluation of carotid artery stenosis. It is an investigative tool that is widely available, is inexpensive, and carries no risk to patients. In addition to stenosis severity it permits visualization of vessel wall thickenings and the echogenity of the plaque *(3,5,6)*. This study has two components (thus the name duplex): the first uses B-mode US technique with superimposed color Doppler (Fig. 1); the second includes a spectral analysis measuring systolic and diastolic blood flow velocities. DUS is ideal for evaluation of the carotid artery bifurcation, which is relatively superficial. However, the ostium and proximal portion of the common carotid artery (CCA), as well as the mid-distal ICA will not be visualized, because sound waves poorly penetrate bone- and air-containing structures.

The major limitations of DUS are the fundamental dependence on technician skills, the wide variation in performance methods, and the nonstandardized interpretation of the results. Although the accreditation of Vascular Laboratories has improved standardization of DUS interpretation, this has not abolished the wide variation in practice pattern. Thus, there are ongoing concerns about the potential inconsistencies between laboratories, and also regrettably within a given laboratory. Further, it is appalling that an estimated 80% of patients in the United States underwent CEA based solely on DUS results, without confirmation with adjunctive tests *(7)*. As the efficacy of CEA has been established based on carotid stenosis severity (≥50% for symptomatic patients and ≥60% for asymptomatic patients) derived largely from angiographic imaging in randomized-controlled trials *(1–3)*, such treatment algorithm based solely on duplex

US (which may be inaccurate based on the above) may subject patients to unnecessary surgery. Thus, the Society of Radiologists in Ultrasound had convened and published a consensus addressing the performance and interpretation of DUS, with hopes that such a document would improve the consistency between and within laboratories *(7)*.

Recommendations on Technical Performance of Duplex US

According to this consensus *(7)*, all ICA imaging should be determined using (a) gray-scale ultrasound, (b) color Doppler, and (c) spectral Doppler. The Doppler waveform should be obtained with an angle of insonation ≤60°. In addition, the sample volume should be positioned within the area of greatest stenosis (after a thorough search through the stenotic plaque for the site of highest velocity) *(7)*.

Recommendations on the Interpretation of Duplex US

The interpretation of ICA stenosis severity should be primarily based on the ICA peak systolic velocity (PSV) and the presence of plaque on grayscale and/or color Doppler. The reliance on PSV is because this measurement is easy to obtain with good reproducibility. If there are clinical or technical concerns about the reliability of the ICA PSV (e.g., tandem lesions, severe contralateral carotid stenosis, discrepancy between visual plaque volume and velocity, hyperdynamic or low cardiac output), then the ICA–CCA PSV ratio and ICA end diastolic velocity (EDV) may also be used. The category of stenosis severity should be stratified into: normal (no stenosis), <50% stenosis, 50–69% stenosis, ≥70% to near occlusion, near occlusion, and total occlusion *(7)*. The consensus criteria for each category are listed in Table 1.

Limitations of DUS

Despite its wide availability and relatively low cost, carotid US has several limitations. Depending on the technical skills and experience of the operator, lesions can be either over- or underestimated for a variety of reasons: any extensive or calcified disease may obstruct distal visualization; some lesions may be inaccessible if they are higher than the second cervical vertebrae or if they are below the clavicle. Likewise, tortuous vessels and severe contralateral disease (resulting from increased collateral flow) may result in an increase in velocity measurement, falsely reflecting more severe disease than is present *(8,9)*. The North American Symptomatic Carotid Endarterectomy Trial (NASCET) showed that carotid US had a low sensitivity (68%) and specificity (67%) *(2,10)*; the protocol, however, used only the visual characteristics alone to characterize the degree of stenosis. In the Asymptomatic Carotid Atherosclerosis Study (ACAS) the specificity increased to 95% by adopting a protocol correlating Doppler measurements with carotid angiography (Fig. 2) *(3)*.

DUS and Bilateral Carotid Stenosis

It has been established that in patients with severe carotid artery stenosis, the flow velocity in the contralateral carotid artery is frequently elevated, as a result of shunting of blood flow from the stenosed vessel to the other carotid, and/or decrease compliance of the diseased contralateral artery *(9,11,12)*. Therefore, DUS may falsely interpret severe ipsilateral carotid stenosis as significant bilateral disease. Revascularization of the severe ipsilateral carotid stenosis either by CEA or carotid artery stenting (CAS) has been shown to reduce the contralateral carotid velocity *(9,11,13)*. In the study by Henderson et al. CEA of one carotid artery in patients

Table 1
Consensus Document Criteria for Stenosis Category

ICA stenosis category	ICA PSV	Plaque estimate	ICA/CCA PSV	ICA EDV
Normal	<125 cm/s	None	<2.0	<40 cm/s
<50%	<125 cm/s	Visible plaque ≤50% or intimal thickening	<2.0	<40 cm/s
50–69%	125–230 cm/s	Visible plaque ≥50%	2.0–4.0	40–100 cm/s
≥70% to near occlusion	>230 cm/s	Lumen narrowing with plaque ≥50%	<4.0	>100 cm/s
Near occlusion	Flow high, low or undetectable	Markedly narrowed lumen	Variable	Variable
Total occlusion	No flow	No detectable lumen	NA	NA

Adapted from ref. 7.
CCA, Common carotid artery; EDV, end diastolic velocity; ICA, internal carotid artery; NA, not applicable; PSV, peak systolic velocity.

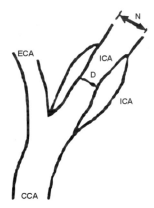

NASCET CRITERIA: Luminal diameter on 2 views at the point of greatest stenosis and the normal part of the artery beyound the carotid bulb. The percent stenosis was determined by calculating the ratio of these 2 measurements.

ACAS ANGIOGRAPHIC CRITERIA: Stenosis of at least 60% using the minimal residual lumen and the distal lumen defined as the first point distal to the minimal residual lumen at which the arterial walls became parallel.

ACAS UL TRASOUND PROTOCOL: It established a cut point for US devices and techniques by comparing Doppler ultrasonography toarteriograms. Dopper cut points were computed for peak systolic frequency or end diastolic frequency.

Fig. 2. NASCET and ACAS criteria to evaluate carotid artery stenosis.

(n = 386) with severe bilateral carotid stenosis resulted in a mean PSV drop of 84 cm/s on the contralateral side (11). Likewise, in the study by Sachar et al. which evaluated 49 patients with bilateral carotid stenosis based on pre-CAS DUS, there was a significant drop in the contralateral PSV (by 60.3 cm/s, p = 0.005) and EDV (by 15.1 cm/s,

$p = 0.03$) after ipsilateral CAS (9). In fact, 71% of patients thought to have significant contralateral carotid stenosis based on DUS pre-CAS did not have significant stenosis on angiography (9). Therefore, patients thought to have bilateral carotid stenosis on DUS should always undergo an additional noninvasive imaging prior to CEA, or confirmation by DSA prior to CAS.

DUS After Carotid Artery Stenting

DUS is routinely performed following CAS to evaluate for development of in-stent restenosis, which may present with asymptomatic elevation of carotid velocity readings. However, such interpretations are often confounded by the increased stiffness in the stented segment, which can produce elevated blood velocities. In the retrospective analysis by Stanziale et al. which included 118 patients who underwent both DUS and DSA after CAS, the PSV and ICA/CCA ratio are significantly higher in stented carotid arteries compared with nonstented arteries (14). Based on their analysis, the authors recommended using the criteria of PSV $\geq$350 cm/s or ICA/CCA ratio $\geq$4.75 to diagnose in-stent restenosis $\geq$70%, and the combined criteria of PSV $\geq$225 cm/s and ICA/CCA ration $\geq$2.5 to diagnose in-stent restenosis $\geq$50% (see Table 5 in Chapter 12) (14).

Carotid Artery Intimal–Medial Thickness

DUS capable of visualizing the arterial wall has also been used as a marker of atherosclerosis. Carotid arterial intimal–medial thickness (IMT) measured with B-mode US is used as an end point in epidemiologic studies and clinical trials to evaluate progression and regression of atherosclerosis (15,16). IMT is assessed by scanning longitudinal views of the CCA. The near and far wall views of the CCA are scanned and measured with an automated computerized edge-detection algorithm (17). Cross-sectional associations have been reported between IMT and cardiovascular risk factors (18,19); in addition, increased IMT has been described to be associated with ischemic stroke (20).

Correlation of DUS to DSA

The literature is replete with studies comparing DUS to other imaging modalities (most often to DSA), as individual laboratories attempt to evaluate the reliability and accuracy of their DUS results. It is impractical to summarize all these individual studies; thus we will only concentrate on meta-analyses.

Nederkoorn et al. reviewed 63 studies published between 1994 and 2001, which compared MRA and/or DUS to DSA as the reference standard. For DUS, the pooled sensitivity and specificity of diagnosing stenosis severity 70–99% was 86% (95% confidence interval [CI]: 84–89%) and 87% (95% CI: 84–90%), respectively. For diagnosing occlusion, DUS has a pooled sensitivity and specificity of 96% (95% CI: 94–98%) and 100% (95% CI: 99–100%), respectively (21).

Jahromi et al. reviewed 47 studies published between 1966 and 2003, which compared DUS to DSA based on the NASCET criteria. As this study was executed after the consensus document publication, the authors tried to evaluate similar criteria that were recommended by the consensus. To identify stenosis $\geq$50%, PSV of $\geq$130 cm/s had a pooled sensitivity and specificity of 98% and 88%, respectively. To identify stenosis $\geq$70%, pooled sensitivities and specificities were 90% and 85% for PSV of $\geq$230 cm/s, 80% and 88% for ICA/CCA ratio $\geq$4, and 82% and 90% for EDV $\geq$100 cm/s (Table 2) (22).

Readers need to keep in mind that these values are derived from heterogeneous studies and may not be applicable to their own laboratory. For more reliable correlation,

Table 2
Pooled Weighted Means of Sensitivities and Specificities of Duplex Ultrasound

DUS Category	N	Sensitivity (%)	95% CI (%)	Specificity (%)	95% CI (%)
For angiographic stenosis ≥50%					
PSV ≥120 cm/s	3001	96	91–100	82	72–93
PSV ≥130 cm/s	1716	98	97–100	88	76–100
For angiographic stenosis ≥70%					
PSV ≥150 cm/s	1996	96	93–98	80	71–90
PSV ≥200 cm/s	2140	90	84–94	94	88–97
PSV ≥230 cm/s	2108	90	83–96	85	77–92
PSV ≥250 cm/s	1904	76	63–89	93	88–98
ICA/CCA ≥3	999	89	81–96	84	77–92
ICA/CCA ≥4	1933	80	70–90	88	83–93
EDV ≥70 cm/s	1419	89	84–94	80	66–93
EDV ≥100 cm/s	1607	82	70–93	90	82–99
EDV ≥120 cm/s	1478	79	71–87	92	86–98

Adapted from the meta-analysis by Jahromi et al. *(22)*.
CCA, Common carotid artery; CI, confidence interval; DUS, duplex ultrasound; EDV, end diastolic velocity; ICA, internal carotid artery; PSV, peak systolic velocity.

individual laboratories are encouraged to perform their own comparative analyses between their institutions' DUS and DSA data, if possible.

CT ANGIOGRAPHY

With older CT equipment, the evaluation of carotid arteries was limited by movement artifacts and thick scanning sections; this resulted in either over or underestimation of stenoses leading to a poor (~50%) correlation with DSA *(23,24)*. However, newer multisection, helical CT scanners can perform angiography via the acquisition of 1.0- to 2.0-mm axial images within a single breath hold. Intravenous contrast material (120–150 mL of nonionic contrast) is injected at 30–40 mL/s to achieve a contrast density of 150 Hounsfield units (HU). All images are first reviewed in the axial plane and measurements are made across the lumen through the narrowest portion of the proximal ICA and across the area of the normal ICA segment just above the stenosis. The degree of stenosis is calculated according to the NASCET criteria.

CTA data can be processed and rendered graphically in several ways (axial, multiplanar reformatted, 3D volume maximum intensity projection [MIP], shaded surface display [SSD] and volume rendering [VR]-model images) that contribute substantially to the sensitivity and accuracy of multisection CTA (Fig. 3). The VR technique creates a stack of parallel planes to create a high-definition image *(25)*. SSD and MIP are both 3D display techniques. SSD is generated by selecting a CT value above a defined density threshold. The threshold must be carefully chosen on the basis of contrast material attenuation in the area of interest. Then a surface is calculated as if the structure is illuminated by a light source to achieve the 3D impression through shading. MIP is a VR method. The intensity of each pixel in the resulting image is the maximum intensity encountered along parallel rays traced through the volume and projected in the desired

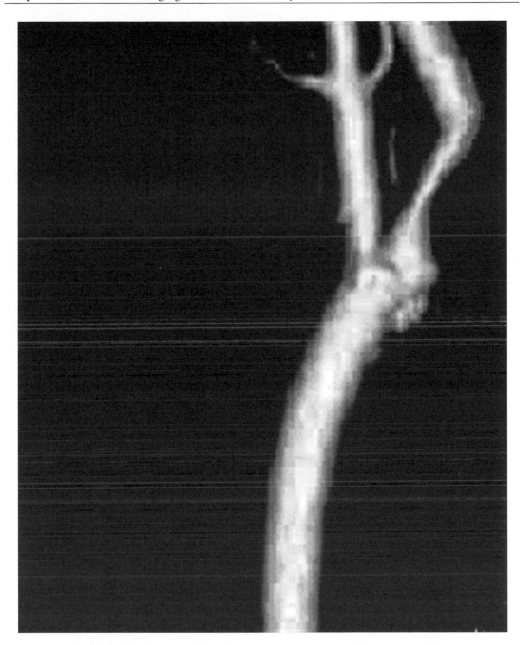

Fig. 3. CT angiography demonstrating an internal carotid artery stenosis.

viewing direction. With this technique the depth information is lost, but the density information is retained *(26)*.

Overall accuracy for carotid CTA exceeds 95% *(27)* and in some studies has a 96% correlation with DSA with a 100% sensitivity. The high sensitivity comes at the cost of only a 63% specificity with a negative predictive value of 70% *(28)*. For intracranial stenoses, the sensitivity reaches 87% with a specificity of 98% and a negative predictive value of 99.5% *(29)*. These recent data are in contradiction with previous articles reporting that CTA is limited in its ability to evaluate the petrous or cavernous ICA *(30,31)*.

CTA imaging quality is technique dependent, and the observed discrepancies may be explained by differences in data acquisition, processing, and postprocessing software performance. These elements are critically important for accurate CTA interpretation.

Limitations of CTA

CTA imaging has several limitations: the use of iodinated contrast restricts its indication in patients with renal disease; metallic objects such as dental implants, vascular clips, or endovascular coils create excessive artifact that may completely obscure nearby vessels; motion artifacts (such as breathing or swallowing) as well as poor technique due to operator error can also affect image quality. The latter occurs if the timing of the scan is premature or delayed relative to the arrival of the IV contrast bolus to the area of interest. In either case poor opacification of the arteries or excessive opacification of venous structures may occur, leading to false-positive results. Dense vascular calcifications, as with US, may also limit the ability of the interpreter to identify severe lesions. False-negative results may occur if the vessels of the carotid bulb are tortuous or dilated, or superimposed jugular veins may hide a stenosis. Another limitation of spiral CTA is the inability to characterize plaque composition and morphology *(32)*. However, in comparison to MRA scan time is much less and claustrophobic patients can tolerate CTA without difficulty. Moreover, there are no contraindications to CTA for patients with pacemakers or implanted devices.

CTA After Carotid Stenting

After carotid stenting, CTA may be a useful adjunct to DUS for follow-up. DUS provides both morphologic and hemodynamic data, but the rostral portion of the stent may be difficult to evaluate because of anatomic factors. With other noninvasive techniques such as contrast-enhanced MRA (CE-MRA), susceptibility artifacts may hinder complete visualization of the stent. CTA with VR can allow differentiation between the enhanced arterial lumen and the wall of the stent *(33)*. Even though this technique may lead to an overestimation of the thickness of the stent, it may be useful for monitoring the carotid artery after stenting to detect restenosis in the long-term follow-up.

MR ANGIOGRAPHY

MR imaging is a high-resolution imaging modality widely used for imaging intracranial and cervical vessels *(34,35)* that does not use ionizing radiation, but rather strong magnetic fields to image tissues. This modality is less susceptible to calcium artifact compared to DUS and CTA.

The first technique is two-dimensional (2D) time-of-flight (TOF) MR angiographic (MRA) imaging, which is performed by the acquisition of multiple 1.5-mm sections. The images are stacked to make a volume set. A three-dimensional (3D) TOF technique is also available; this method is similar to 2D TOF except that the data is collected as a 3D volume set rather than individual slices. The 3D technique allows for the acquisition of 0.7-mm slices and offers better resolution than 2D TOF *(36)*. Both of these modalities are flow-based, that is, they are not luminograms. Although TOF is an extremely sensitive technique, it is not specific as the data acquired are susceptible to turbulence. Furthermore poststenotic decreases in flow velocity can result in signal loss. The length of the resulting signal loss correlates with the degree of velocity elevation within the stenosis; increasing peak velocity increases the length of the signal void *(37,38)*. With this technique, vessels appear with high signal intensity due to the inflow effect of blood during its passage through the acquisition volume, whereas the background tissue appears dark due to the short repetition time that prevents stationary tissue relaxation. Motion artifacts are also responsible for image degradation due to the long time required for data acquisition. Finally, this technique does not allow assessment of the anterior and posterior circulation from the aortic arch to the circle of Willis.

The second technique, the CE-MRA, is performed by using a timed and rapid injection of gadolinium dimeglumine (15–20 mL). The gadolinium injection rate and volume influences the arrival time in the CCA and the jugular vein as well as the arteriovenous transit time. These factors may affect the optimal quality of the MRA *(39)*. The underlying effect of CE-MRA is the T1 shortening caused by the presence of gadolinium chelates, which produce excellent signal-to-noise ratio, bypassing the relatively poor resolution of the 2D TOF technique. The images are obtained using a short TR, short echo time (TE), and T1-weighted technique. A 3D TOF image or a contrast-enhanced short-TE sort-TR image is interpreted as an angiogram according to the NASCET criteria (Fig. 4). A great advantage of CE-MRA is that a greater volume of the body can be imaged in a shorter time, allowing simultaneous evaluation of the entire vasculature from the aortic arch to the circle of Willis, which can be viewed in multiple planes. Both the carotid and the vertebral arteries may be assessed throughout their cervical and intracranial portions with a uniform high signal intensity providing angiographic images similar to those obtained with conventional catheter angiography *(33)*.

Limitations with MRA

Despite the great recent advances in this technique, it has several limitations: pseudo-stenosis secondary to turbulent flow particularly in severely angulated vessels; exaggeration of the stenosis length due to a tight focal stenosis; and metal and movement artifacts (e.g., swallowing). The overall sensitivity of MRA is 75% and specificity is 88% *(40,41)*. Based on a meta-analysis study, MRA appears to be effective for detecting 70–99% stenosis as defined by conventional angiography, with a sensitivity and specificity of 99%. However, the use of MRA does not seem appropriate to select patients for treatment when the degree of stenosis is <70% *(42)*.

MR imaging is contraindicated in patients who have cardiac pacemakers, early generation cerebral aneurysm clips, or in those who have undergone certain other medical procedures. Additional limitations include the potential for data degradation if data acquisition is not perfectly timed with the arrival of the contrast bolus, although effective methods have been described to overcome this *(43,44)*. Current limitations, including timing errors and artifacts, will be probably be resolved in the near future. However, specific equipment and software, including tracking pulse sequences, MR fluoroscopy, larger coil configuration, and higher gradient strength are required to improve image quality to reach the excellent resolution of X-ray angiography.

In a research perspective, high-resolution, multicontrast, MR can image and characterize vulnerable plaques in terms of lipid and fibrous content, and identify the presence of thrombus or calcium *(45)*. The clinical application of this technique may enhance the understanding of the progression and regression of atherosclerotic disease and in the future may be a useful marker of treatment efficacy.

TRANSCRANIAL DOPPLER

TCD was first introduced in 1982 *(46)*, whereby a Doppler ultrasound probe (low-frequency 2-MHz transducer) placed in the temporal area just above the zygomatic

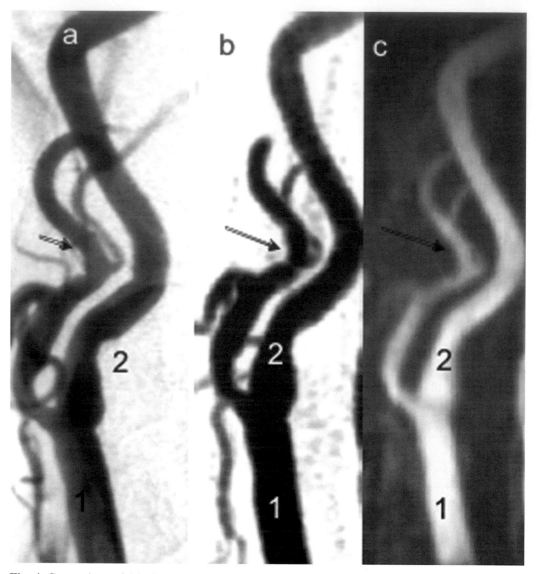

Fig. 4. Comparison of **(a)** digital substraction angiography (DSA), **(b)** gadolinium enhanced MRA, and **(c)** TOF MRA. Notice the definition of the carotid bulb in the DSA and the enhanced MRA, whereas in the TOF it cannot be completely defined (possible stenosis). The external carotid artery is normal in the DSA, but it shows a narrowing in the gadolinium enhanced MRA *(arrow)*. *1,* Common carotid artery; *2,* internal carotid artery.

arch allowed flow velocities in the anterior cerebral artery (ACA), middle cerebral artery (MCA), and posterior cerebral artery (PCA) to be measured. TCD utilizes the Doppler principle that ultrasound waves reflected off red blood cells demonstrate a change in frequency in proportion to the velocity. It is a noninvasive technique that allows measurement of blood flow velocity and direction in major cerebral arteries at the base of the brain. It is a simple, inexpensive, and readily available bedside test. However, image acquisition depends on adequate acoustic windows (roughly 15% of patients have insufficient windows) *(47)*, and data interpretation is very much operator

Table 3
Accuracy of Conventional Transcranial Doppler in Identifying Intracranial
Stenosis, Using Angiography as the Reference Standard

Indication	Sensitivity (%)	Specificity (%)
Intracranial stenotic lesions		
Anterior circulation	70–90	90–95
Posterior circulation	50–80	80–96
Intranial occlusive lesions		
MCA	85–95	90–98
ICA, VA, BA	55–81	96
Extracranial ICA stenosis	49–95	42–100

Adapted from ref. *51.*
BA, Basilar artery; ICA, internal carotid artery; MCA, middle cerebral artery; VA, vertebral artery.

dependent. Only large proximal intracranial vessels may be imaged; for instance, the distal M1 segment and the M2 segment of the MCA are poorly visualized, and significant stenosis in these segments may be missed in 50% of patients *(47).*

In the setting of acute ischemic stroke, intracranial arterial occlusions detected by TCD are associated with poor neurological recovery, disability, or death after 90 d *(48),* whereas normal results predict early improvement *(49).* The responsible artery of an acute cerebral infarction may be detected with TCD with a sensitivity and specificity reaching 90% *(50).* However, the sensitivity and specificity values may vary with the vessel of concern (Table 3) *(51).* In general TCD is inadequate as the sole vascular imaging modality because of its lower sensitivity compared to the other noninvasive imaging modalities and it is best used in conjunction with one of the other studies such as MRA or CTA. Critical (i.e., flow-limiting) extracranial ICA stenosis can sometimes be detected by TCD with findings such as reversal of the direction of ophthalmic artery flow, presence of collateral flow patterns via the anterior or posterior communicating arteries, absence of ophthalmic or carotid siphon flow, and reduced MCA flow velocity and pulsatility *(52).* TCD is also an accurate indicator of blood flow status and correlates well with MRA abnormalities in acute stroke *(53).* The relative value of TCD compared with MRA or CTA remains to be determined. Use of single TCD measurements or a battery of TCD measurements has variable sensitivity and specificity, but when highly specific carotid duplex criteria are added, sensitivity and specificity are considerably improved *(54,55).*

High-Intensity Transient Signals (Microembolic Signals)

A few years after the introduction of TCD, it was discovered that high-intensity transient signals (HITS) can be observed with TCD *(56).* These signals are due to increased ultrasound signals reflected and scattered from microemboli compared to the surrounding blood (Fig. 5). These microembolic signals may be liberated spontaneously (e.g., ICA stenosis, prosthetic heart valves, cardiomyopathy, myocardial infarction, atrial fibrillation, aortic arch atheroma, fat embolization syndrome, and retinal or general cerebral vascular disease) *(57),* or during cerebrovascular and cardiovascular procedures. Until recently, TCD was not able to differentiate between solid (e.g., platelet thrombus, cholesterol emboli) or gaseous signals. However, a multifrequency TCD system is now

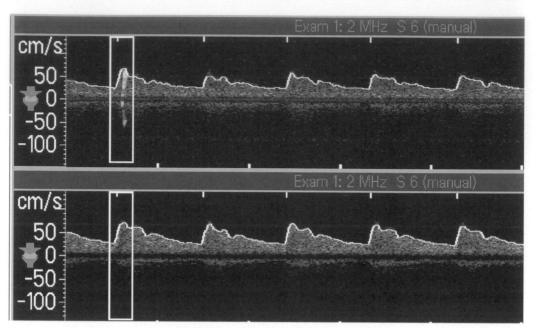

Fig. 5. Transcranial Doppler of the MCA shows one high-intensity transient signal HITS *(arrow)* consistent with an embolus in a patient with a symptomatic ICA stenosis.

available *(58)*, which allows automatic discrimination between solid and gaseous microemboli by insonating emboli with two different frequencies *(59)*. A solid embolus would reflect more ultrasound with the higher frequency, whereas a gaseous embolus would reflect more ultrasound with the lower frequency.

In patients with high-grade carotid stenosis, sources of asymptomatic microembolic signals may include ulcerated plaques *(60)* and microscopic platelet aggregates and fibrin clots *(61)*. Asymptomatic cerebral microembolization is associated with an increased risk of further cerebral ischemia in this setting *(60)*.

Limitations of TCD

As with any ultrasonographic technique, TCD is operator dependent and requires training and experience to perform and interpret results. TCD can be performed at the bedside and repeated as needed or applied for continuous monitoring. Its chief limitation is that it is a blind technique in that the target vessels cannot usually be visualized as with DUS and the need for ultrasonic windows (orbital, transtemporal, and foramen magnum) that allow transmission of the ultrasound signal through the calvarium. The latter restrict the area of insonation to the major cerebral arteries and the proximal part of their branches, lower the spatial resolution, and in the case of the transtemporal window, may prevent insonation of the anterior circulation if the temporal bone is too thick (20–30% of individuals).

Transcranial Color-Coded Duplex Sonograhy (TCCS)

TCCS is a bedside noninvasive technique that shows a real-time two-dimensional depiction of the intracranial vascular structures *(62,63)*. Compared with conventional TCD, there is more accurate demonstration of vascular anatomy. In general, flow velocity measurements are highly reproducible. As with conventional TCD, a major limitation of TCCS is insufficient transtemporal US beam penetration due to hyperostosis of the skull

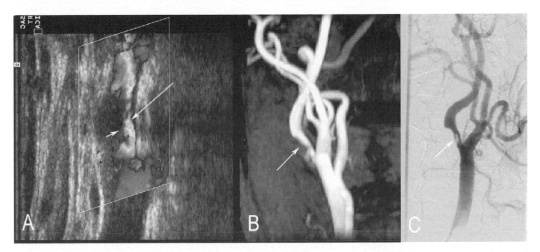

Fig. 6. Three imaging studies of a right internal carotid artery stenosis causing recurrent strokes and retinal TIAs. **(A)** Color Doppler ultrasound image showing the homogenous "plaque" *(short arrow)* and the area of stenosis with Doppler shift *(long arrow)*. A contrast-enhanced MRA **(B)** shows the same stenosis *(arrow)* but does not give any information about the plaque. A catheter angiographic image also shows the stenosis but discloses the presence of an intraluminal filling defect *(arrow)* consistent with thrombus. Although all three studies clearly define the location of the stenosis, angiography revealed the thrombus and shows that the degree of stenosis is actually not as severe as the >70% value reported by ultrasound and MRA. What the noninvasive studies were measuring as stenosis was actually the thrombus, which likely formed on top of the moderate 30–40% stenosis after plaque rupture.

(62,63). The use of transpulmonary echocontrast agents (ECA) may increase the Doppler signal intensity and improve the signal-to-noise ratio for transcranial insonation permitting insonation through otherwise impenetrable temporal bone windows *(64)*. However, ECA has not been approved by the US Food and Drug Administration. In patients with ischemic cerebrovascular disease, contrast-enhanced TCCS may detect the presence of hemodynamically significant ICA stenosis or occlusion, with improvement of diagnostic confidence (65–67).

PITFALLS OF NONINVASIVE IMAGING

Noninvasive techniques provide high-quality imaging of the carotid artery with low risk and at a lower cost. However, some pitfalls can lead to errors in clinical decisions. Misreading the degree of stenosis (either over- or underestimating), or misinterpreting a critical stenosis for an occlusion are not uncommon situations with noninvasive imaging. The inability to detect intraluminal filling defects or accurately analyze flow patterns are also important limitations (Fig. 6). Therefore, for complex lesions and in situations in which there is a discrepancy between two noninvasive studies, DSA remains the gold standard.

CONCLUSIONS

Recent advances in noninvasive imaging enable physicians to accurately evaluate the cerebral arteries and in particular the carotid arteries. The current techniques have excellent sensitivity and specificity. The choice of which technique to use varies by center, characteristics, and prevalence of disease in the study population, diagnostic criteria, and technical expertise. The need for DSA may be restricted to patients who need an invasive treatment or those with equivocal noninvasive diagnosis.

REFERENCES

1. North American Symptomatic Carotid Endarterectomy Trial Collaborators. Beneficial effect of carotid endarterectomy in symptomatic patients with high-grade carotid stenosis. N Engl J Med 1991;325: 445–453.
2. MRC European Carotid Surgery Trial: interim results for symptomatic patients with severe (70-99%) or with mild (0-29%) carotid stenosis. European Carotid Surgery Trialists' Collaborative Group. Lancet 1991;337:1235–1243.
3. Endarterectomy for asymptomatic carotid artery stenosis. Executive Committee for the Asymptomatic Carotid Atherosclerosis Study. JAMA 1995;273:1421–1428.
4. Kuntz KM, Skillman JJ, Whittemore AD, Kent KC. Carotid endarterectomy in asymptomatic patients—is contrast angiography necessary? A morbidity analysis. J Vasc Surg 1995;22:706–714; discussion 714–716.
5. Chang YJ, Golby AJ, Albers GW. Detection of carotid stenosis. From NASCET results to clinical practice. Stroke 1995;26:1325–1328.
6. Erdoes LS, Marek JM, Mills JL, et al. The relative contributions of carotid duplex scanning, magnetic resonance angiography, and cerebral arteriography to clinical decisionmaking: a prospective study in patients with carotid occlusive disease. J Vasc Surg 1996;23:950–956.
7. Grant EG, Benson CB, Moneta GL, et al. Carotid artery stenosis: grayscale and Doppler ultrasound diagnosis—Society of Radiologists in Ultrasound consensus conference. Ultrasound Q 2003;19: 190–198.
8. Sidhu PS. Ultrasound of the carotid and vertebral arteries. Br Med Bull 2000;56:346–366.
9. Sachar R, Yadav JS, Roffi M, et al. Severe bilateral carotid stenosis: the impact of ipsilateral stenting on Doppler-defined contralateral stenosis. J Am Coll Cardiol 2004;43:1358–1362.
10. Eliasziw M, Rankin RN, Fox AJ, Haynes RB, Barnett HJ. Accuracy and prognostic consequences of ultrasonography in identifying severe carotid artery stenosis. North American Symptomatic Carotid Endarterectomy Trial (NASCET) Group. Stroke 1995;26:1747–1752.
11. Henderson RD, Steinman DA, Eliasziw M, Barnett HJ. Effect of contralateral carotid artery stenosis on carotid ultrasound velocity measurements. Stroke 2000;31:2636–2640.
12. van Everdingen KJ, van der Grond J, Kappelle LJ. Overestimation of a stenosis in the internal carotid artery by duplex sonography caused by an increase in volume flow. J Vasc Surg 1998;27:479–485.
13. Williamson WK, Abou-Zamzam AM, Jr., Moneta GL, et al. Prophylactic repair of renal artery stenosis is not justified in patients who require infrarenal aortic reconstruction. J Vasc Surg 1998;28:14–20; discussion 20–22.
14. Stanziale SF, Wholey MH, Boules TN, Selzer F, Makaroun MS. Determining in-stent stenosis of carotid arteries by duplex ultrasound criteria. J Endovasc Ther 2005;12:346–353.
15. Blankenhorn DH, Hodis HN. George Lyman Duff Memorial Lecture. Arterial imaging and atherosclerosis reversal. Arterioscler Thromb 1994;14:177–192.
16. Mack WJ, Selzer RH, Hodis HN, et al. One-year reduction and longitudinal analysis of carotid intima-media thickness associated with colestipol/niacin therapy. Stroke 1993;24:1779–1783.
17. Selzer RH, Hodis HN, Kwong-Fu H, et al. Evaluation of computerized edge tracking for quantifying intima-media thickness of the common carotid artery from B-mode ultrasound images. Atherosclerosis 1994;111:1–11.
18. Bonithon-Kopp C, Scarabin PY, Taquet A, Touboul PJ, Malmejac A, Guize L. Risk factors for early carotid atherosclerosis in middle-aged French women. Arterioscler Thromb 1991;11:966–972.
19. O'Leary DH, Polak JF, Kronmal RA, et al. Distribution and correlates of sonographically detected carotid artery disease in the Cardiovascular Health Study. The CHS Collaborative Research Group. Stroke 1992;23:1752–1760.
20. Touboul PJ, Elbaz A, Koller C, et al. Common carotid artery intima-media thickness and brain infarction: the Etude du Profil Genetique de l'Infarctus Cerebral (GENIC) case-control study. The GENIC Investigators. Circulation 2000;102:313–318.
21. Nederkoorn PJ, van der Graaf Y, Hunink MG. Duplex ultrasound and magnetic resonance angiography compared with digital subtraction angiography in carotid artery stenosis: a systematic review. Stroke 2003;34:1324–1332.

22. Jahromi AS, Cina CS, Liu Y, Clase CM. Sensitivity and specificity of color duplex ultrasound measurement in the estimation of internal carotid artery stenosis: a systematic review and meta-analysis. J Vasc Surg 2005;41:962–972.

23. Castillo M. Diagnosis of disease of the common carotid artery bifurcation: CT angiography vs catheter angiography. AJR Am J Roentgenol 1993;161:395–398.

24. Cumming MJ, Morrow IM. Carotid artery stenosis: a prospective comparison of CT angiography and conventional angiography. AJR Am J Roentgenol 1994;163:517–523.

25. Verhoek G, Costello P, Khoo EW, Wu R, Kat E, Fitridge RA. Carotid bifurcation CT angiography: assessment of interactive volume rendering. J Comput Assist Tomogr 1999;23:590–596.

26. Leclerc X, Godefroy O, Pruvo JP, Leys D. Computed tomographic angiography for the evaluation of carotid artery stenosis. Stroke 1995;26:1577–1581.

27. Berg M, Zhang Z, Ikonen A, et al. Multi-detector row CT angiography in the assessment of carotid artery disease in symptomatic patients: comparison with rotational angiography and digital subtraction angiography. AJNR Am J Neuroradiol 2005;26:1022–1034.

28. Josephson SA, Bryant SO, Mak HK, Johnston SC, Dillon WP, Smith WS. Evaluation of carotid stenosis using CT angiography in the initial evaluation of stroke and TIA. Neurology 2004;63:457–460.

29. Bash S, Villablanca JP, Jahan R, et al. Intracranial vascular stenosis and occlusive disease: evaluation with CT angiography, MR angiography, and digital subtraction angiography. AJNR Am J Neuroradiol 2005;26:1012–1021.

30. Skutta B, Furst G, Eilers J, Ferbert A, Kuhn FP. Intracranial stenoocclusive disease: double-detector helical CT angiography versus digital subtraction angiography. AJNR Am J Neuroradiol 1999;20: 791–799.

31. Hirai T, Korogi Y, Ono K, et al. Prospective evaluation of suspected stenoocclusive disease of the intracranial artery: combined MR angiography and CT angiography compared with digital subtraction angiography. AJNR Am J Neuroradiol 2002;23:93–101.

32. Walker LJ, Ismail A, McMeekin W, Lambert D, Mendelow AD, Birchall D. Computed tomography angiography for the evaluation of carotid atherosclerotic plaque: correlation with histopathology of endarterectomy specimens. Stroke 2002;33:977–981.

33. Leclerc X, Gauvrit JY, Pruvo JP. Usefulness of CT angiography with volume rendering after carotid angioplasty and stenting. AJR Am J Roentgenol 2000;174:820–822.

34. Huston J, 3rd, Lewis BD, Wiebers DO, Meyer FB, Riederer SJ, Weaver AL. Carotid artery: prospective blinded comparison of two-dimensional time-of-flight MR angiography with conventional angiography and duplex US. Radiology 1993;186:339–344.

35. Mittl RL, Jr., Broderick M, Carpenter JP, et al. Blinded-reader comparison of magnetic resonance angiography and duplex ultrasonography for carotid artery bifurcation stenosis. Stroke 1994;25:4–10.

36. Scarabino T, Carriero A, Magarelli N, et al. MR angiography in carotid stenosis: a comparison of three techniques. Eur J Radiol 1998;28:117–125.

37. Polak JF, Bajakian RL, O'Leary DH, Anderson MR, Donaldson MC, Jolesz FA. Detection of internal carotid artery stenosis: comparison of MR angiography, color Doppler sonography, and arteriography. Radiology 1992;182:35–40.

38. Heiserman JE, Drayer BP, Keller PJ, Fram EK. Intracranial vascular stenosis and occlusion: evaluation with three-dimensional time-of-flight MR angiography. Radiology 1992;185:667–673.

39. Herold T, Paetzel C, Volk M, et al. Contrast-enhanced magnetic resonance angiography of the carotid arteries: influence of injection rates and volumes on arterial-venous transit time. Invest Radiol 2004;39:65–72.

40. Clifton AG. MR angiography. Br Med Bull 2000;56:367–377.

41. JM UK-I, Trivedi RA, Graves MJ, et al. Contrast-enhanced MR angiography for carotid disease: diagnostic and potential clinical impact. Neurology 2004;62:1282–1290.

42. Westwood ME, Kelly S, Berry E, et al. Use of magnetic resonance angiography to select candidates with recently symptomatic carotid stenosis for surgery: systematic review. BMJ 2002;324:198.

43. Isoda H, Takehara Y, Isogai S, et al. Technique for arterial-phase contrast-enhanced three-dimensional MR angiography of the carotid and vertebral arteries. AJNR Am J Neuroradiol 1998;19:1241–1244.

44. Foo TK, Saranathan M, Prince MR, Chenevert TL. Automated detection of bolus arrival and initiation of data acquisition in fast, three-dimensional, gadolinium-enhanced MR angiography. Radiology 1997;203:275–280.

45. Fayad ZA, Fuster V. Characterization of atherosclerotic plaques by magnetic resonance imaging. Ann N Y Acad Sci 2000;902:173–186.

46. Aaslid R, Markwalder TM, Nornes H. Noninvasive transcranial Doppler ultrasound recording of flow velocity in basal cerebral arteries. J Neurosurg 1982;57:769–774.

47. Suwanwela NC, Phanthumchinda K, Suwanwela N. Transcranial doppler sonography and CT angiography in patients with atherothrombotic middle cerebral artery stroke. AJNR Am J Neuroradiol 2002;23:1352–1355.

48. Baracchini C, Manara R, Ermani M, Meneghetti G. The quest for early predictors of stroke evolution: can TCD be a guiding light? Stroke 2000;31:2942–2947.

49. Kushner MJ, Zanette EM, Bastianello S, et al. Transcranial Doppler in acute hemispheric brain infarction. Neurology 1991;41:109–113.

50. Zanette EM, Fieschi C, Bozzao L, et al. Comparison of cerebral angiography and transcranial Doppler sonography in acute stroke. Stroke 1989;20:899–903.

51. Sloan MA, Alexandrov AV, Tegeler CH, et al. Assessment: transcranial Doppler ultrasonography: report of the Therapeutics and Technology Assessment Subcommittee of the American Academy of Neurology. Neurology 2004;62:1468–1481.

52. Molina CA, Montaner J, Abilleira S, et al. Timing of spontaneous recanalization and risk of hemorrhagic transformation in acute cardioembolic stroke. Stroke 2001;32:1079–1084.

53. Razumovsky AY, Gillard JH, Bryan RN, Hanley DF, Oppenheimer SM. TCD, MRA and MRI in acute cerebral ischemia. Acta Neurol Scand 1999;99:65–76.

54. Wilterdink JL, Feldmann E, Furie KL, Bragoni M, Benavides JG. Transcranial Doppler ultrasound battery reliably identifies severe internal carotid artery stenosis. Stroke 1997;28:133–136.

55. Can U, Furie KL, Suwanwela N, et al. Transcranial Doppler ultrasound criteria for hemodynamically significant internal carotid artery stenosis based on residual lumen diameter calculated from en bloc endarterectomy specimens. Stroke 1997;28:1966–1971.

56. Padayachee TS, Gosling RG, Bishop CC, Burnand K, Browse NL. Monitoring middle cerebral artery blood velocity during carotid endarterectomy. Br J Surg 1986;73:98–100.

57. Ringelstein EB, Droste DW, Babikian VL, et al. Consensus on microembolus detection by TCD. International Consensus Group on Microembolus Detection. Stroke 1998;29:725–729.

58. Brucher R, Russell D. Automatic online embolus detection and artifact rejection with the first multifrequency transcranial Doppler. Stroke 2002;33:1969–1974.

59. Russell D, Brucher R. Online automatic discrimination between solid and gaseous cerebral microemboli with the first multifrequency transcranial Doppler. Stroke 2002;33:1975–1980.

60. Molloy J, Markus HS. Asymptomatic embolization predicts stroke and TIA risk in patients with carotid artery stenosis. Stroke 1999;30:1440–1443.

61. Stork JL, Kimura K, Levi CR, Chambers BR, Abbott AL, Donnan GA. Source of microembolic signals in patients with high-grade carotid stenosis. Stroke 2002;33:2014–2018.

62. Bogdahn U, Becker G, Winkler J, Greiner K, Perez J, Meurers B. Transcranial color-coded real-time sonography in adults. Stroke 1990;21:1680–1688.

63. Martin PJ, Evans DH, Naylor AR. Transcranial color-coded sonography of the basal cerebral circulation. Reference data from 115 volunteers. Stroke 1994;25:390–396.

64. Postert T, Federlein J, Przuntek H, Buttner T. Insufficient and absent acoustic temporal bone window: potential and limitations of transcranial contrast-enhanced color-coded sonography and contrast-enhanced power-based sonography. Ultrasound Med Biol 1997;23:857–862.

65. Baumgartner RW, Arnold M, Gonner F, et al. Contrast-enhanced transcranial color-coded duplex sonography in ischemic cerebrovascular disease. Stroke 1997;28:2473–2478.

66. Gerriets T, Postert T, Goertler M, et al. DIAS I: duplex-sonographic assessment of the cerebrovascular status in acute stroke. A useful tool for future stroke trials. Stroke 2000;31:2342–2345.

67. Zunker P, Wilms H, Brossmann J, Georgiadis D, Weber S, Deuschl G. Echo contrast-enhanced transcranial ultrasound: frequency of use, diagnostic benefit, and validity of results compared with MRA. Stroke 2002;33:2600–2603.

7

Cerebrovascular Angiography

J. Emilio Exaire, MD, Jacqueline Saw, MD, and Christopher Bajzer, MD

CONTENTS

INTRODUCTION
PROCEDURAL PREPARATIONS
DIAGNOSTIC ANGIOGRAPHY
COMPLICATIONS
CONCLUSIONS
REFERENCES

Summary

Digital subtraction angiography remains the gold standard to assess both the severity and the characteristics of cerebrovascular stenoses. A full four-vessel cerebral angiography allows accurate evaluation of both extracranial and intracranial, carotid, and vertebral arteries. A comprehensive carotid diagnostic angiography is necessary as part of the carotid artery stenting procedure to provide anatomic details for strategizing the interventional approach and for anticipating potential challenges.

Key Words: Carotid artery angiography, digital subtraction angiography, vertebral artery angiography.

INTRODUCTION

Digital subtraction angiography (DSA) remains the gold standard to assess both the severity and the characteristics of cerebrovascular stenoses. A full four-vessel cerebral angiography allows accurate evaluation of both extracranial and intracranial, carotid, and vertebral arteries. Although it provides only a two-dimensional representation of the vessel lumen, it has several advantages over noninvasive imaging. It allows high-resolution assessment of the entire cerebrovascular circulation, differentiation between critical stenosis and complete occlusion, characterization of the Circle of Willis, and detailed visualization of plaque characteristics (e.g., ulceration, length, calcification, and thrombus). A comprehensive carotid diagnostic angiography is necessary as part of the carotid artery stenting (CAS) procedure to provide anatomic details for strategizing the interventional approach and for anticipating potential challenges. Typically, the vertebral circulation need not be evaluated prior to CAS, unless intracranial vertebral stenosis is suspected, or the collateral circulation needs to be scrutinized (especially

From: *Contemporary Cardiology: Handbook of Complex Percutaneous Carotid Intervention*
Edited by: J. Saw, J. E. Exaire, D. S. Lee, and S. Yadav © Humana Press Inc., Totowa, NJ

with the use of balloon occlusion emboli protection device). Although DSA is not necessary prior to carotid endarterectomy, a confirmatory computed tomography (CT) or magnetic resonance (MR) angiography is recommended in addition to Duplex ultrasonagraphy prior to surgery.

This chapter provides a detailed discussion on performing carotid, vertebral, and intracerebral angiography. Including discussions of techniques, equipment used, angiographic projections, and complications. Cerebrovascular anatomy is reviewed separately in Chapter 5, although radiographic cerebrovasculature is shown in this chapter.

PROCEDURAL PREPARATIONS

Arterial Access

Vascular access is typically obtained from the common femoral artery, as catheter manipulation to engage the great vessels is most natural from this location. Brachial and radial approaches to engage the carotid or vertebral arteries can be extremely challenging (especially engaging the ipsilateral carotid artery or contralateral vertebral artery); however, they may be necessary in patients with severe aortoiliac peripheral artery disease. We do not recommend direct percutaneous puncture of the common carotid artery (CCA) because of potential complications (e.g., carotid dissection, thrombosis, local hematoma compression of trachea, stent compression during carotid hemostasis) and the need for general anesthesia. A 5 Fr sheath is typically used for diagnostic cerebral angiography, as 5 Fr diagnostic catheters are preferred. The choice of a 5 Fr system allows adequate visualization of the cerebral vasculature, while lowering the risk of catheter manipulation in the carotid arteries (e.g., dissection and embolization). Although a 4 Fr system may be used successfully as well, it requires stronger injection for adequate opacification of the vessels.

Anticoagulation and Catheter Preparations

As a precautionary measure against thrombus formation in catheters, we routinely administer intravenous heparin (50 U/kg) prior to diagnostic cerebral angiography. We take extreme care to avoid air or thrombus embolism (which should be a routine caution throughout the carotid interventional procedure). Following each catheter connection to the transducer, air bubbles are suctioned and evacuated. We minimize blood contamination of the contrast syringe to avoid clot formation. Further, each contrast injection is performed with at least 45° angulation of the syringe, to avoid inadvertent injection of air. We also recommend routine monitoring of arterial pressure with a transducer, which allows constant hemodynamic assessment of patients (as blood pressure control is critical during CAS, and reflex bradycardia and hypotension is frequent) and provides warning to operators with catheter pressure dampening (which indicates catheter is lodged against atherosclerotic plaque or vessel wall).

Contrast Agent

An isoosmolar, nonionic contrast agent (e.g., Iodixanol [Visipaque®, GE Healthcare, Buckinghamshire, UK]) is routinely used for cerebral angiography. This reduces the discomfort that patients may experience with cerebral contrast injection. The use of high-osmolar ionic contrast may cause a warmth sensation, discomfort, and headache with cerebral angiograms. An alternative is Ioxaglate (Hexabrix®, Mallinckrodt, St. Louis, MO), which is a low-osmolar ionic dimmer that is also well tolerated.

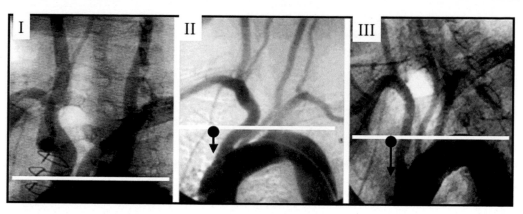

Fig. 1. Aortic arch angiogram of all three types of aortic arch anatomy. (Modified from Myla, CAROTID INTERVENTION. 3:1, 2000, REMEDICA.)

Table 1
Diagnostic Carotid and Cerebral Angiographic Views

Anatomy	Angiographic views
Aortic arch	45° LAO, large field of view to include aortic arch, great vessels, and carotid bifurcations.
Right carotid bifurcation	Routine ipsilateral oblique (30° RAO) and lateral (90% LAO). Sometimes PA or LAO (30°–60°) projections. Center imaging close to mandible.
Left carotid bifurcation	Routine ipsilateral oblique (30° LAO) and lateral (90° LAO). Sometimes PA or RAO (30°–60°) projections. Center imaging close to mandible.
Intracerebral carotid vessels	PA and lateral (90° LAO) intracranial views of both ICA. Include visualization of vessels above cervical ICA, and terminal vessels of ACA, MCA, and PCA.
Vertebral arteries (ostium and proximal vessel)	Nonselective injections of VA in contralateral oblique projections (i.e., 30° LAO for right VA).
Intracerebral vertebral artery	PA cranial (20–30°), and lateral (90° LAO) projections. Sometimes PA caudal (20–30°) with mouth wide open.

ACA, Anterior cerebral artery; ICA, internal carotid artery; LAO, left anterior oblique; MCA, middle cerebral artery; PA, posteroanterior; PCA, posterior cerebral artery; RAO, right anterior oblique; VA, vertebral artery.

DIAGNOSTIC ANGIOGRAPHY

Aortic Arch Angiogram

A thoracic aortic arch angiogram is routinely performed prior to selective carotid angiography, to allow classification of the aortic arch and visualize proximal great vessel stenosis and tortuosity (Fig. 1). This step is extremely useful to facilitate planning of catheter selection and interventional strategy. With large image intensifiers, the arch angiogram would also allow visualization of the carotid bifurcation, and vertebral artery patency and dominance. A 5 Fr pigtail catheter is advanced into the ascending aorta, and the arch angiogram performed in the 45° LAO projection (Table 1). This angulation allows proper separation of the origin of supra-aortic vessels and the bilateral carotid

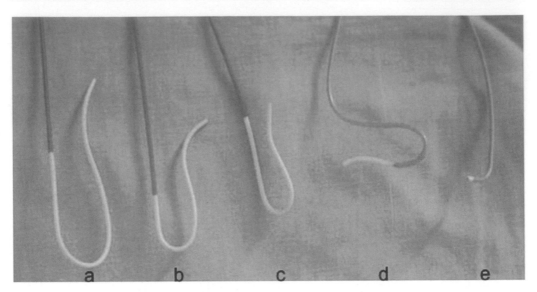

Fig. 2. Catheters used for cerebral angiography: **(a)** Simmons 1, **(b)** Simmons 2, **(c)** Simmons 3, **(d)** VTK catheter, **(e)** JR4 catheter.

bifurcation. The patient's head is turned to the right, and the field of view set to include the aortic arch, the great vessels, and the carotid bifurcations if possible (usually at the level of the angle of the mandible). The injector is programmed to 15 cc/s for 30 cc at 600 psi. The arch angiogram, as with selective cerebral angiography, should be performed under digital subtraction. Thus, the patient is given strict instructions during cine acquisition to hold his or her breath (preferably at mid- or end-expiration), not to move, and not to swallow.

Selective Carotid Angiography

Depending on the anatomy of the aortic arch, several catheters can be used for selective angiograms (Fig. 2). For the vast majority of type 1 or II arches, a 5 Fr JR4 catheter will suffice. Alternatives include Berenstein, angle taper Glidecath®, or headhunter catheters. With a type III aortic arch, a reverse-curved catheter is often necessary for selective engagement of the common carotid artery (CCA). Examples are the VTK catheter (Cook) or Simmons catheters (Fig. 2). Simmons catheters are not recommended for novice operators, as they need to be "reformed" at the aortic arch and need more aggressive maneuvering than the VTK catheter (see discussion later). This may potentially dislodge atherosclerotic plaques or cause great vessels dissections.

We typically begin with the CCA that is not planned for CAS (i.e., we engage the right CCA first if the left one needs CAS), followed by the contralateral CCA. This allows transition from the diagnostic procedure to the interventional procedure without having to re-engage the CCA of interest. The JR4 catheter is advanced over a Wholey wire (Mallinckrodt Hazelwood, MO) or an angled Glidewire® (Terumo Medical, Somerset, NJ) (Fig. 3) up to the ascending aorta; the wire is then withdrawn and the catheter is flushed with care. The JR4 catheter is then rotated counterclockwise to engage the innominate artery. A shallow RAO (20°–30°) is used to obtain a roadmap. This projection allows separation of the right CCA from the right vertebral artery origin (in the LAO projection, the right CCA and vertebral artery usually overlap). A stiff angled Glidewire® is then advanced into the mid segment of the CCA and the catheter is then

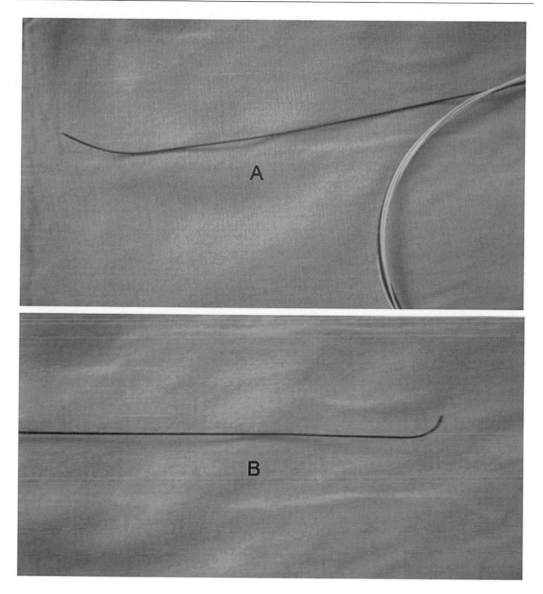

Fig. 3. Wires used for cerebral angiography: **(A)** Wholey wire, **(B)** stiff angled Glidewire®.

tracked over-the-wire to the mid-distal CCA. Selective cine angiograms of the right carotid bifurcation are then routinely obtained in RAO 30° and cross-table LAO 90° projections, with centering of the image at about the level of the mandible (since the bifurcation is typically located at C4–5 level). If necessary, PA and LAO 30–60° may be used to separate the internal carotid artery (ICA) from the external carotid artery (ECA). Intracerebral angiograms are then obtained in the PA (with 10–15° cranial angulation) and cross-table LAO 90° (Figs. 4 and 5). To obtain good-quality DSA images, the patients are again instructed to hold their breaths, not move, and not swallow.

To engage the left CCA, a similar approach is utilized. Although, in the setting of a bovine aortic arch, often a reverse-curve VTK catheter is necessary (see Fig. 3 in

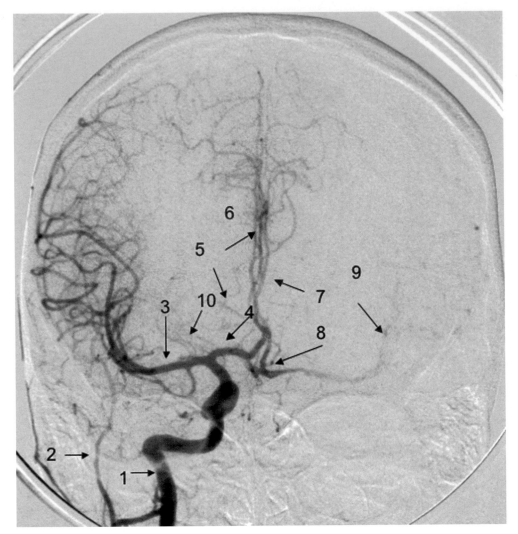

Fig. 4. Intracerebral angiography in the PA projection: *1*, internal carotid artery; *2*, facial artery; *3*, right middle cerebral artery (MCA); *4*, right anterior cerebral artery (ACA); *5*, callosomarginal artery; *6*, right pericallosal artery; *7*, left pericallosal artery; *8*, left ACA; *9*, left MCA; *10*, lenticulostrate arteries.

Chapter 9). Using the JR4 catheter from the aorta, a counter-clockwise turn is used to engage the left CCA. Often, a roadmap is necessary in the LAO 30° projection to enable a Glidewire® to facilitate catheter advancement into the mid-distal left CCA. For the left CCA bifurcation, routine cine angiograms are performed in the LAD 30° and 90° projections (Fig. 6). If necessary, RAO 30° or PA projections may be used.

Nonselective Vertebral Artery Angiography

The vertebral artery is of a smaller caliber and is less resilient than the carotid artery; thus, selective engagement is not recommended for fear of dissection. Furthermore, vertebral artery stenosis typically involves the origin of the vessel, and engagement with a catheter may result in pressure dampening and possible dissection. A 5 Fr JR4 is almost

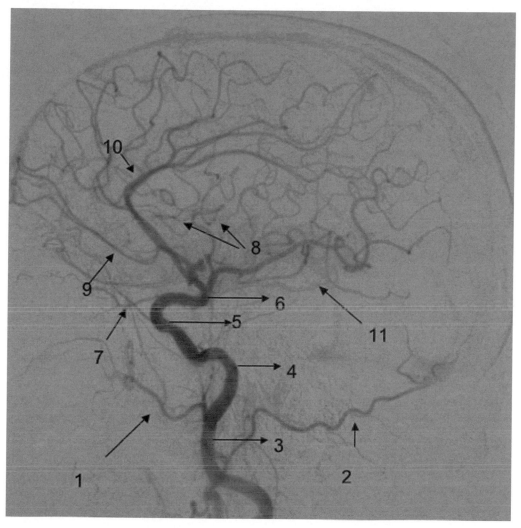

Fig. 5. Intracerebral angiography in the cross-table 90° LAO lateral projection: *1*, lingual artery from the external carotid artery (ECA); *2*, occipital artery from ECA; *3*, Prepetrous segment of the internal carotid artery (ICA); *4*, petrous segment of ICA; *5*, cavernous segment of ICA; *6*, supraclinoid segment of ICA; *7*, ophthalmic artery off ICA; *8*, posterior frontal and frontal parietal branches of the middle cerebral artery; *9*, callosomarginal branch of the anterior cerebral artery; *10*, pericallosal branch of the anterior cerebral artery; *11*, anterior choroidal artery.

always sufficient to engage the innominate or left subclavian arteries (occasionally, a VTK catheter is needed for the innominate artery in type III arch). The JR4 is advanced over a wire close to the proximity of the vertebral artery origin. An ipsilateral blood pressure cuff is then inflated above the systolic pressure to maximize contrast filling of the vertebral system. The contralateral 30° projection is ideal to visualize the vertebral artery origin (i.e., LAO 30° for right vertebral origin, and the RAO 30° for left vertebral origin). Cine angiograms in the PA (with 20–30° cranial) projection and LAO 90° projection are then performed for the intracranial vertebral circulation (Figs. 7 and 8). Often, a caudal PA projection (~30° caudal) is necessary with the patient's mouth open to visualize the vertebrobasilar junction without bony interference. If nonselective angiography

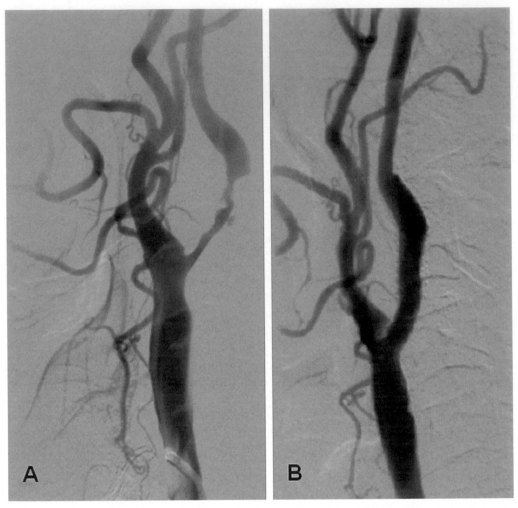

Fig. 6. Left carotid bifurcation: **(A)** prestenting in the LAO 30° projection, **(B)** poststenting in the lateral (90° LAO) projection.

is inadequate to visualize the intracranial vessels, a 5 Fr angle taper Glidecath® may be used to selectively engage the vertebral origin with minimal trauma. In approx 6% of cases, the left vertebral artery arises directly from the aortic arch, which then requires selective engagement from the aorta *(1)*. Classification of the vertebral artery segments is described in Fig. 9.

Special Instructions on the Use of Reverse-Curved Catheters

The technique is more demanding when a VTK or Simmons catheter is necessary. For the VTK catheter, the 0.035-in. guidewire is advanced into the ascending aorta and the catheter is advanced into the descending aorta. The wire is then withdrawn and the catheter flushed. The VTK is then re-formed with a counter-clockwise maneuver to orient the tip upwards pointing into the origin of the supra-aortic vessels (see Fig. 4 in Chapter 9). It is then pushed into the desired artery (i.e., the left subclavian, left CCA, or innominate artery). To engage the right CCA, once the VTK catheter is in the origin of the innominate artery, the catheter is pulled backwards, which allows the secondary curve to force the primary curve into the right CCA. This maneuver is frequently

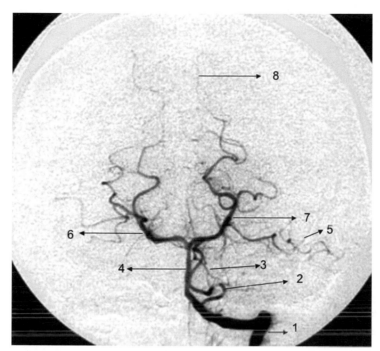

Fig. 7. Vertebrobasilar angiography in the PA cranial projection: *1*, vertebral artery; *2*, posterior inferior cerebellar artery; *3*, anterior inferior cerebellar artery; *4*, basilar artery; *5*, superior cerebellar artery; *6*, right posterior cerebral artery; *7*, left posterior cerebral artery; *8*, calcarine branch of the posterior cerebellar artery.

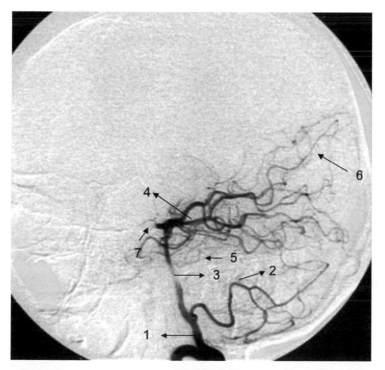

Fig. 8. Vertebrobasilar angiography in the cross-table 90° LAO lateral projection: *1*, vertebral artery; *2*, posterior inferior cerebellar artery; *3*, basilar artery; *4*, posterior cerebral arteries; *5*, anterior inferior cerebellar artery; *6*, calcarine branch of the posterior cerebral artery; *7*, posterior communicating artery.

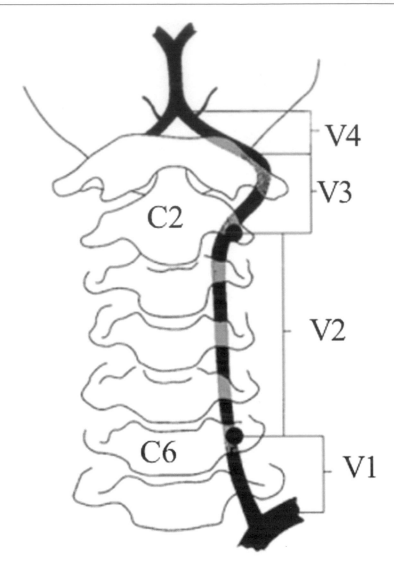

Fig. 9. Vertebral artery segments (adapted from ref. *1*). V1 starts from the origin of the vertebral artery to the fifth or sixth cervical vertebra where it enters the transverse foramina. V2 courses within the intervertebral foramina and exits as V3 behind the atlas. V4 pierces the dura and arachnoid mater at the base of the skull and ends as it meets its opposite vertebral artery to form the midline basilar artery.

sufficient to engage the right CCA, although at times roadmapping and advancement of a stiff angled Glidewire® is necessary. To disengage the VTK catheter, the catheter tip is pushed forward and given a clockwise rotation. This turns the catheter tip downwards (opposite the supra-aortic vessels), and a wire is then advanced out into the ascending aorta to straighten the pronounced primary and secondary curves before it is withdrawn through the descending aorta.

COMPLICATIONS

There are some inherent risks in performing DSA, namely neurological complications of transient ischemic attacks (0.5%), minor strokes (0.5%), major strokes (0.8%), and death (0.3%) *(2–6)*. In the Asymptomatic Carotid Atherosclerosis Study *(7)*, the risk of stroke or death with diagnostic cerebral angiography was 1.2%. In more contemporary experience, with the routine use of heparin and particular attention to avoid air and thrombotic complications, much lower complication rates can be achieved in high-volume centers by experienced operators. For instance, at the Cleveland Clinic, the periprocedural stroke incidence was 0.3% among approx 700 cerebral angiographies, with no incidence of death (unpublished data). In a study evaluating cerebral angiography by cardiologists, neurologic complication rate was 0.52% (minor stroke) *(2)*.

Arterial complications may occur as with coronary angiography. The incidence is approx 1% with diagnostic angiography, including major or minor bleeding, hematoma, pseudo-aneurysm, arteriovenous fistula, and retroperitoneal bleeding *(8)*. Complications associated with brachial and radial arterial access sites are typically related to thrombosis, with a complication rate similar to that for femoral access. Other complications include contrast-induced nephropathy, cholesterol embolization, and contrast allergy.

CONCLUSIONS

Carotid and cerebral angiography remains the gold standard to evaluate the anatomy of the supra-aortic vessels and intracerebral vasculature. A comprehensive diagnostic angiography with intracerebral evaluation should be performed prior to any carotid or vertebral artery stenting. In the hands of experienced operators who take extreme precautions during angiography, it can be performed safely with very low complications.

REFERENCES

1. Cloud GC, Markus HS. Diagnosis and management of vertebral artery stenosis. QJM 2003;96(1): 27–54.
2. Fayed AM, White CJ, Ramee SR, Jenkins JS, Collins TJ. Carotid and cerebral angiography performed by cardiologists: cerebrovascular complications. Catheter Cardiovasc Interv 2002;55(3):277–280.
3. Hankey GJ, Warlow CP. Symptomatic carotid ischaemic events: safest and most cost effective way of selecting patients for angiography, before carotid endarterectomy. BMJ 1990;300(6738):1485–1491.
4. Hankey GJ, Warlow CP, Molyneux AJ. Complications of cerebral angiography for patients with mild carotid territory ischaemia being considered for carotid endarterectomy. J Neurol Neurosurg Psychiatry 1990;53(7):542–548.
5. Heiserman JE, Dean BL, Hodak JA, et al. Neurologic complications of cerebral angiography. AJNR Am J Neuroradiol 1994;15(8):1401–1407; discussion 1408–1411.
6. Davies KN, Humphrey PR. Complications of cerebral angiography in patients with symptomatic carotid territory ischaemia screened by carotid ultrasound. J Neurol Neurosurg Psychiatry 1993;56(9):967–972.
7. ACAS Investigators. Endarterectomy for asymptomatic carotid artery stenosis. Executive Committee for the Asymptomatic Carotid Atherosclerosis Study. JAMA 1995;273(18):1421–1428.
8. Exaire JE, Dauerman HL, Topol EJ, et al. Triple antiplatelet therapy does not increase femoral access bleeding with vascular closure devices. Am Heart J 2004;147(1):31–34.

8 Indications for Carotid Artery Stenting

Cameron Haery, MD, Sharat Koul, DO, and Deepak L. Bhatt, MD

CONTENTS

INTRODUCTION
HISTORY
THE PRESENT
CONSIDERATIONS FOR CAS
FUTURE DIRECTIONS
REFERENCES

Summary

Indications for carotid artery stenting (CAS) have continued to evolve since carotid artery balloon angioplasty was first introduced in the early 1980s. Indeed, with the ongoing development of endovascular techniques and hardware (including stent design, emboli protection devices, and delivery systems) designed to reduce the risks of CAS, coupled with emerging data demonstrating the long-term safety and durability of CAS; accepted indications for CAS hold promise to emerge as a standard alternative to traditional carotid endarterectomy across a wider array of patient populations.

Key Words: Carotid artery stenting, carotid endarterectomy, indications.

INTRODUCTION

Indications for carotid artery stenting (CAS) have continued to evolve since carotid artery balloon angioplasty was first introduced in the early 1980s. Indeed, with the ongoing development of endovascular techniques and hardware (including stent design, emboli protection device [EPD], and delivery systems) designed to reduce the risks of CAS, coupled with emerging data demonstrating the long-term safety and durability of CAS; accepted indications for CAS hold promise to emerge as a standard alternative to traditional carotid endarterectomy (CEA) across a wider array of patient populations (Tables 1 and 2).

Patient selection to determine the most appropriate means of carotid stenosis management, whether CAS, surgical CEA, or lone pharmacologic management, is a complex one. Currently CAS is an attractive alternative to CEA in many patient populations,

From: *Contemporary Cardiology: Handbook of Complex Percutaneous Carotid Intervention*
Edited by: J. Saw, J. E. Exaire, D. S. Lee, and S. Yadav © Humana Press Inc., Totowa, NJ

Table 1
Medicare Approved Indications for Carotid Artery Stenting

1. Patients at high risk for CEA with symptomatic carotid artery stenosis ≥70%

2. Patients at high risk for CEA with symptomatic carotid artery stenosis between 50% and 70%, in accordance with the Category B IDE clinical trials regulation (42 CFR 405.201), as a routine cost under the clinical trials policy (Medicare National Coverage Determination (NCD) Manual 310.1), or in accordance with the NCD on CAS post-approval studies (Medicare NCD Manual 20.7)

3. Patients at high risk for CEA with asymptomatic carotid artery stenosis ≥80%, in accordance with the Category B IDE clinical trials regulation (42 CFR 405.201), as a routine cost under the clinical trials policy (Medicare National Coverage Determination (NCD) Manual 310.1), or in accordance with the NCD on CAS post-approval studies (Medicare NCD Manual 20.7)

Adapted from CMS Manual System, Pub.100-04 Medicare Claims processing, Department of Health & Human Services.
CAS, Carotid artery stenting; CEA, carotid endarterectomy.

Table 2
Current Accepted Indications for Carotid Artery Stenting

Congestive heart failure NYHA class III/IV
Left ventricular ejection fraction <30%
Unstable angina
Contralateral carotid occlusion
Recent myocardial infarction (within 30 d)
Previous carotid endarterectomy with recurrent stenosis
Prior radiation of the neck
Age >80 yr
Severe Pulmonary disease with:
    A. FEV 1 <50% or
    B. Resting PO_2 of <60 or
    C. Baseline hematocrit >50% or
    D. Chronic O_2 therapy
Requirement for staged coronary artery bypass surgery, cardiac valve replacement, or abdominal aortic aneurysm repair after index procedure (in 30 d)
Multivessel coronary artery disease:
    A. Two or more major coronary arteries >70% occluded with angina
    B. Abnormal stress test that would place the patient at increased risk for surgical procedures
History of radical neck surgery or current tracheotomy/stoma or spinal immobility.
Contralateral laryngeal nerve paralysis.
Anatomic lesion criteria:
    A. Bilateral stenosis of >60% or
    B. Surgically inaccessible lesion (above C2 or below clavicle) or
    C. Tandem lesion >70%
Major organ dysfunction such as:
    A. Currently on the list for major organ transplant
    B. History of liver failure with elevated prothrombin time
    C. Renal failure requiring dialysis

and currently is reserved as standard therapy for patients determined to be traditionally at elevated risk for CEA. The decision regarding the optimal mode of revascularization (CEA or CAS) must be determined on an individual patient-by-patient basis. The inherent risks of each treatment modality, anatomic considerations, medical comorbidities, and individual patient preference after thorough informed discussions are critical components in determining the appropriateness of CAS for any individual patient. In addition, as new data become available, the indications for CAS are likely to expand.

HISTORY

The rationale behind CAS is based on the currently well-established practice of surgical CEA to relieve carotid artery stenosis. CEA has been shown to reduce the overall risk of stroke in both symptomatic and asymptomatic patients (1). The initial CEA trials, although well designed, excluded large populations of patients with varying comorbid conditions, in order not to confound the cardiovascular outcomes and potential benefits of CEA itself. In the North American Symptomatic Carotid Endarterectomy Trial (NASCET), 659 patients with a high-grade internal carotid stenosis (70–99%) and a history of ipsilateral hemispheric, nondisabling stroke or retinal transient ischemic attack (TIA) were randomized to either medical management or medical management plus CEA. During a 2-yr follow-up, the risk of ipsilateral stroke was 26% in the medical therapy arm and 9% in the CEA arm ($p < 0.001$) (2,3). These findings were further strengthened in the European Carotid Surgery Trialists' (ECST) Collaborative group study (4). After correction for differences in technique of quantifying severity of carotid stenosis and redefining outcome events, the overall risk reduction in stroke in symptomatic patients with significant carotid stenosis was very comparable to that found in NASCET, with CEA reducing the 5-yr risk of any stroke or surgical death by 5.7% in patients with 50–69% stenosis ($p = 0.05$) and by 21.2% in patients with 70–99% stenosis without "near occlusion" ($p < 0.0001$) (5). A recent reanalysis of the pooled data from the NASCET, ECST, and Veterans Affairs Trial 309 confirmed these findings by showing some surgical benefit in symptomatic lesions 50–69% in severity and significant benefit for symptomatic lesions 70% or greater in severity (6).

Indications for CEA have subsequently been extended to certain asymptomatic patients populations with significant carotid stenosis primarily with the results of two landmark trials. In the Asymptomatic Carotid Atherosclerosis Study (ACAS), 1662 patients with 60% or greater carotid stenosis with no history of ipsilateral neurologic events were randomized to either a medical arm (325 mg of aspirin daily) or a surgical arm (aspirin plus CEA). Although less robust than the risk reductions seen in the trials involving symptomatic patients, analysis revealed that the aggregate risk over 5 yr for ipsilateral stroke and any perioperative stroke or death was estimated to be 5.1% for surgical patients and 11.0% for medically treated patients (aggregate risk reduction 53%, 95% confidence interval [CI] 22–72%, $p < 0.001$) (7). More recently, in the Asymptomatic Carotid Surgery Trial (ACST) collaborative group, 3120 asymptomatic patients with 60% or greater carotid stenosis with no associated neurologic symptoms within 6 mo were randomized equally to immediate CEA vs indefinite deferral for CEA. Analysis of the 5-yr follow-up revealed that after exclusion of perioperative events, the 5-yr stroke risk was 3.8% for the surgical arm and 11% for the medical arm ($p < 0.0001$). Benefit was demonstrated across age groups, in both gender groups, and across the spectrum of carotid stenosis severity (8).

Table 3
Conditions that Define the High-Risk Surgical Patient

- Congestive heart failure NYHA class III/IV
- Left ventricular ejection fraction <30%
- Unstable angina
- Contralateral carotid occlusion
- Recent myocardial infarction
- Previous carotid endarterectomy with recurrent stenosis
- Prior radiation treatment to the neck
- Other conditions that were used to determine patients at high risk for carotid endarterectomy in prior carotid artery stenting studies, such as ARCHER, CABERNET, SAPPHIRE, BEACH, and MAVERIC II.

Adapted from CMS Manual System, Pub.100-04 Medicare Claims processing, Department of Health & Human Services.

THE PRESENT

A recent Cochrane Systematic Review of the randomized trials comparing CEA with carotid angioplasty and/or stenting was published, and despite the wide confidence intervals, no significant difference in the major risks of the respective treatments was found (9). An updated review of the Global Carotid Artery Stent registry published in 2003 reported that in the total number of CAS performed worldwide ($n = 12,392$), technical success was achieved in 98.9% with a 30-d complication rate of 3.67%, 2.14%, 1.20%, and 0.64% for TIA, minor stroke, major stroke, and death, respectively (10). The major concern regarding the use of CAS stems from potential atheroembolization to the brain that may occur during the procedure. Zahn et al. reported results from a prospective CAS registry of 1483 patients. Of these, EPD was used in 668 (45%) cases, translating into a lower rate of ipsilateral stroke (1.4% vs 4.1%, $p = 0.007$) and a lower rate of all nonfatal strokes and all deaths (2.1% vs 4.9%, $p = 0.004$) (11). Other studies have confirmed the relatively low complication rates seen with the use of EPD (12–14) (Table 3). These reports and others suggest that with the described levels of success and medical complications, CAS may become a more viable option for treatment of carotid disease (15).

As with any invasive procedure, the judgment and skill of the operator are paramount in deciding whether CAS should be performed. As seen in the large surgical trials, CEA is an acceptable form of treatment as long as the procedure can be performed with only a very narrow margin for error. In a systematic review of 25 trials of CEA in both symptomatic and asymptomatic patients, Rothwell et al. reported that the overall risk for stroke and/or death within 30 d in symptomatic patients was 5.18% (95% CI 4.30–6.06) compared with 3.35% (95% CI 2.38–4.31) in asymptomatic patients (16). The risk to benefit ratio that is based on these analysis is beneficial only when surgical 30-d stroke and death rate does not exceed 5% in patients with transient ischemic attack, 7% for those with stroke, and 3% for those who are asymptomatic (1). Unfortunately, the relatively low complication rates that were seen in the large surgical trials have been difficult to duplicate in the community hospital setting. The perioperative mortality rate for Medicare patients undergoing CEA at nonstudy sites was 1.7% for high-volume institutions, 1.9% for average-volume institutions, and 2.5% for low-volume institutions (17).

These data highlight the importance of ensuring a high level of competency among CAS operators. To ensure the abilities of operators performing CAS, strict guidelines have been recommended. These recommendations have focused on both fundamental knowledge and skills as well as technical requirements such as proper equipment and support staff *(18,19)*. Rigorous certification standards seem to have translated into competent performance of CAS in the community setting. Bush et al. described the experience of a team of interventionalists at a nonclinical trial center using a standard CAS protocol *(20)*. Despite the lack of EPD use in this series, CAS was performed with a high degree of success and safety. As suggested by these and similar reports, CAS can be performed with a very high degree of safety in most environments, community- and university-based laboratories alike.

Recent clinical trials have established CAS as a primary therapy in patients requiring carotid revascularization but deemed to be at high a surgical risk for traditional CEA.

In the NASCET trial, specific exclusion criteria were established, defining the high-risk surgical patient. The short list of exclusion criteria included (but are not limited to) age older than 80 yr, intracranial atherosclerosis worse than cervical lesion, unstable neurologic condition, surgically inaccessible lesion, previous CEA, cancer with life expectancy <5 yr, unstable congestive heart failure, unstable angina, failure to visualize both intracranial carotid arteries, and other intracranial vascular pathology *(2)*. Such descriptions have created a generally accepted set of CEA risk factors.

Factors favoring CAS over CEA may be categorized broadly by surgical and medical variables (Table 4). Surgical risk variables relate to inherent anatomic and patient characteristics that make the CEA more difficult. Anatomic characteristics include carotid lesions that are difficult to access during the surgical procedure. Distal type lesions such as a carotid bifurcation above C2 or a lesion more than 3 cm into the internal carotid artery require a more extensive dissection with possible mobilization of the mandible *(21)*. Proximal type lesions such as proximal or ostial common carotid lesions can also require a more aggressive dissection that can include mobilizing the clavicle. These procedures will require a longer general anesthesia time as well as run the risk of nerve damage or prolonged healing time. Specific patient characteristic that also make traditional CEA more technically challenging include short obese necks as well as limited cervical mobility. These procedures usually require a more extensive dissection as well *(21)*.

The unique characteristics of radiation-induced carotid artery disease (CAD) make traditional CEA difficult. In this population, lesions tend to exist in a more proximal location, often involving the common carotid artery with sparing of the bifurcation. During the surgical procedure, alterations in the architecture of the arterial intima occur that makes delineation of anatomic planes difficult. Periarterial fibrosis and weakened arterial walls often necessitate reconstruction after CEA. In addition, the quality of the skin and soft tissues is altered after radiation treatment, making delayed healing and increased risk of wound infection a hazard for CEA *(22)*.

Similarly, restenosis after CEA poses elevated surgical anatomic risk, including cranial nerve injury and delayed wound healing. This group was excluded from the major CEA trials *(2–4,7,8)*. The nature of the myointimal hyperplasia that occurs with post-CEA restenosis likely makes it less prone to embolization during CAS. Two additional patient populations that have been shown to pose higher anatomic surgical risk are those with fibromuscular dysplasia *(18,23–25)* and those with inflammatory arteritis such as Takayasu *(18)*. Carotid disease in fibromuscular dysplasia tends to present in unfavorable surgical locations with relatively longer segments of disease. Takayasu's

Table 4
Current CAS Clinical Trials

Study	Sponsor	Stent	EPD	Study design	Status
ACT I	Abbot Vascular Devices	Xact Carotid Stent	Emboshield	Randomized multicenter trial of asymp. pts at standard risk for CEA	Enrolling
ARCHeR 1 and 2	Guidant	OTW Acculink	ARCHeR 2– OTW Accunet	High-risk registry	FDA approval 8/04
ARCHeR 3	Guidant	RX Acculink	RX Accunet	High-risk registry	FDA approval 8/04
BEACH	Boston Scientific	Carotid Wallstent Monorail	Filterwire EX and EZ	High-risk registry	Enrollment complete; in long-term follow-up
CABERNET	EndoTex	Nexstent Monorail	FilterWireEX And EZ	High-risk registry	Enrollment complete; currently in long-term follow-up
CASES	Cordis	Precise	Angioguard XP	Multicenter, high-risk, post marketing surveillance study	Enrolling
CREATE	ev3	Protégé	Spider OTW	High-risk registry	Enrollment complete; 1 yr results at TCT
CREATEII	ev3	Guidant Acculink	Spider RX	High-risk registry	Enrollment complete
CREST	NIH/Guidant	RX Acculink	RX Accunet	Randomized multicenter trial for symp. and asymp. CEA eligible patients	Enrolling
CAPTURE	Guidant	RX Acculink	RX Accunet	Multicenter, postapproval study including sequential enrollment of all patients receiving ACCULINK Stent	Enrolling

Trial	Industry partner	Stent	EPD	Design	Status
MAVErIC Internt'l	Medtronic	Exponent	Interceptor	High-risk registry	CE Mark approved
MAVErIC I & II	Medtronic	Exponent	GuardWire	High-risk registry	Enrollment complete
MAVErIC III	Medtronic	Exponent	Interceptor plus	High-risk registry	Enrolling
MO.MA	Invatec	Any	MO.MA	Multicenter EU registry	Completed; 30-d all CVA/death = 5.7%, 30-d MI = 0%
PRIAMUS	Invatec	Any	MO.MA	Multicenter Italian registry	Completed; 30-d all CVA/death = 4.5%, 30-d MI = 0%
PASCAL	Medtronic	Exponent	Any CE Mark-approved device	Outside U.S. high-risk registry	Enrollment complete
RULE-Carotid	Rubicon Medical	Any	Rubicon Filter	Multicenter EU sympt/asympt CE	CE Mark approved
SAPPHIRE	Cordis	Precise	AngioGuard-XP	Randomized multicenter trial of high-risk patients	Trial complete. 3-yr results at TCT 2005
SECuRITY	Abbot	Xact carotid stent	EmboShield	High-risk registry	1 yr results at TCT 2004
TACIT	N/A	N/A	N/A	Randomized, three-arm prospective trial	Enrollment to begin 2006
VIVA	Bard	Vivexx carotid stent	Industry partner	High-risk registry	IDE conditionally approved

Adapted from Endovascular Today 2005:4(9).
CEA, Carotid endarterectomy; EPD, emboli protection device; N/A, not available.

arteritis often involves the entire thickness of the vessel wall, making identification of an adequate plane of cleavage technically difficult or impossible (26).

Medical variables associated with high surgical risk include patients with significant CAD. Many patients who undergo CEA have concomitant CAD. Elevated risk of CEA related complications in patients with concomitant CAD are well documented (27–30). Likewise, those with depressed left ventricular ejection fraction <35% have a significantly elevated risk of the combined end point of death and myocardial infarction when compared to those with left ventricular ejection fraction (LVEF) >35% (43% vs 9%; $p = 0.036$).

Patients with significant pulmonary disease are also at elevated risk for surgical complications. Without need for general anesthesia or mechanical ventilatory support, potential increased risk for cardiopulmonary complications can be avoided effectively with CAS. A third medical variable is the presence of a contralateral carotid occlusion. In the NASCET trial, contralateral carotid occlusion increased risk for periprocedural stroke to 14.3% (31,32).

The unique qualities of CAS that make it a potential first-line therapy for carotid intervention in high surgical risk patients have been formally addressed in the landmark Stenting and Angioplasty with Protection in Patients at High Risk for Endarterectomy investigators (SAPPHIRE) trial (33). In SAPPHIRE, 334 patients with both symptomatic and asymptomatic carotid stenoses and conditions that potentially increased the risk posed by CEA (Table 5) were randomized to either CAS (Precise™ stent [Cordis Corporation, Warren, NJ]) with the use of an EPD (AngioGuard XP™ [Cordis Corporation, Warren, NJ]) vs CEA. The primary end point, which included the cumulative incidence of a major cardiovascular event at 1 yr, was seen in 20 patients (12.2%) randomized to CAS and in 32 patients (20.1%) randomized to CEA. The study demonstrated noninferiority of CAS as compared to CEA in this patient population ($p = 0.004$) (33).

To date, two carotid stent with EPD systems have been approved by the US Food and Drug Administration for CAS. They are the AccuLink™ and AccuNet™ system (Guidant, Santa Clara, CA) and Xact® and EmboShield™ system (Abbott Vascular Devices, Redwood City, CA). Based on the ARCHeR registry trials whereby high surgical risk patients underwent CAS with the AccuLink™ and AccuNet™ system, both devices have been approved for the following indications: patients with neurologic symptoms and ≥50% stenosis of common or internal carotid artery by ultrasound or angiogram **OR** patients without neurologic symptoms and ≥80% stenosis of the common or internal carotid artery by ultrasound or angiogram **AND** patients must have reference vessel diameter within the range of 4.0 mm and 9.0 mm at target lesion (34,35).

In the SECuRITY trial, a registry of 305 high surgical risk patients underwent CAS using the Xact® and EmboShield™ carotid stent system (36,37). As a result, the two devices have also been approved for similar indications: patients with symptomatic CAD of ≥50% by ultrasound or angiography or asymptomatic disease of ≥80% located between the origin of the common carotid and the intracranial segment of the internal carotid artery with the reference vessel diameter within the range of 4.8 mm and 9.1 mm (36,37).

CONSIDERATIONS FOR CAS

Endovascular carotid artery intervention poses unique risks. Multiple risk factors have been clearly identified in CAS. In review of the NASCET study, the following variables have been defined as indicating a higher surgical risk: hemispheric vs retinal

Table 5
Eligibility Criteria for Major Carotid Artery Stenting Trials

Trial	Inclusion criteria	Exclusion criteria

SAPPHIRE	General
	  Age ≥18 yr
	  Unilateral or bilateral
	    atherosclerotic or restenotic lesion
	    in native carotid arteries
	  Symptoms plus stenosis ≥50%
	  No symptoms plus stenosis >80%
		Ischemic stroke within previous
		  48 h
		Presence of intraluminal thrombus
		Total occlusion of target vessel
		Vascular disease precluding use of
		  catheter based technique

	Criteria for high risk (at least 1)
	  Clinically significant cardiac
	    disease (congestive heart failure,
	    abnormal stress test or need for
	    open heart surgery)
	  Severe pulmonary disease
	  Contralateral carotid occlusion
	  Contralateral laryngeal-nerve palsy
	  Previous radical neck surgery or
	    radiation therapy to neck
	  Recurrent stenosis after CEA
	  Age >80 yr
		Intracranial aneurysm >9 mm in
		  diameter
		Need for more than two stents
		History of bleeding disorder
		Percutaneous or surgical
		  intervention planned within
		  next 30 d
		Life expectancy <1 yr
		Ostial lesions of common carotid
		  or brachiocephalic artery

ARCHeR 1, 2, 3	Symptoms within 180 d of enrollment plus stenosis ≥50% No symptoms plus stenosis ≥80%	

	Two or more of the following criteria:
	Two or more proximal or diseased
	  coronary arteries with ≥70% with no
	  revascularization
	Unstable/rest angina with ECG changes
	MI within the previous 30 d
	Concurrent requirement for CABG or
	  cardiac valve surgery within 30 days
	Contralateral occlusion of internal carotid	

	Or one or more the following criteria:
	  Being evaluated for major organ transplant
	  LVEF <30% or NYHA ≥Class III
	  FEV1 <30%
	  Hemodialysis
	  Uncontrolled diabetes
	  Restenosis after previous CEA
	  Status post radiation treatment to neck
	  Status post radical neck surgery
	  Surgically inaccessible lesions
	  Spinal immobility
	  Presence of tracheostomy
	  Contralateral laryngeal nerve paralysis	

Adapted from ref. *32* and www.guidant.com.

TIA as the qualifying event, contralateral carotid occlusion, ipsilateral ischemic lesion on CT scan, and an irregular or ulcerated ipsilateral plaque *(31)*. *Many of the same factors that increase the risk of CEA also increase the risk of CAS.*

Despite the many obvious advantages of CAS, many variables must be considered before performing the procedure to produce an overall risk–benefit evaluation that can be shared with the patient when considering CAS. These variables may be categorized as anatomic and physiologic.

When proceeding with CAS, thorough understanding of the patient's cerebrovascular arterial anatomy must be obtained. The overall condition of the aorta and the arterial supply of the lower extremities should also be carefully considered. Significant atherosclerotic disease may make arterial access difficult, if not limb threatening. In addition, the presence of significant disease in the aortic arch may lead to atheroembolic complications. A recent study by Schluter et al. described elective CAS in 42 consecutive patients using 6 different types of EPD *(38)*. All patients underwent MRI examination before and after the procedure. In this series, one patient experienced a major stroke with subsequent MRI exam revealing 12 ischemic foci exclusively in the contralateral hemisphere *(38)*. These findings suggest that despite the use of distal protection devices, manipulation of endoluminal equipment in the supra-aortic vessels is a major risk factor for cerebral embolism during CAS *(38,39)*. A complete knowledge of the relevant anatomy can limit the amount of manipulation and catheter exchanges so as to minimize these possible disruptions. Likewise, severe lower extremity and descending aortic disease lends itself to elevated risk of lower extremity atheroembolism, renal failure, and limb ischemia.

The overall structure of the aortic arch and great vessels should be reviewed to assess for the potential "hostile" arch. As detailed elsewhere, the description of the arch as either type I, II, or III will affect both equipment used as well as risk of aortic trauma. Typical arch anatomy is seen in about 70% of patients, but the incidence of shared origin of brachiocephalic trunk and left common carotid is seen in approx 10% of cases (bovine arch) *(40)*. With hypertension, atherosclerosis, aortic valve disease, and increasing age, the aorta sinks and elongates into the thoracic cavity while simultaneously pulling the great vessels with it. This can make cannulation and exchange of catheters difficult. To reduce the risk of complications resulting from endoluminal manipulation, complete diagnostic angiography prior to CAS is essential; including arch aortography, and four-vessel cervicocerebral angiography. This includes anatomy of the internal carotid anatomy, vertebral artery dominance, angiographic characteristics of the target lesion, and an understanding of the intracerebral circulation along with coexisting collateral circulation.

Significant tortuosity of the common carotid as well as internal carotid artery poses unique challenges for CAS. Significant tortuosity in the common carotid artery (proximal to the target lesion) may limit the ability to deliver a guide catheter or guiding sheath for delivery of EPD and stent devices. Likewise, once a guiding catheter or guide sheath has been successfully positioned in a very tortuous common carotid artery, the vessel may elongate or be displaced upward ("accordion"), altering the natural configuration of the vessel and the target lesion. This circumstance may also result in angiographic appearance of "pseudostenosis" or even mimic vessel dissection or spasm. Discerning true vessel injury from such angiographic aberrations due to vessel manipulation is essential to reduce procedural complications. In this case, special care must be taken to ensure appropriate stent length and diameter, to treat the lesion in its "naturally occurring state" once the interventional devices have been removed. Severe tortuosity in the distal cervical segment (and below the carotid siphon) of the internal carotid artery also increases the risk of procedural stroke and reduces procedural success rates. Tortuosity can reduce the ability to deliver the EPD, complicate tracking of the stent delivery system and may require specific equipment for proper deployment *(40)*. Severe loops and tortuosity in the proximal ICA near the carotid bulb may also be a nidus for distal stent edge dissection if the stent edge is deployed near such a stress point in the vessel. Severe loops, tortuosity, and kinks in the target internal carotid artery are contraindications to CAS.

Heavy calcification of the target lesion, increasing length of lesion and greater plaque burden, as well as presence of an acute thrombus, pose a greater risk of cerebral embolization and slow reflow when performing CAS. In addition, recent studies have suggested that with the use of specific technologies, characterization of lesion echolucency may be ascertained and aid in determining risk of embolization during the procedure. In the Imaging in Carotid Angioplasty and Risk of Stroke (ICAROS) study *(41)*, an echographic evaluation of carotid plaque was performed using a computer-assisted index grayscale median (GSM) before performing CAS with embolic protection. The onset of neurologic deficits during and after the procedure was recorded. There were 11 of 155 strokes (7.1%) in patients with GSM ≤25 and 4 of 263 (1.5%) in patients with GSM >25 ($p = 0.005$). This study suggested that carotid plaque echolucency, as measured by GSM ≤25, increases the risk of stroke in CAS *(41)*. Heavy target lesion calcification may inhibit stent delivery to the target lesion, preclude complete stent expansion, and increase risk of carotid dissection during post-stent dilation. Severe target lesion calcification should be considered a relative contraindication to CAS.

Hyperperfusion syndrome is a well-known complication of CEA and may be seen in patients with significant carotid disease. With chronic hypoperfusion of the cerebral circulation, autoregulation and vasomotor function of the cerebral circulation are impaired *(42,43)*. With sudden restoration of perfusion, patients may experience headache, seizure, altered mental status, stupor, neurologic deficits, hypertension, intracranial hemorrhage, or death. Evaluation of the intracranial circulation and the network of intracranial collateral arterial flow is important for considering the presence of the "isolated hemisphere." Henderson et al. reviewed all angiographic data for all patients entered in the NASCET study and performed Kaplan-Meier event-free survival analysis for all patients demonstrating angiographic filling through either anterior communicating and posterior communicating arteries and retrograde filling through ophthalmic arteries *(44)*. The 2-yr risk of hemispheric stroke in medically treated patients with severe internal carotid artery stenosis was reduced in the presence of collaterals: 27.8% to 11.3% ($p = 0.005$). The 2-yr stroke risk for surgical patients with and without collaterals were 5.9% vs 8.4%, respectively *(44)*.

The initial definition of hyperperfusion syndrome has seen some evolution, and the suggestion of defining the syndrome as presentation with the above detailed signs and symptoms without evidence of new infarction on MRI exam has been made *(42,43)*. In a recent series by Abou-Chebl et al., a prospective database of 450 patients who underwent CAS with embolic protection demonstrated a 1.1% incidence of hyperperfusion syndrome. *These patients all shared the characteristics of having concurrent contralateral stenosis >80% or contralateral occlusion and periprocedural hypertension (43).* Although the exact incidence of hyperperfusion syndrome with intracranial hemorrhage after CEA is not known, it is estimated to be between 0.75% and 3.0%

(45,46). The risk factors for hyperperfusion syndrome after CAS described by Abou-Chebl et al., in addition to history of previous stroke, poor intracranial collateral blood flow, and the presence of critical carotid stenosis, have been corroborated as factors predisposing to hyperperfusion following CEA *(42,43)*.

Other physiologic factors that elevate CAS risk include impaired renal function and intolerance for aggressive antiplatelet regimens. As with all invasive angiographic procedures, significant renal impairment aggressively limits the quantities of iodinated or noniodinated contrast that can be used while also placing the patient at risk for the need for contrast-induced nephropathy and hemodialysis *(47)*.

Regarding the use of intraarterial antiplatelet agents, there currently is no clear indication for their use in routine CAS. With concerns for intracranial hemorrhage or hyperperfusion syndrome, their use has been limited. Other hematologic disorders including coagulopathies, bleeding diatheses, or platelet disorders make the use of various agents such as glycoprotein IIB/IIIa antagonist, heparin products, and direct thrombin inhibitors risky in this patient population *(48)*. Likewise, patient intolerance or inability to take aspirin or thienopyridine platelet antagonists (clopidogrel or ticlopidine) is a contraindication to carotid artery stent deployment.

Timing of CAS in relation to the sentinel neurological event in the symptomatic patient has been a subject of debate. In the SAPPHIRE trial, patients who presented within 48 h of the neurologic event were excluded *(27)*. In the ARCHeR trials, patients were excluded if they had stroke within 7 d. In the SECuRITY trial, patients were excluded if there was evidence of stroke within 30 d.

Surgical databases have shown that the presence of intraluminal thrombus is associated with poorer outcomes. Biller et al. reported that 9 of 2250 patients with cerebral ischemia had carotid artery stenosis with intraluminal thrombus identified by cerebral angiography *(49)*. The NASCET study reported that 53 (1.8%) of 2863 patients had intraluminal thrombus identified by angiography *(2,50)*, and the 30-d risk of stroke or death for these patients was 12.0% and 10.7% treated with surgery or medical therapy, respectively *(50)*. In regard to CAS, this same situation has been defined as a contraindication to the procedure. Tsumoto et al. described their experience with the performance of CAS with EPD for 6 patients with carotid artery stenosis and an intraluminal thrombus where satisfactory patency of the carotid artery was achieved *(51)*. Despite the technically challenging nature of this procedure, experiences such as that of Tsumoto et al. suggest that with appropriate use of EPD, this scenario can be dealt with using CAS. Regarding the optimum timing of carotid intervention, there is no general consensus as to safety with early intervention. Two recent series described the experience at three separate university hospitals where CAS was performed emergently for either acute internal carotid artery occlusion or acute stroke. These procedures were characterized by a high rate of recanalization *(52,53)*. These reports seem to suggest that carotid disease that presents acutely with either acute carotid obstruction or a stuttering pattern of evolving neurologic events may also be managed with using CAS.

Understanding periprocedural hemodynamic fluctuations associated with CAS poses unique circumstances and contraindications. Patients who are not likely to tolerate potential significant hypotension and bradycardia typically seen from carotid sinus activation should be approached with caution. For example, a patient undergoing CAS with concomitant severe aortic valve stenosis (with or without left ventricular systolic dysfunction), may experience potentially catastrophic cardiopulmonary decompensation if the baroreceptor reflex is profound during CAS. Patients with severe vertebrobasilar insufficiency, contralateral carotid occlusion, or significant intracranial disease should be approached with similar awareness. Although rarely required, prophylactic temporary transvenous pacemaker placement, atropine administration, or adrenergic agonist infusions may be indicated.

FUTURE DIRECTIONS

The role of CAS has thus far been defined by the limitations of CEA, in that patients that may be inappropriate surgical candidates may be revascularized with CAS *(54)*. From a practical standpoint, there are some distinct limitations for CAS. However, a growing body of literature argues that CAS may be performed with relative safety even in patients who have been traditionally labeled as high risk.

With the high incidence of significant concomitant disease in both the carotid and coronary vasculature, the approach to these patients has been a challenge. The precise rate of outcomes after combined CEA/CABG has not been well established. In a recently published review of a multistate community-based US Medicare database, it was reported that patients undergoing simultaneous CEA and coronary artery bypass (CABG) had a combined stroke and death rate of 17.7%, with 80% of nonfatal strokes being disabling *(27)*. Some recent reviews of single-center series have looked at overall success rates in a combined CAS/CABG approach. Muller et al. reviewed the courses of 23 patients who did not meet eligibility by NASCET criteria who underwent CAS before planned CABG. Despite the use of EPD in only 10 of the 26 procedures, the overall rate of death, persistent stroke or myocardial infarction was 5% *(55)*. Although the bulk of such studies looking at this combined approach have lacked large patient population or rigorous, standardized evaluation *(55–57)*, these reports suggest that a hybrid approach with CAS and either traditional CABG or percutaneous coronary intervention can be done with relative safety.

As seen in the large surgical databases, the occurrence of significant carotid disease concurrent with contralateral carotid disease is rare but associated with significant risk. Management of this clinical situation is a challenge for clinicians. Chen et al. recently described the outcome of simultaneous bilateral carotid stenting in 10 patients at a single center. These procedures were notable for successful stenting of all but one lesion with no reported procedural complications *(58)*. Gonzalez et al. reported a review of a single center registry that identified 96 patients with significant carotid disease and contralateral occlusion that underwent CAS. Total neurological complications including transient ischemic attacks, minor and major stroke occurred in four patients (4.1%) *(59)*. Although these reports are generally from small, single-center registries, there is an indication that CAS may be a reasonable approach to the patient with significant bilateral disease.

Potential indications for CAS are in evolution. *Nevertheless, at this point in time, CAS is primarily indicated for patients who pose elevated risk for traditional CEA.* However, with the apparent advantages of CAS as compared to CEA, there is much speculation as to whether CAS may serve as a primary choice in treatment of carotid atherosclerotic disease.

To address this point, multiple studies are being conducted currently to compare the overall safety and longevity of the results seen with CAS compared to CEA in patients at low CEA risk. Sherif et al. recently reported a propensity score-adjusted analysis of the long-term risks for stroke after CAS compared to medical therapy in patients with asymptomatic high-grade carotid stenosis. In a total of 946 patients with 525 patients treated medically and 421 patients treated with CAS, the risk of stroke increased in parallel with the degree of stenosis in conservatively treated patients, but remained unchanged in patients undergoing CAS *(60)*. Although based on a single-center study, this suggests that future studies may confirm the long-standing efficacy of CAS for asymptomatic high-grade stenosis.

In one of the largest CAS trials to date, the currently ongoing Carotid Revascularization Endarterectomy vs Stent Trial (CREST), both symptomatic and asymptomatic patients deemed to be CEA eligible are being randomized to either CAS with the AccuLink™ and AccuNet™ system or CEA. Primary outcomes to be assessed are death, stroke, or myocardial infarction at 30 d postoperatively *(61)*.

The Asymptomatic Carotid Stenosis (ACT I) trial is a prospective, randomized multicenter trial where asymptomatic patients at standard risk for CEA will be randomized 1:3 to either CEA or CAS using the Xact® and EmboShield™ system *(62)*. The Stenting versus Endarterectomy trial and the International Carotid Stenting study (ICSS) is a prospective, randomized multicenter trial in which symptomatic patients suitable for both CAS and CEA will be accordingly randomized between the two modalities *(63)*.

These and other studies will provide a significant amount of information regarding appropriateness for expanding future indications for CAS. How the use of current pharmacologic therapies directed to reduce the risk of cardiovascular events will influence the natural course of carotid disease is yet to be fully determined. In addition, how will the concept of the diagnosing "vulnerable" plaque play into the treatment of carotid disease? In an analysis of the ESCT database, Rothwell et al. developed two prognostic models based on data from the patients with 0–69% carotid stenosis. From these models, the authors developed a prognostic score based on seven clinical variables that would identify the patient group with a high risk of stroke on medical treatment but a low surgical risk. When the algorithm was applied to patients with 70–99% carotid artery stenosis, it was suggested that the 5-yr total risk of ipsilateral stroke, operative major stroke, or death was lowered by 33% in only the 16% of patients with a score of 4 or more ($p < 0.0001$) *(64)*. This type of analysis highlights the need to accurately identify patients who would benefit most from CAS in the future.

Carotid artery revascularization is recognized to reduce the risk of stroke and subsequent neurologic events beyond pharmacologic therapy alone. Determining the optimal mode of treatment (CAS vs CEA) must ultimately be made based on careful individual assessment of patient clinical risk profiles. Indications for CAS are sure to evolve as eagerly anticipated data from ongoing trials are completed.

REFERENCES

1. Biller J, et al. Guidelines for carotid endarterectomy: a statement for healthcare professionals from a special writing group of the Stroke Council, American Heart Association. Stroke 1998;29:554–562.
2. Beneficial effect of carotid endarterectomy in symptomatic patients with high-grade carotid stenosis. North American Symptomatic Carotid Endarterectomy Trial Collaborators. N Engl J Med 1991;325:445–453.
3. Barnett HJ, et al. Benefit of carotid endarterectomy in patients with symptomatic moderate or severe stenosis. North American Symptomatic Carotid Endarterectomy Trial Collaborators. N Engl J Med 1998;339:1415–1425.
4. Randomised trial of endarterectomy for recently symptomatic carotid stenosis: final results of the MRC European Carotid Surgery Trial (ECST). Lancet 1998;351:1379–1387.

5. Rothwell PM, Gutnikov SA, Warlow CP. Reanalysis of the final results of the European Carotid Surgery Trial. Stroke 2003;34:514–523.
6. Rothwell PM, et al. Analysis of pooled data from the randomised controlled trials of endarterectomy for symptomatic carotid stenosis. Lancet 2003;361:107–116.
7. Endarterectomy for asymptomatic carotid artery stenosis. Executive Committee for the Asymptomatic Carotid Atherosclerosis Study. JAMA 1995;273:1421–1428.
8. Halliday A, et al. Prevention of disabling and fatal strokes by successful carotid endarterectomy in patients without recent neurological symptoms: randomised controlled trial. Lancet 2004;363: 1491–1502.
9. Coward LJ, Featherstone RL, Brown MM. Safety and efficacy of endovascular treatment of carotid artery stenosis compared with carotid endarterectomy: a Cochrane systematic review of the random-ized evidence. Stroke 2005;36:905–911.
10. Wholey MH, Al-Mubarek N. Updated review of the global carotid artery stent registry. Catheter Cardiovasc Interv. 2003;60:259–266.
11. Zahn R, et al. Embolic protection devices for carotid artery stenting: better results than stenting with-out protection? Eur Heart J 2004;25:1550–1558.
12. Cosottini M, et al. Silent cerebral ischemia detected with diffusion weighted imaging in patients treated with protected and unprotected carotid artery stenting. Stroke 2005;36:2389–2393.
13. Reimers B, et al. Routine use of cerebral protection during carotid artery stenting: results of a multi-center registry of 753 patients. Am J Med 2004;116:217–222.
14. Cremonesi A, et al. Protected carotid stenting: clinical advantages and complications of embolic pro-tection devices in 442 consecutive patients. Stroke 2003;34:1936–1941.
15. Roubin GS, et al. Immediate and late clinical outcomes of carotid artery stenting in patients with symptomatic and asymptomatic carotid artery stenosis: a 5-year prospective analysis. Circulation 2001;103:532–537.
16. Rothwell PM, Slattery J, Warlow CP. A systematic comparison of the risks of stroke and death due to carotid endarterectomy for symptomatic and asymptomatic stenosis. Stroke 1996;27:266–269.
17. Wennberg DE, et al. Variation in carotid endarterectomy mortality in the Medicare population: trial hospitals, volume, and patient characteristics. JAMA 1998;279:1278–1281.
18. Barr JD, et al. Quality improvement guidelines for the performance of cervical carotid angioplasty and stent placement. AJNR Am J Neuroradiol 2003;24:2020–2034.
19. Rosenfield K, et al. Clinical competence statement on carotid stenting: training and credentialing for carotid stenting—multispecialty consensus recommendations: a report of the SCAI/SVMB/SVS Writing Committee to develop a clinical competence statement on carotid interventions. J Am Coll Cardiol 2005;45:165–174.
20. Bush RL, et al. Carotid artery stenting in a community setting: experience outside of a clinical trial. Ann Vasc Surg 2003;17:629–634.
21. Dangas G, et al. Carotid artery stenting in patients with high-risk anatomy for carotid endarterectomy. J Endovasc Ther 2001;8:39–43.
22. Ziada KM, Yadav JS. In Expanding the Indications for Carotid Stenting: Radiation-Induced Extracranial Carotid Artery Disease. Carotid Intervention, 2001;3:34–45.
23. Osborn A. Diagnostic Cerebral Angiography. Philadelphia: Lippincott Williams & Wilkins, 1999.
24. Finsterer J, et al. Bilateral stenting of symptomatic and asymptomatic internal carotid artery stenosis due to fibromuscular dysplasia. J Neurol Neurosurg Psychiatry 2000;69:683–686.
25. Gomez CR. The role of carotid angioplasty and stenting. Semin Neurol 1998;18:501–511.
26. Liang P, Hoffman GS. Advances in the medical and surgical treatment of Takayasu arteritis. Curr Opin Rheumatol 2005;17:16–24.
27. Brown KR, et al. Multistate population-based outcomes of combined carotid endarterectomy and coronary artery bypass. J Vasc Surg 2003;37:32–39.
28. Naylor R, et al. A systematic review of outcome following synchronous carotid endarterectomy and coronary artery bypass: influence of surgical and patient variables. Eur J Vasc Endovasc Surg 2003; 26:230–241.
29. Bass A, et al. Combined carotid endarterectomy and coronary artery revascularization: a sobering review. Isr J Med Sci 1992;28:27–32.
30. Paciaroni M, et al. Medical complications associated with carotid endarterectomy. North American Symptomatic Carotid Endarterectomy Trial (NASCET). Stroke 1999;30:1759–1763.
31. Ferguson GG, et al. The North American Symptomatic Carotid Endarterectomy Trial: surgical results in 1415 patients. Stroke 1999;30:1751–1758.

32. Nicosia A, et al. Carotid artery stenting in the presence of contralateral carotid occlusion: mind the hyperperfusion syndrome! Ital Heart J 2004;5:152–156.

33. Yadav JS, et al. Protected carotid-artery stenting versus endarterectomy in high-risk patients. N Engl J Med 2004;351:1493–1501.

34. www.strokecenter.org, Stroke Trials Directory—ARCHeR.

35. www.fda.gov, New Device Approval—ACCULINK Carotid Stent System.

36. www.fda.gov, New Device Approval—Xact Carotid Stent System.

37. www.abbott.com, Abbott Laboratories Press Releases (614).

38. Schluter M, et al. Focal ischemia of the brain after neuroprotected carotid artery stenting. J Am Coll Cardiol 2003;42:1007–1013.

39. Hammer FD, et al. Cerebral microembolization after protected carotid artery stenting in surgical high-risk patients: results of a 2-year prospective study. J Vasc Surg 2005;42:847–853; discussion 853.

40. Myla S. Carotid Access Technique: An Algorithmic Approach.

41. Biasi GM, et al. Carotid plaque echolucency increases the risk of stroke in carotid stenting: the Imaging in Carotid Angioplasty and Risk of Stroke (ICAROS) study. Circulation, 2004;110:756–762.

42. Coutts SB, Hill MD, Hu WY. Hyperperfusion syndrome: toward a stricter definition. Neurosurgery 2003;53:1053–1058; discussion 1058–1060.

43. Abou-Chebl A, et al. Intracranial hemorrhage and hyperperfusion syndrome following carotid artery stenting: risk factors, prevention, and treatment. J Am Coll Cardiol 2004;43:1596–1601.

44. Henderson RD, et al. Angiographically defined collateral circulation and risk of stroke in patients with severe carotid artery stenosis. North American Symptomatic Carotid Endarterectomy Trial (NASCET) Group. Stroke 2000;31:128–132.

45. Jansen C, et al. Prediction of intracerebral haemorrhage after carotid endarterectomy by clinical criteria and intraoperative transcranial Doppler monitoring: results of 233 operations. Eur J Vasc Surg 1994;8:220–225.

46. Penn AA, Schomer DF, Steinberg GK. Imaging studies of cerebral hyperperfusion after carotid endarterectomy. Case report. J Neurosurg 1995;83:133–137.

47. Baim D. Grossma's Cardiac Catheterization, Angiography, and Intervention, 7th ed. Philadelphia: Lippincott Williams & Wilkins, 2006.

48. Kapadia SR, et al. Initial experience of platelet glycoprotein IIb/IIIa inhibition with abciximab during carotid stenting: a safe and effective adjunctive therapy. Stroke 2001;32:2328–2332.

49. Biller J, et al. Intraluminal clot of the carotid artery. A clinical-angiographic correlation of nine patients and literature review. Surg Neurol 1986;25:467–477.

50. Villarreal J. Prognosis of patients with intraluminal thrombus in the internal carotid artery. Stroke 1998;29:276.

51. Tsumoto T, et al. Carotid artery stenting for stenosis with intraluminal thrombus. Neuroradiology 2005;1–6.

52. Jovin TG, et al. Emergent stenting of extracranial internal carotid artery occlusion in acute stroke has a high revascularization rate. Stroke 2005;36:2426–2430.

53. Zaidat OO, et al. Early carotid artery stenting and angioplasty in patients with acute ischemic stroke. Neurosurgery 2004;55:1237–1242; discussion 1242–1243.

54. Malek AM, et al. Stent angioplasty for cervical carotid artery stenosis in high-risk symptomatic NASCET-ineligible patients. Stroke 2000;31:3029–3033.

55. Kovacic JC, et al. Staged carotid artery stenting and coronary artery bypass graft surgery: initial results from a single center. Catheter Cardiovasc Interv 2006;67:142–148.

56. Lopes DK, et al. Stent placement for the treatment of occlusive atherosclerotic carotid artery disease in patients with concomitant coronary artery disease. J Neurosurg 2002;96:490–496.

57. Ziada KM, et al. Comparison of results of carotid stenting followed by open heart surgery versus combined carotid endarterectomy and open heart surgery (coronary bypass with or without another procedure). Am J Cardiol 2005;96:519–523.

58. Chen MS, et al. Feasibility of simultaneous bilateral carotid artery stenting. Catheter Cardiovasc Interv 2004;61:437–442.

59. Gonzalez A, et al. Safety and security of carotid artery stenting for severe stenosis with contralateral occlusion. Cerebrovasc Dis 2005;20(Suppl 2):123–128.

60. Sherif C, et al. Neurological outcome of conservative versus endovascular treatment of patients with asymptomatic high-grade carotid artery stenosis: a propensity score-adjusted analysis. J Endovasc Ther 2005;12:145–155.

61. www.strokecenter.org, Stroke Trials Directory—CREST.

62. www.ClinicalTrials.gov, Carotid Stenting vs. Surgery for the Treatment of Severe Carotid Artery Disease and the Prevention of Stroke in Asymptomatic Patients (ACT I).

63. Featherstone RL, Brown MM, Coward LJ. International carotid stenting study: protocol for a randomised clinical trial comparing carotid stenting with endarterectomy in symptomatic carotid artery stenosis. Cerebrovasc Dis 2004;18:69–74.

64. Rothwell PM, Warlow CP. Prediction of benefit from carotid endarterectomy in individual patients: a risk-modelling study. European Carotid Surgery Trialists' Collaborative Group. Lancet 1999;353: 2105–2110.

II

TECHNIQUES OF CAROTID AND VERTEBRAL ARTERY STENTING

9 The Approach to Extracranial Carotid Artery Stenting

Jacqueline Saw, MD *and Jay S. Yadav,* MD

CONTENTS

INTRODUCTION
PREPROCEDURAL MANAGEMENT
CAROTID ARTERY STENTING PROCEDURE
POSTPROCEDURAL MONITORING
CONCLUSIONS
REFERENCES

Summary

Carotid artery stenting is a high-risk procedure that requires meticulous techniques to avoid potentially devastating complications. Performance of this procedure should be limited to experienced endovascular specialist with good catheter-based techniques. This chapter guides readers through a step-by-step approach to carotid stenting.

Key Words: Carotid artery stenting, technical approach.

INTRODUCTION

Carotid artery stenting (CAS) is a high-risk procedure that requires meticulous techniques to avoid potentially devastating complications. Performance of this procedure should be limited to experienced endovascular specialists with good catheter-based techniques. Extra precautions are necessary to reduce the risk of embolic stroke and intracranial hemorrhage. Several committees and governing bodies have collaborated to produce consensus recommendations for minimum training and credentialing necessary to perform CAS *(1,2)*. The cognitive and technical competencies recommended by SCAI/SVMB/SVS are listed in Table 1 *(1)*, and should serve as guidelines for operators to achieve.

Prior to embarking on CAS, the operator should ensure that patients meet accepted indications (outlined in Chapter 8) and lack contraindications (Table 2). Detailed explanation to patients on the potential risks and complications is necessary preprocedure. Reported periprocedural event rates associated with CAS vary and are generally lower in patients who are asymptomatic, considered low risk for surgery, and whom an emboli protection device (EPD) is used. The 30-d death or stroke (major or minor) event rate is

From: *Contemporary Cardiology: Handbook of Complex Percutaneous Carotid Intervention*
Edited by: J. Saw, J. E. Exaire, D. S. Lee, and S. Yadav © Humana Press Inc., Totowa, NJ

Table 1
SCAI/SVMB/SVS Recommendations on Cognitive and Technical Competencies Required
to Perform Carotid Artery Stenting

Cognitive requirements	Technical requirements

Including the fund of knowledge regarding cerebrovascular disease, its natural history, pathophysiology, diagnostic methods, and treatment alternatives.
 	
1. Pathophysiology of carotid artery disease and stroke
  a. Causes of stroke: embolization (cardiac, carotid, aortic, other), vasculitis, arteriovenous malformation, intracranial bleeding (subdural, epidural), space-occupying lesion
  b. Causes of carotid artery narrowing: atherosclerosis, fibromuscular dysplasia, spontaneous dissection, other
  c. Atherogenesis (pathogenesis and risk factors)
2. Clinical manifestations of stroke
  a. Knowledge of stroke syndromes (classic and atypical)
  b. Distinction between anterior and posterior circulation events
3. Natural history of carotid artery disease
4. Associated pathology (e.g., coronary and peripheral artery disease)
5. Diagnosis of stroke and carotid artery disease
  a. History and physical examination: neurologic, non-neurologic (cardiac, other)
  b. Noninvasive imaging and appropriate use thereof: duplex ultrasound, MRA, CTA
6. Angiographic anatomy (arch, extracranial, intracranial, basic collateral circulation, common anatomic variants, and nonatherosclerotic pathologic processes)
7. Knowledge of alternative treatment options for carotid stenosis and their results (immediate success, risks, and long-term outcome)
  a. Pharmacotherapy (e.g., antiplatelet agents, anticoagulation, lipid-lowering agents)
  b. Carotid endarterectomy: results from major trials (NASCET, ACAS, ECST, ACST), results in patients with increased surgical risk
  c. Stent revascularization: results with and without distal embolic protection
	Minimum numbers of procedures to achieve competence:
	
	1. Diagnostic cervicocerebral angiograms—30 (half as primary operator)[a]
	2. Carotid stent procedures—25 (half as primary Operation)[a]
	
	Technical elements for competence in both diagnostic angiography and interventional techniques:
	
	1. High level of expertise with antiplatelet therapy and procedural anticoagulation
	2. Angiographic skills:
	  a. Vascular access skills
	  b. Selection of guidewires and angiographic catheters
	  c. Appropriate manipulation of guidewires and catheters
	  d. Use of "closed system" manifold
	  e. Knowledge of normal angiographic anatomy and common variants
	  f. Knowledge of Circle of Willis and typical/atypical collateral pathways
	  g. Proper assessment of aortic arch configuration, as it affects carotid intervention
	  h. Familiarity with use of angulated views and appropriate movement of the X-ray gantry
	3. Interventional skills:
	  a. Guide catheter/sheath placement
	  b. Deployment and retrieval of embolic protection devices
	  c. Pre- and post-dilation
	  d. Stent positioning and deployment
	4. Recognition and management of intra-procedural complications:
	  a. Cerebrovascular events: stroke or cerebrovascular ischemia, embolization, hemorrhage, thrombosis, dissection, seizure and loss of consciousness
	  b. Cardiovascular events: arrhythmias, hypotension, hypertension, myocardial ischemia/infarction
	  c. Vascular access events: bleeding, ischemia, thrombosis
	5. Management of vascular access
	  a. Proper sheath removal and attainment of hemostasis
	  b. Closure device utilization

(*Continued*)

Table 1 (*Continued*)

Cognitive requirements	Technical requirements

8. Case selection
   a. Indications and contraindications
      for revascularization to prevent stroke
   b. High risk criteria for carotid endarterectomy
   c. High risk criteria for percutaneous intervention
9. Role of postprocedure follow-up and surveillance

Adapted from ref. *1*.

[a]Angiograms and stenting procedures may be performed in the same sitting (e.g., in the same patients), provided that one performs 15 angiograms as primary operator before performing the first stent as primary operator.

Table 2

Contraindications to Extracranial Carotid Artery Stenting

Absolute contraindications

1. Thrombus in the internal carotid artery bifurcation plaque
2. Severe atherosclerotic disease in the aortic arch with friable plaque
3. Total occlusion of the internal carotid artery
4. Inability to obtain vascular access
5. Active septicemia

Relative contraindications

1. Heavily calcified carotid artery plaque
2. Severe type III aortic arch with difficult catheter access
3. Severe tortuosity in the distal internal carotid artery
4. Critical stenosis with string sign
5. Intolerance to aspirin or thienopyridine

approx 2% to 4%; and the 30-d death, stroke, or myocardial infarction (MI) *event-rate* is approx 2% to 5% (*3–5*). This chapter guides readers through a step-by-step approach to CAS.

PREPROCEDURAL MANAGEMENT

Noninvasive Imaging

A routine baseline carotid Doppler is performed to gauge the severity of stenosis and for contralateral disease. A routine CT head to document baseline neurologic pathology is also useful for postprocedural comparisons if complications arise. CT or magnetic resonance (MR) angiography is helpful, but not a necessity because diagnostic carotid and cerebral angiography will be performed as part of CAS.

Neurology Assessment

A baseline neurologic evaluation is performed (e.g., assessing mentation, motor, sensory, speech, and vision), which will allow for postprocedural comparisons if neurologic deficits arise.

Antiplatelet Therapy

All patients should be pretreated with aspirin and clopidogrel. Clopidogrel should be given at least 5 d prior to CAS at 75 mg/d, or loading with 300 mg the day before the procedure followed by 75 mg/d. If inadequate pretreatment time is available, 600 mg clopidogrel may be administered 2 h prior to CAS.

Other Medications

Antihypertensive medications (especially diuretics and β-blockers) are usually held the morning of the procedure, because of anticipated stimulation of carotid baroreceptors. Sedation should be avoided before, during, and after the procedure to allow prompt recognition of neurologic changes.

CAROTID ARTERY STENTING PROCEDURE

Arterial Access

The femoral artery is the preferred access site. If severe lower extremity peripheral arterial disease is present, the brachial artery may be accessed. In such cases, the contralateral arm is typically used (i.e., left brachial artery access for right carotid stenosis), which facilitates guide engagement. In modern-day practice, direct carotid arterial puncture has been abandoned because of higher complications (e.g., carotid dissection, thrombosis, neck hematoma), especially with equipment improvements that enabled over 98% technical success via the femoral approach.

Anticoagulation

Following arterial access, intravenous heparin (50–100 U/kg) is given to achieve an optimal activated clotting time between 250 and 300 s (6). Alternatively, bivalirudin (at the dosage given during percutaneous coronary intervention: 0.75 mg/kg bolus, and 1.75 mg/kg/h infusion) may be used, although this regimen has not been tested against heparin during CAS. The use of routine GP IIb/IIIa inhibitors are avoided because of higher risk of intracranial hemorrhage and strokes (7). The exceptions are patients presenting with large thrombotic acute stroke, or patients who are not eligible for EPD use (8).

Diagnostic Carotid and Cerebral Angiography

Diagnostic carotid angiography is performed as part of the CAS procedure to provide anatomic details, enable strategizing the interventional approach and to anticipate potential challenges. We start with a thoracic arch angiogram at about 45° angle to evaluate the arch anatomy and proximal great vessels. The presence of type III arch (Fig. 1) or proximal arterial stenoses portend additional challenges that the operator has to anticipate. A 5 Fr diagnostic catheter is then used to engage the right and left common carotid arteries, starting with either a JR4 or an angle taper Glidecath® (Terumo Medical) (see Fig. 1 in Chapter 10) for patients with type I or II aortic arches. With type III arches, we frequently start with a VTK catheter (Cook), progressing to Simmons catheters (Cook) for particularly challenging cases. In patients with a bovine arch, catheters tend to prolapse into the ascending aorta, especially when trying to engage the left common carotid artery (CCA) (Fig. 2), and thus, the VTK catheter is often necessary. These reverse-curved catheters need to be reformed in the descending aorta prior to engaging the CCA (Fig. 3). See Chapter 7 for details on cerebral angiography. Vertebral angiography is not compulsory prior to CAS, unless the operator suspects

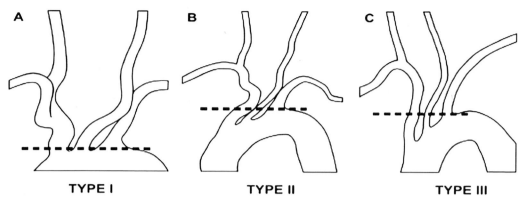

Fig. 1. Aortic arch classification.

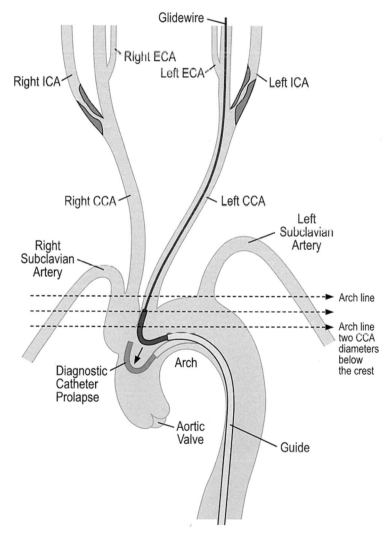

Fig. 2. With bovine arch, catheters tend to prolapse into the ascending aorta during engagement of the left common carotid artery (CCA).

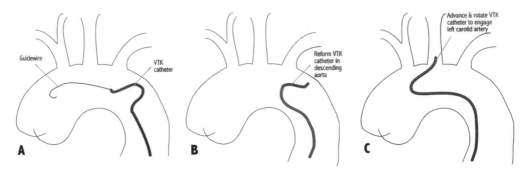

Fig. 3. Reforming of reverse-curve catheters (e.g., VTK catheter) in the descending aorta. **(A)** VTK catheter is advanced over a guidewire into the descending aorta. **(B)** Guidewire is removed, and the VTK catheter is reformed in the descending aorta. **(C)** VTK catheter is advanced and rotated to engage the left common carotid artery.

Table 3
Sheath vs Guide Catheter Approach

Sheath approach	Guide catheter approach
• Smaller arterial access (6 Fr)	• Larger arterial access (8 Fr)
• Requires multiple steps: sheath insertion, diagnostic catheter to engage and then track sheath into common carotid artery	• One-step access to engage common carotid artery using a 5 French catheter telescoping set-up within the 8 French guide
• Sheath dilator allows smooth transition and advancement into carotid artery, lower chance of scrapping plaque debris	• Abrupt transition at the tip may scrape plaque debris. A 5 French telescoping set-up is required to improve transition and advancement into common carotid artery
• Potential for sheath kinking with angulated vessels and steep aortic arch	• Less potential of kinking
• No torque control	• Good torque control
• Less support for advancing balloons, stents, and filters	• More support for tortuous vessels and difficult aortic arch
• Difficult to advance sheath higher without reinserting the dilator	• Ability to advance guide to a higher position during procedure

symptomatic vertebral stenosis, or needs to assess the Circle of Willis (especially if Percusurge® GuardWire™ use is intended). During contrast injection, operators should be extremely vigilant to avoid air or atherothrombotic embolism.

Sheath or Guide Approach

The choice of sheath or guide catheter approach depends on the perceived technical difficulty of the procedure (Table 3). The guide approach is preferred for more challenging cases that require more support, such as steep aortic arch (types II or III), tortuous carotid artery, or extremely stenotic or calcified carotid lesions.

GUIDE APPROACH

Several different guide catheters may be used for CAS (see Fig. 2 in Chapter 10), although we typically start with an 8 Fr 100-cm H1 guide (Cook). We favor the

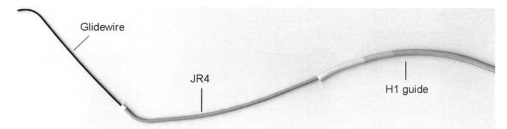

Fig. 4. Telescoping setup: a 5 Fr JR4 diagnostic catheter is telescoped within an 8 Fr H1 guiding catheter.

telescoping technique to advance the guide catheter into the CCA. Either a 5 Fr 125 cm length diagnostic JR4 or VTK catheter is telescoped within the guide (100 cm length) (Fig. 4). Once the 5 Fr diagnostic catheter engages the innominate or left CCA, a 0.035-in. stiff angled Glidewire® (Terumo Medical) is then advanced into the external carotid artery (ECA) under roadmap guidance. If the ostial ECA has a significant stenosis, the Glidewire® may be parked in the distal CCA. The diagnostic catheter is then advanced over the Glidewire® into the distal CCA, followed by tracking along the guide catheter into the mid-distal CCA, with a counter-clockwise torque when advancing across the origin of the great vessel (Fig. 5). The diagnostic catheter and Glidewire® are then removed, and the Tuohy-Borst adaptor opened to expel blood that may contain atherosclerotic debris from catheter manipulation.

SHEATH APPROACH

A 6 Fr 90-cm Shuttle sheath is typically used for this technique. Either a 5 Fr diagnostic JR4 or VTK catheter can be used to engage the innominate or left common carotid artery. Under roadmap guidance, a 0.0350-in. stiff angled Glidewire® is advanced into the ECA, followed by tracking the diagnostic catheter into the ECA. The Glidewire® is then replaced with a long stiff Amplatz wire. The diagnostic catheter is carefully backed out over the stiff Amplatz wire under fluoroscopy. The sheath and its dilator are then advanced over the stiff Amplatz wire into the mid-distal CCA. Once in position, the diagnostic catheter and stiff Amplatz wire are removed, and the Tuohy-Borst adaptor opened to expel blood.

DIRECT GUIDE APPROACH

Rarely, a type III arch may be so challenging that the guide catheter cannot be advanced beyond the origin of the CCA. In these cases, inexperienced operators should probably abandon the procedure; experienced operators may proceed with an 8 Fr AL1 guide, engaging only the origin of the CCA (Fig. 6). Such a guide position may not provide enough support for challenging anatomy (tortuous artery or heavily calcified lesions), and the operator may need an additional support 0.014-in. guidewire (e.g., Ironman, Balance Heavy Weight) in the ECA. Alternatively, a 0.035-in. stiff guidewire may be placed in the ECA, but this will require a 9 Fr AL1 guide catheter to enable CAS with such additional support.

Emboli Protection Device (EPD)

Once the guide or sheath is in position, an EPD is used to cross the lesion. We prefer a filter EPD (as opposed to balloon occlusion devices), as some patients may not tolerate

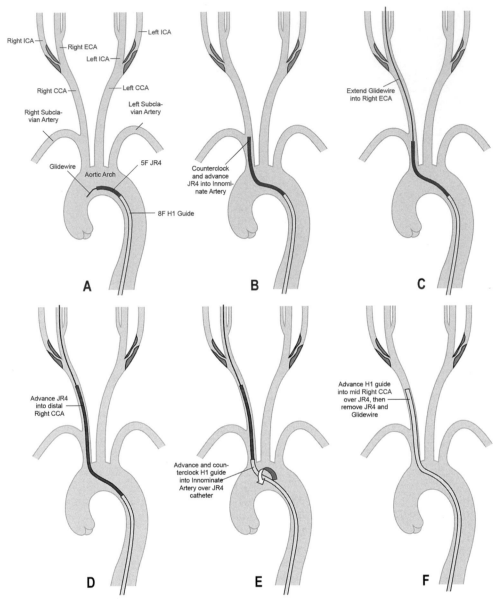

Fig. 5. Schematic representation of steps of carotid artery stenting: **(A)** The telescoped setup (in Fig. 4) is advanced over an 0.035-in. guidewire into the aortic arch. **(B)** The 5 Fr JR4 diagnostic catheter is rotated counterclockwise to engage the innominate artery. **(C)** A stiff-angled Glidewire® is advanced into the right external carotid artery (ECA) under roadmap guidance. **(D)** The JR4 catheter is advanced into the distal right common carotid artery (CCA). **(E)** The H1 guide is advanced and rotated counterclockwise into the right CCA over the JR4 catheter. **(F)** The Glidewire® and JR4 are removed, leaving the H1 guide in the distal right CCA.

temporary obstruction to cerebral blood flow, especially those with contralateral stenosis or incomplete cerebral collateral circulation. The types of EPD available for CAS are described in Chapter 11. To advance the EPD across the stenosis, both primary and secondary curves are shaped on the floppy tip of the 0.014-in. guidewire. The primary curve is shaped to reflect the severity and angle of the stenosis, and the secondary curve

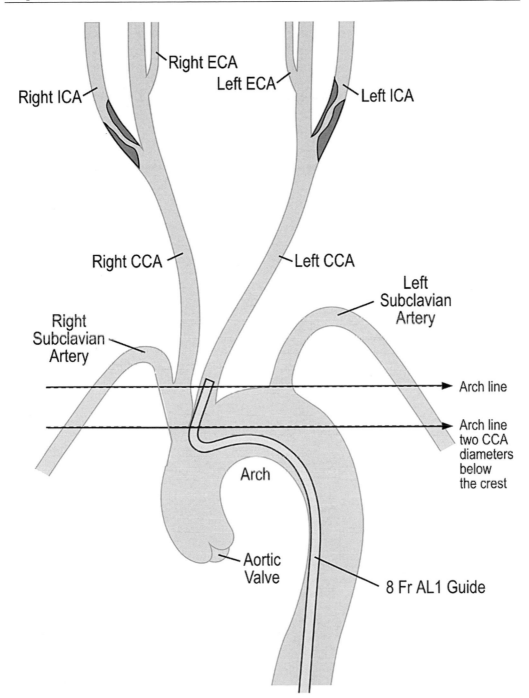

Fig. 6. With a type III aortic arch, sometimes a direct guide approach is necessary, with placement of an 8 Fr AL1 guide engaging the origin of the common carotid artery (CCA).

to reflect the diameter of the CCA (Fig. 7). The filter is then advanced across the stenosis carefully, as this portion of the procedure is not protected. The floppy tip of the guidewire is positioned in the petrous portion of the internal carotid artery (ICA), and the filter basket is deployed proximal to the petrous bone in the straight portion of the cervical ICA

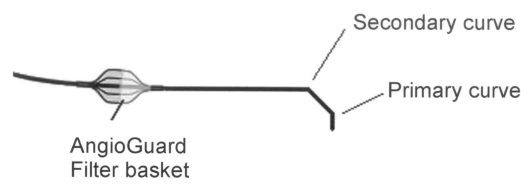

Fig. 7. The use of primary and secondary curves on the guidewire of filter emboli protection device.

(Fig. 8). After deployment, angiographic assessment is performed to ensure that the basket is well apposed to the vessel wall.

Balloon Predilatation

Before stent placement, balloon predilatation is typically performed using a coronary 4.0/20-mm balloon (e.g., Maverick™ [Boston Scientific), CrossSail™ (Guidant]) at 6–8 atm for 5–10 s. If significant bradycardia or hypotension occurs during this predilatation, atropine (0.6–1 mg) may be administered prior to repeat balloon dilatation following stent placement.

Stent Placement

A self-expanding nitinol or stainless-steel stent is favored for the carotid artery. Balloon-expandable stents are no longer used because of problems with stent deformation as the extracranial carotid is a superficial artery *(9)*. Many self-expanding stents are commercially available for peripheral indications (e.g., biliary, lower extremities) and have been used for CAS in studies (Chapter 10). The AccuLink™ stent and AccuNet™ device (Guidant, Santa Clara, CA), and the Xact® and EmboShield™ system (Abbott Vascular Devices, Redwood City, CA) were FDA approved for CAS in August 2004 and September 2005, respectively. The FDA's Circulatory System Devices Panel also had recommended approval of the Precise™ stent and AngioGuard XP™ (Cordis Corporation, Warren, NJ), although this system has not received final FDA approval.

The length of stent selected depends on the lesion length (usually 20–40 mm); in general, operators should avoid unnecessary long stents. As most carotid stenoses involve the ostium of the ICA, the carotid stents have to be placed from the ICA into the distal CCA. In these cases, the diameter of the self-expanding stent should match the distal CCA (we most commonly use an 8 mm diameter stent). For nontapered stents, we try to avoid overexpansion of the ICA with stents >8 mm, which may risk dissection and intramural hematoma. In general, a stent-to-artery ratio of 1.1:1 to 1.4:1 for the ICA is considered appropriate. For patients with a large size-mismatch between the ICA and CCA, tapered stents would be ideal (e.g., AccuLink™ stent, 6–8 mm or 7–10 mm diameters). It is important not to have the edge of the stent struts "hanging" in the CCA, or be at an angle to the CCA, which may potentially obstruct the movements of balloon and retrieval catheters after stent deployment (Fig. 9A). If the carotid stenosis does not involve the ostium of the ICA, then the stent can be placed exclusive in the ICA (we generally use a 7 mm diameter in these cases) (Fig. 9B).

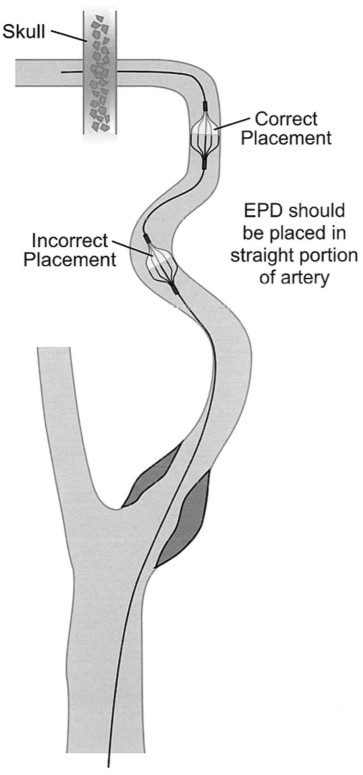

Fig. 8. Proper placement of a filter emboli protection device should be in the straight portion of the cervical internal carotid artery, just before the petrous bone of the skull.

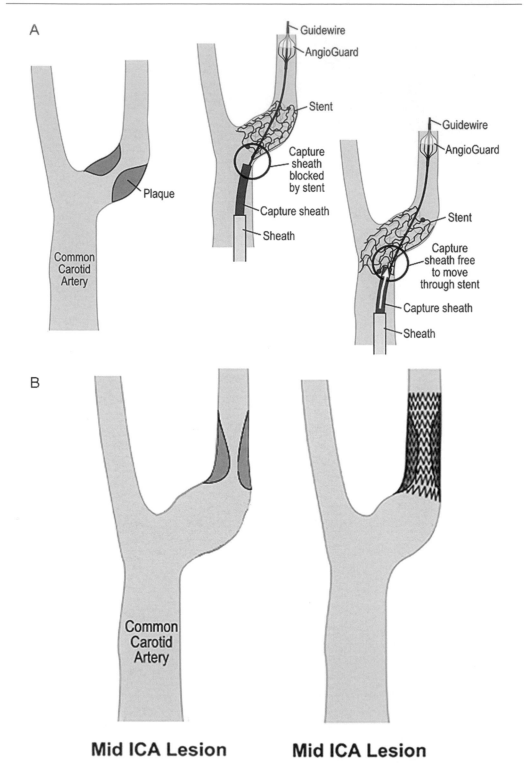

Fig. 9. (A) For ostial common carotid artery (CCA) lesion, it is best to place stent across the internal carotid artery (ICA) origin into the distal CCA. Improper stent placement, with stent edge "floating" at the distal end of CCA or at an angle to the CCA can obstruct catheter movements within stent lumen. **(B)** For mid-ICA lesion, stent can be positioned solely in the ICA.

Table 4
Maneuvers to Facilitate Advancement of Filter Retrieval Catheter Across Stented Segment
to Recapture Emboli Protection Device

- Pull back catheter from stent, rotate the catheter, and readvance.
- Rotate the guiding catheter to change orientation of the catheter tip.
- Rotate patient's head to alter carotid artery orientation (turning to the side, or flexion/extension).
- Remove the retrieval catheter and modify the distal shape of catheter (if catheter tip shape is fixed, consider using a different retrieval catheter with modifiable tip).
- Postdilate the stent to enlarge stent lumen or alter stent configuration.
- Use a buddy wire to straighten the carotid artery.

Before deploying the stent, the undeployed self-expanding stent is advanced slightly beyond the stenosis and then pulled back into the desired position (to prevent forward "jumping"). This is to release the stored energy from longitudinal compression of the delivery system inner core, which is built up during advancement of the stent into the carotid artery. The unsheathing of the self-expanding stent should be done slowly and carefully; sometimes repositioning the stent during deployment is necessary.

Balloon Postdilatation

We almost always postdilate the self-expanding stent with a 5.0–6.0 mm diameter by 20 mm length peripheral balloon (e.g., Amiia™ [Cordis, Miami, FL], Viatrac™ [Guidant, Indianapolis, IN]) to 6–8 atm for 5–10 s. High-pressure inflations are avoided because of the risk of carotid perforation and distal embolization. Care should be taken not to protrude the balloon outside of the stented region to minimize risk of edge dissection. Up to 20% residual stenosis is acceptable as an adequate result. The self-expanding stents will tend to progressively expand to its intended diameter with time. We do not recommend the use of noncompliant balloon, unless the lesion is heavily calcified and the residual stenosis is >20% after the usual postdilatation. Activation of the carotid sinus reflex most frequently occurs during postdilatation, particularly if the lesion is situated in the carotid bulb. Prophylactic atropine administration is typically not required, as this reflex is usually transient and responds to coughing, although occasionally intravenous atropine and/or dopamine may be necessary for prolonged bradycardia and hypotension.

Removal of EPD

After postdilatation, carotid angiography is performed to evaluate blood flow up to the filter EPD. If slow flow is demonstrated, suctioning of the stagnant column of blood is essential, using either the Percusurge Export® aspiration catheter (Medtronic) or a 5 Fr 125-cm multipurpose catheter. Approximately 40–100 cc of blood should be removed before retrieval of the filter EPD. Occasionally, the operator may encounter difficulties in advancing the retrieval catheter to retrieve the EPD device, due to calcified lesions, tortuous and angulated vessels, or stent position. In such situations, a number of maneuvers can be attempted as detailed in Table 4.

Final Angiography

After EPD retrieval, angiography of the bifurcation and the intracranial circulation should be repeated (Fig. 10). Operators must vigilantly assess for distal embolization cutoff signs. Patients are also examined for neurologic deficit. If large embolization to the M1 or M2 middle cerebral artery territory has occurred, a mechanical approach to

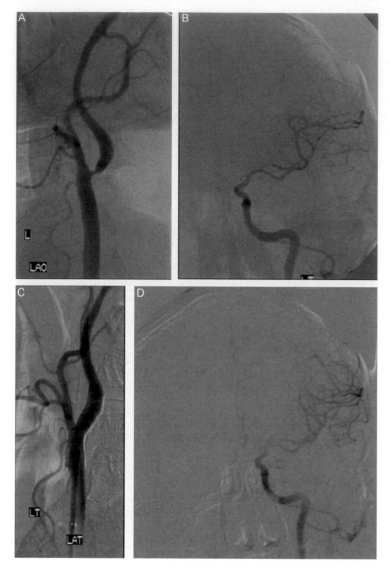

Fig. 10. Angiography image of a severe left internal carotid artery stenosis: **(A)** bifurcation lesion prestenting, **(B)** intracranial angiography prestenting, **(C)** bifurcation angiography poststenting, **(D)** intracranial angiography poststenting.

establish patency is necessary. This may be achieved by crossing the embolus with a hydrophilic wire, with or without using coronary angioplasty balloon or a snare device *(10)*. In refractory cases, intraarterial tissue plasminogen activator (PA) or glycoprotein (GP) IIb/IIIa inhibitors can be administered. On the contrary, small distal embolization beyond the M2 segment are generally tolerated, causing only transient ischemic symptoms and need not be chased.

POSTPROCEDURAL MONITORING

Hemodynamic Monitoring

Postprocedure, patients are closely monitored in a telemetry ward overnight. Blood pressure and heart rate are checked q15 min for 4 h, then q1 h for 4 h, then q4 h overnight. Blood pressure needs to be tightly controlled with systolic pressure <140 mmHg, to prevent the development of hyperperfusion syndrome. Intravenous beta-blockers or infusion with nitroglycerin may be necessary for persistent hypertension, especially if hyperperfusion headache occurs (see Chapter 12). On the opposite spectrum, patients may be hypotensive as a consequence of prolonged vasodilatory response to the carotid baroreceptor reflex. Patients are typically asymptomatic; however, if their systolic pressure is persistently <90 mmHg despite saline infusion, oral pseudoephedrine (30–60 mg q4 h prn) can be administered. Very rarely, intravenous vasoconstrictor support (e.g., dopamine, norepinephrine) may be required.

Neurologic Assessments

Patients are closely monitored post-CAS, at the same frequency as blood pressure monitoring. Nursing staffs assess patients for development of neurologic symptoms (e.g., headache, visual loss, speech disturbance, sensory change, motor deficit), changes in mentation and motor function. A full neurologic assessment (NIH stroke scale, Rankin score, and Barthel index) by a neurologist should be performed the following day.

Carotid Duplex Ultrasound

A carotid ultrasound should be performed the following day post-CAS to have a baseline for future comparison. We then perform repeat ultrasound at 1 mo, 6 mo, and 1 y routinely to assess for restenosis.

Discharge Medications

We routinely discharge patients on a regimen of aspirin (indefinite duration), clopidogrel (for at least 1 mo), and a statin. In a Cleveland Clinic prospective carotid registry ($n = 616$), patients discharged on a statin had a lower 30-d death or stroke event-rate (3.4% statin vs 9.0% no statin, $p = 0.005$) (11). There are no prospective data evaluating the optimal duration of clopidogrel therapy following CAS.

Postdischarge Follow-Up

Patients return for clinical follow-up at 1 mo, 6 mo, and 1 yr following CAS to evaluate for neurologic events. Repeat carotid ultrasounds are performed at each of these time points to assess for increased velocity, which may indicate in-stent restenosis. However, velocity readings are notoriously elevated because of increased stiffness in the stented segment of the carotid artery. A higher threshold of peak systolic velocity and internal carotid artery/common carotid artery ratio should be used to correctly identify the presence of restenosis (see Chapter 12) (12). It is also important to assess the change in contralateral ICA velocities following CAS among patients with bilateral carotid artery stenosis. Data from the Cleveland Clinic have shown a significant drop in contralateral peak systolic velocity (by 60.3 cm/s, $p = 0.005$) and end-diastolic velocity (by 15.1 cm/s, $p = 0.03$) after ipsilateral CAS among patients with bilateral stenosis (13).

Contralateral Carotid Stenosis

For patients who have significant bilateral carotid stenosis for which bilateral CAS is required, it is usually recommended to stage the contralateral procedure (several days to 1 mo apart). Some small case series suggest that simultaneous bilateral CAS may be safe (14,15). However, this simultaneous approach unnecessarily exposes patients to higher risk of cerebral hyperperfusion, hemodynamic compromise, and ischemic complications. Thus, unless the patient requires relatively urgent surgeries (e.g., coronary bypass surgery), a staged approach is preferred.

CONCLUSIONS

In summary, carotid artery stenting is a challenging procedure that requires meticulous techniques to ensure success and patient safety. We have detailed a basic step-by-step approach to guide operators through this procedure, and provided anecdotes to potential problems that may arise during carotid stenting. Readers are encouraged to review cases in Part II for more complicated high-risk carotid stenting procedures.

REFERENCES

1. Rosenfield KM. Clinical competence statement on carotid stenting: training and credentialing for carotid stenting—multispecialty consensus recommendations. J Vasc Surg 2005;41:160–168.
2. Creager MA, Goldstone J, Hirshfeld JW, Jr., et al. ACC/ACP/SCAI/SVMB/SVS clinical competence statement on vascular medicine and catheter-based peripheral vascular interventions: a report of the American College of Cardiology/American Heart Association/American College of Physician Task Force on Clinical Competence (ACC/ACP/SCAI/SVMB/SVS Writing Committee to develop a clinical competence statement on peripheral vascular disease). J Am Coll Cardiol 2004;44:941–957.
3. Yadav JS, Wholey MH, Kuntz RE, et al. Protected carotid-artery stenting versus endarterectomy in high-risk patients. N Engl J Med 2004;351:1493–1501.
4. Kastrup A, Groschel K, Kraph H, Brehm B, Dichgans J, Schulz J. Early outcome of carotid angioplasty and stenting with and without cerebral protection devices. A systematic review of the literature. Stroke 2003;34:813–819.
5. Wholey MH, Al-Mubarek N. Updated review of the global carotid artery stent registry. Catheter Cardiovasc Interv 2003;60:259–266.
6. Saw J, Casserly I, Sachar R, et al. Evaluating the optimal activated clotting time during percutaneous carotid interventions. Am J Cardiol 2006;97:1657–1660.
7. Wholey MH, Eles G, Toursakissian B, Bailey S, Jarmolowski C, Tan WA. Evaluation of glycoprotein IIb/IIIa inhibitors in carotid angioplasty and stenting. J Endovasc Ther 2003;10:33–41.
8. Kopp CW, Steiner S, Nasel C, et al. Abciximab reduces monocyte tissue factor in carotid angioplasty and stenting. Stroke 2003;34:2560–2567.
9. Mathur A, Dorros G, Iyer SS, Vitek JJ, Yadav SS, Roubin GS. Palmaz stent compression in patients following carotid artery stenting. Cathet Cardiovasc Diagn 1997;41:137–140.
10. Yadav JS. Technical aspects of carotid stenting. EuroPCR. Version 3 ed. Paris, 2003:1–18.
11. Saw J, Exaire J, Lee D, et al. Statins reduce early death or stroke events following carotid artery stenting. Circulation 2004;110:III–646.
12. Lal BK, Hobson RW, 2nd, Goldstein J, Chakhtoura EY, Duran WN. Carotid artery stenting: is there a need to revise ultrasound velocity criteria? J Vasc Surg 2004;39:58–66.
13. Sachar R, Yadav JS, Roffi M, et al. Severe bilateral carotid stenosis: the impact of ipsilateral stenting on Doppler-defined contralateral stenosis. J Am Coll Cardiol 2004;43:1358–1362.
14. Chen MS, Bhatt DL, Mukherjee D, et al. Feasibility of simultaneous bilateral carotid artery stenting. Catheter Cardiovasc Interv 2004;61:437–442.
15. Al-Mubarak N, Roubin GS, Vitek JJ, Gomez CR. Simultaneous bilateral carotid stenting for restenosis after endarterectomy. Cathet Cardiovasc Diagn 1998;45:11–15.

10 Equipment for Extracranial Carotid Artery Stenting

Jacqueline Saw, MD
and J. Emilio Exaire, MD

CONTENTS

Summary

Since the first carotid angioplasty performed in 1980, the equipment available has evolved dramatically. This chapter reviews the modern equipment available for carotid angiography and stenting.

Key Words: Balloon angioplasty, balloon-expandable stents, carotid stenting, catheters, guidewires, self-expanding stents.

INTRODUCTION

Since the first carotid angioplasty that was performed in 1980, the equipment available have evolved dramatically. Numerous catheters with different shapes for engagement of specific vessels have been introduced. Catheter and sheath construction has improved, with larger inner luminal diameter achievable without increasing the outer diameter. Thus, smaller arterial puncture may be made with lower risk of access site complications. A wide selection of guidewires have been introduced, some with hydrophilic coating and others with either flexible or stiff support for a variety of uses. Balloon catheters and stents have also evolved with lower profile, greater flexibility, and ease of deliverability. The technique of carotid artery stenting (CAS) has also progressed to routine use of emboli protection device (EPD) and self-expanding nitinol stents. These and other technological advances have improved the success and safety of CAS, with reported technical success rate of approx 99% *(1)*, and estimated periprocedural death and stroke rate of approx 2% (see Chapter 12).

From: *Contemporary Cardiology: Handbook of Complex Percutaneous Carotid Intervention*
Edited by: J. Saw, J. E. Exaire, D. S. Lee, and S. Yadav © Humana Press Inc., Totowa, NJ

Table 1
Recommended Peripheral Guidewires Commonly Used for Carotid Stenting

Guidewires	Company	Characteristics
Flexible guidewires		
Wholey Hi-Torque Floppy	Mallinckrodt	0.035-in., 260-cm length
Magic Torque™	Boston Scientific	0.035-in., 260-cm length
Hydrophilic guidewire		
Glidewire®	Terumo Medical	0.035-in., angle tip, stiff shaft, 260-cm length
Stiff guidewires		
Amplatz Super Stiff™	Boston Scientific	0.035-in., 260-cm length, 3.5-cm shapeable straight-tip
Amplatz Extra Stiff	Cook Incorporated	0.035-in., 260-cm length, shapeable straight-tip

This chapter reviews the modern equipment available for carotid angiography and stenting, with the exception of EPDs (reviewed in Chapter 11). The approach to using this equipment for CAS is reviewed in Chapter 9.

PERIPHERAL GUIDEWIRES

We limit our discussion of peripheral guidewires to those used routinely with CAS (Table 1). Coronary 0.014-in. wires are not discussed, as they are not often used in CAS since the routine use of EPDs (most of which are packaged with their 0.014-in. guidewires, discussed in Chapter 11). Peripheral guidewires used with CAS are typically 0.035-in. in caliber, and several wires, each with unique characteristics, are often required for CAS.

Flexible Guidewires

Patients with carotid artery stenosis often have associated peripheral artery disease (up to one third) *(2)*. Thus, the use of flexible and soft-tipped 0.035-in. guidewires is often necessary for advancing across diseased aortoiliac and iliofemoral arteries, for introducing catheters up to the aortic arch, and sometimes for wiring into subclavian or carotid arteries to anchor catheters. The two most common flexible peripheral guidewires we use are the 0.035-in. Wholey Hi-Torque Floppy (Mallinckrodt, Hazelwood, MO) and Magic Torque™ (Boston Scientific, Natick, MA) guidewires. The Wholey guidewire has a radiopaque gold-tip, a 0.01-in. core over 13 cm distally for added flexibility, and Teflon coating to reduce friction. It comes in 145-cm, 175-cm, and 260-cm lengths. The Magic Torque™ guidewire has a 3-cm shapeable tip, a hydrophilic Glidex™ coating on the distal 10 cm (and polytetrafluoroethylene (PTFE) coating on the distal 11–50 cm), and four distal platinum radiopaque markers 1 cm apart. It comes in 180-cm and 260-cm lengths.

Hydrophilic Guidewires

A stiff-shaft hydrophilic 0.035-in. guidewire is indispensable for CAS. A highly torque-able and hydrophilic wire is needed to advance into the common carotid artery (CCA) and external carotid artery (ECA), which then allows tracking of diagnostic or guide catheters into the mid-distal CCA. It can also be used to track into the ECA, and exchanged out with a stiff Amplatz wire, if a sheath is used (see Chapter 9). Our work-horse hydrophilic wire for CAS is the 0.035-in., 260-cm length, stiff shaft angle tip Glidewire® (Terumo Medical Corporation, Somerset, NJ), with a 3-cm flexible distal tip. It also comes in lengths of 80 cm, 150 cm, and 180 cm. This wire has a lubricious hydrophilic coating allowing smooth passage through vessels and tight lesions, and a superelastic nitinol core that provides flexibility and eliminates wire kinking. We prefer the stiff shaft for CAS, which helps to straighten the CCA and ECA, allowing easy tracking of catheters.

Stiff Guidewires

The Amplatz stiff wires are also frequently used during CAS. We use the exchange length Amplatz wires for stiff and stable support, to exchange diagnostic catheters for guides or sheaths (see Chapter 9). The two commonly available options are the Amplatz Super Stiff™ (Boston Scientific, Natick, MA) and Amplatz Extra Stiff (Cook Incorporated, Bloomington, IN), both with PTFE coating. The exchange-length 260-cm Amplatz Super Stiff™ comes in 0.035-in. or 0.038-in., variable length shapeable straight-tips (1 cm, 3.5 cm, or 6 cm), or J-tip (3-mm curve). The exchange-length straight-tip Amplatz Extra Stiff comes in both 0.035-in. (260-cm length) and 0.038-in. (300-cm length); a 3-mm J-tip 260-cm length version is also available. In general, we prefer the 0.035 in. Amplatz Super Stiff™ 3.5-cm straight-tip, 260-cm length guidewire for CAS (we manually shape the tip to a J-shape configuration).

CATHETERS AND SHEATHS

Diagnostic Catheters

Diagnostic cerebral angiography is most often performed with 5 Fr catheters, although 4 Fr may also be used (see Chapter 7). The simple coronary-shaped JR4 catheter is sufficient to successfully engage CCA in more than two thirds of patients. In those with type II or III aortic arches, a VTK catheter (Cook, Bloomington, IN) is our next option if the JR4 catheter is not successful. With this approach, we have a >99% success rate in performing diagnostic cerebral angiography and subsequent CAS. In the remainder of the cases, a Simmons-shaped catheter may be necessary for the extremely challenging type III arch with tortuous great vessels. We recognize the differences in practice patterns among interventionalists, who may favor alternative catheters as their standard armamentarium. Other diagnostic catheters that are also utilized by interventionalists include angle taper Glidecath® (Terumo Medical Corporation, Somerset, NJ), Berenstein (Boston Scientific, Natick MA), and Headhunter (Cook, Bloomington, IN) catheters. Table 2 lists diagnostic catheters commonly used for cerebral angiography (Fig. 1), divided into simple-curved and reverse-curved catheters. Of note, standard catheter lengths are usually 100 cm. For the telescoping approach (detailed in Chapter 9), a 5 Fr diagnostic catheter length of 125 cm is required to telescope within a 100-cm 8 Fr guide catheter. These 125-cm length catheters (5 Fr JR4 and VTK catheter) can be specially ordered (e.g., from Cordis).

Guide Catheters

The choice of guide catheters is also a matter of interventionalists' preference. An 8 Fr guide catheter (which generally has an 0.088-in. internal lumen) is necessary to

Table 2
Diagnostic Catheters Commonly Used for Cerebral Angiography

Classification	Types of diagnostic catheters
Simple-curved	JR4 catheter
	Angle-tip Glidecath®
	Berenstein catheter
	Headhunter catheter
Reverse-curved	VTK catheter
	Simmons 1, Simmons 2, Simmons 3 catheters

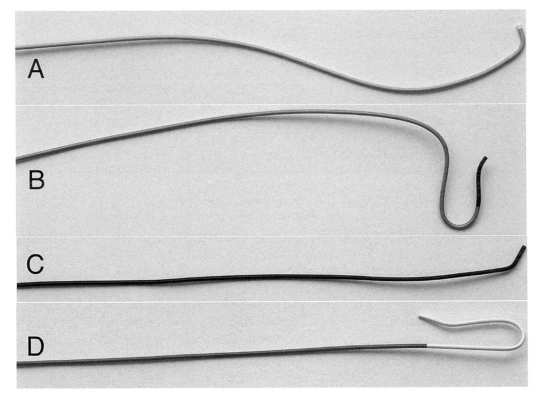

Fig. 1. Commonly used diagnostic catheters for carotid angiography: **(A)** JR4, **(B)** VTK, **(C)** angle taper Glidecath®, **(D)** Simmons.

accommodate the self-expanding nitinol carotid stents. We typically start with an H1 guide (Cordis, Miami, FL), which has a more angulated primary curve, and a gentler secondary curve (Fig. 2). This configuration allows easier engagement of the CCA, and also angulation of the catheter toward the lesion when necessary. Infrequently, a direct guide approach may be required because of an extremely steep type III arch (see Chapter 9); in this case, we would place an Amplatz Left-1 (AL1) guide at the origin of the CCA (Fig. 6 in Chapter 9). To better engage the CCA origin, the AL1 guide can be modified with heat using a hair dryer (Fig. 3).

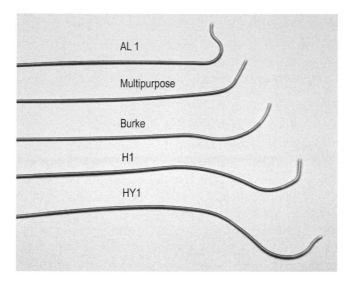

Fig. 2. Commonly used guide catheters for carotid artery stenting.

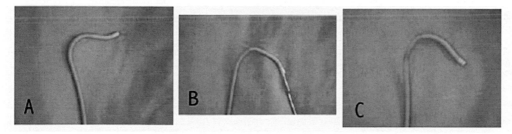

Fig. 3. Steps to modify an AL1 guide: (**A**) AL1 catheter. (**B**) A paper clip is inserted and a hair dryer is directed toward the tip of the catheter to modify the curve. (**C**) Modified AL1 catheter. Note the absence of the primary curve and the soft secondary curve.

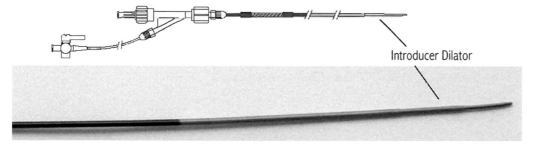

Fig. 4. Shuttle sheath (6 Fr 90 cm).

Sheaths

A sheath approach to CAS is frequently used (see Chapter 9 for the sheath vs guide approach). These sheaths should have a hydrophilic coating, and the length should be approx 90 cm. We favor the Shuttle Sheath (Cook, Bloomington, IN), which provides excellent navigability and support. The 6 Fr sheath has a 0.087-in. internal lumen (equivalent to an 8 Fr guiding catheter), a 7 Fr has a 0.100-in. lumen, and the 8 Fr has a 0.113-in. lumen (equivalent to a 10 Fr guiding catheter). Thus, our standard choice is a 6 Fr 90-cm Shuttle Sheath (Fig. 4).

ANGIOPLASTY BALLOONS

Semicompliant angioplasty balloons compatible with the 0.014-in. or 0.018-in. system are typically used for both predilatation and postdilatation. The monorail system is preferred for ease of use, although some operators still choose over-the-wire system.

Predilatation Balloons

The 0.014-in. coronary balloons are usually used for predilatation, and a wide variety are commercially available. Balloons with low crossing profile (~0.026 in.) and excellent flexibility and trackability are usually preferred. We typically use either the Maverick2™ (Boston Scientific, Natick, MA) or the CrossSail® (Guidant, Indianapolis, IN) balloons, which have the above characteristics. Generally, a 4.0 mm × 20-mm balloon is used for predilatation (6–8 atm for 5–10 s) after crossing with an EPD. Balloon lengths >20 mm are used only for long lesions; we do not find "watermelon seeding" to be an issue with short balloon for CAS, unless we are dealing with restenotic lesions. Infrequently, a 5-mm diameter balloon may be required if difficulty with stent delivery persists after predilatation with the 4-mm balloon.

Postdilatation Balloons

As the internal carotid artery (ICA) is typically 6–7 mm in diameter, peripheral angioplasty balloons are required for postdilatation of self-expanding stents. Transcranial Doppler has demonstrated that postdilatation is the phase in CAS where most emboli are generated *(3–5)*. Thus, aggressive postdilatation is generally not recommended, and residual stenosis up to 20% is considered acceptable for CAS. Peripheral balloons usually have lower nominal pressure than coronary balloons, and have selection choices to track over 0.014-in., 0.018-in. or 0.035-in. wires. We tend to use a 5.0 × 20 mm, 5.5 × 20 mm, or 6.0 × 20 mm balloon, compatible with a 0.014-in. –0.018-in. system, inflating up to 6–8 atm. Examples of semicompliant peripheral balloons suitable for postdilatation are Amiia™ (Cordis, Miami, FL), Viatrac™ (Guidant, Indianapolis, IN), and Gazelle™ (Boston Scientific, Natick, MA) (Table 3). We use only a noncompliant balloon (e.g., Titan™ [Cordis, Miami, FL]) if the lesion is heavily calcified and there is a residual stenosis >20%.

SELF-EXPANDING STENTS

Balloon-expandable stents are no longer used for the carotid bifurcation, because of fractures seen with superficial compression. They are still used for ostial CCA lesions, where good radial strength is desired for aorto-ostial lesions. For the typical carotid bifurcation lesions, self-expanding stents are routinely used, which can be made of nitinol (nickel–titanium) or stainless steel *(6)*. We prefer the nitinol stents as they have minimal foreshortening, are more flexible, and conform better to vessel curvature. The AccuLink™ (Guidant, Santa Clara, CA) and Xact® (Abbott Vascular Devices, Redwood City, CA) stents are now FDA approved for CAS (both devices described in more detail below). The Precise™ (Cordis, Warren, NJ) stent has been recommended for approval by the FDA's Circulatory System Devices Panel, but has not had final FDA approval. Other nitinol stents being evaluated in clinical trials are listed in Table 4. Chapter 9 reviews the appropriate nitinol stent size selection for CAS. The only stainless steel self-expanding stent available for CAS is the Wallstent® (Boston Scientific, Natick, MA). This stent

Table 3
Examples of Peripheral Angioplasty Balloons that May Be Used for Postdilatation for Carotid Stenting

Name	Company	System (in.)	Diameter (mm)	Length (mm)	Sheath size (Fr)	Delivery	Compliance
Amiia™	Cordis	0.014	4–7	15, 20, 30, 40	4–6	RX	Compliant
Viatrac™	Guidant	0.014	4–6.5	20, 30	4–5	RX	Compliant
Agiltrac™	Guidant	0.018	4–7	15, 20, 30, 40	5–7	OTW	Compliant
Gazelle™	Boston Scientific	0.018	2–6	20	4–5	RX	Compliant
Slalom™	Cordis	0.018	3–8	20, 40	4–6	OTW	Compliant
Talon™	Boston Scientific	0.018	4–7	15, 20, 40	5–6	OTW	Noncompliant
Ultra-Soft™ SV	Boston Scientific	0.018	4–7	15, 20	4–5	RX	Compliant

Table 4
Investigational and Approved Self-Expanding Stents for Carotid Stenting

Company	Self-expanding stents	Straight design (mm)	Tapered design (mm)	Studies
Abbott	Xact®	D: 7–10 L: 20, 30	D: 6/8, 7/9, 8/10 L: 30, 40	ACT 1 SECURITY
Bard	Vivexx™	D: 5–12 L: 20, 30, 40	D: 6/8, 7/10, 8/12 L: 30, 40	VIVA
Boston Scientific	Wallstent®	D: 6, 8, 10 L: 20, 30, 40	Not available	BEACH
Cordis	Precise™	D: 5–10 L: 20, 30, 40	Not available	CASES SAPPHIRE
EndoTex	NexStent™	D: 4–9 L: 30	Not available	CABERNET
EV3	Protege™	D: 6–10 L: 20, 30, 40, 60	D: 6/8, 7/10 L: 30, 40	CREATE
Guidant	AccuLink™	D: 5–10 L: 20, 30, 40	D: 6/8, 7/10 L: 30, 40	ARCHER CREATE 2 CREST CAPTURE
Medtronic	Exponent	D: 6–10 L: 20, 30, 40	Not available	MAVerIC 1,2, 3 PASCAL

D, Diameter (For straight design: 5–10 means diameter from 5 to 10 mm at 1-mm intervals; For tapered design: 6/8 means distal diameter 6 mm, and proximal diameter 8 mm); L, length.

can have substantial foreshortening (about 20%), and also reduced radial force; thus it is always oversized (usually a 10-mm diameter × 20 mm length works well for most carotid bifurcation lesions). It is also more rigid than nitinol stents, and does not conform as well to tortuous vessels (Fig. 5).

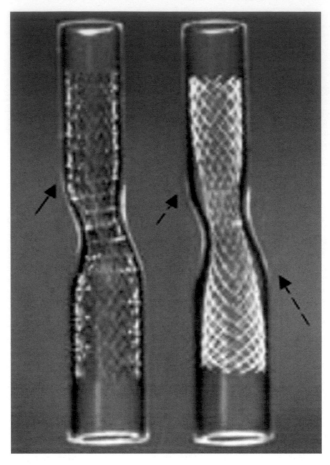

Fig. 5. The nitinol stent (on the **left**) covers the lesion and tortuosity well *(arrow)*, but the stainless steel stent (on the **right**) does not conform as well, leaving uncovered gaps *(dashed arrows)*.

RX AccuLink™

The RX AccuLink™ (Guidant, Santa Clara, CA) is a self-expanding nitinol stent that is premounted on a rapid-exchange (RX) stent delivery catheter (Fig. 6). It is compatible with a 0.014-in. guidewire, and an 8 Fr guide catheter or 6 Fr sheath with a minimal luminal diameter of 0.085-in. It comes in both a straight and tapered configuration. The stent sizes available and the recommended reference vessel diameters are described in Table 5. This stent has minimal foreshortening, reported at 1% with the 7 × 40 mm stent. The delivery catheter has a 132-cm working length compatible with a 100-cm guide catheter, and has a unique handle that allows a one-handed deployment (Fig. 7).

Xact® Carotid Stent System

The Xact® (Abbott Vascular Devices, Redwood City, CA) is a self-expanding nitinol stent that is premounted on an RX delivery system. It has a closed-cell design that creates a tightly knit mesh (with dense scaffolding), promoting a smooth inner vessel surface preventing plaque prolapse, which may reduce distal embolization. The closed-cell design (with no exposed struts) and flared-end design of the stent facilitate un-impeded advancement of balloon or retrieval catheters (Fig. 8). The stent is still

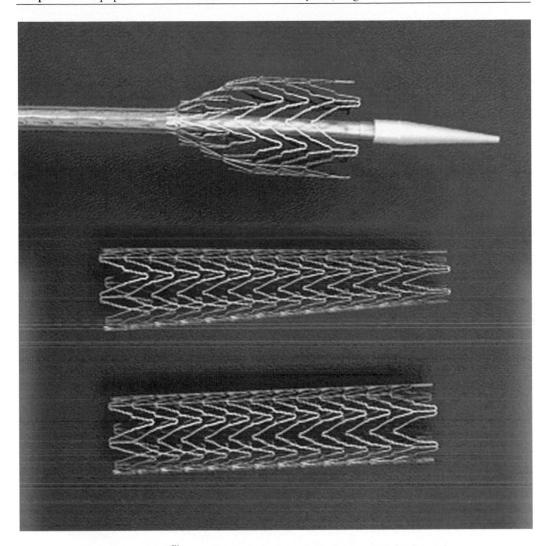

Fig. 6. AccuLink™ stent shown in both straight and tapered configurations.

Table 5
Available Sizes of the RX AccuLink™ Stents and Recommended Reference Vessel Diameters

Stent diameter	Stent lengths		Reference vessel diameter
Straight stents			
5.0 mm	20, 30, 40 mm		3.6–4.5 mm
6.0 mm	20, 30, 40 mm		4.3–5.4 mm
7.0 mm	20, 30, 40 mm		5.0–6.4 mm
8.0 mm	20, 30, 40 mm		5.7–7.3 mm
9.0 mm	20, 30, 40 mm		6.4–8.2 mm
10.0 mm	20, 30, 40 mm		7.1–9.1 mm
Tapered stents			
6–8 mm taper	30, 40 mm	ICA: 4.3–5.4 mm	CCA: 5.7–7.3 mm
7–10 mm taper	30, 40 mm	ICA: 5.0–6.4 mm	CCA: 7.1–9.1 mm

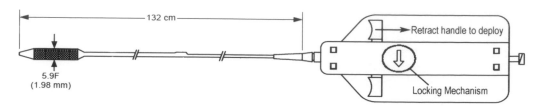

Fig. 7. Schematic diagram of the AccuLink™ stent showing the unique handle design (pull handle back to deploy stent) and locking mechanism.

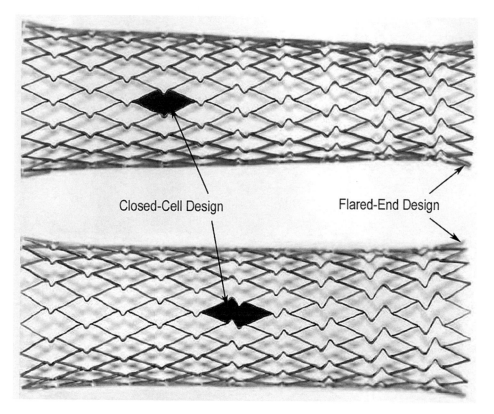

Fig. 8. Xact® stent shown in both straight and tapered configurations, with the closed-cell and flared-end design's.

claimed to be highly flexible despite the closed-cell design. The delivery system has an outer diameter of 5.7 Fr, and thus is compatible with an 8 Fr guide catheter or 6 Fr sheath with a 0.088-in. inner diameter. The delivery system has a working length of 136 cm and is compatible with a 0.014-in. guidewire. The stent is available in both straight and tapered configurations, with diameters ranging from 6 to 10 mm, and lengths of 20–40 mm (Table 6).

CONCLUSIONS

The technical success and procedural safety of carotid artery stenting has improved with advances in technology and equipment. This chapter reviewed the typical modern

Table 6
Available Sizes of the Xact® Stents and Recommended Reference Vessel Diameters

Stent diameter	Stent lengths		Reference vessel diameter
Straight stents			
7.0 mm	20, 30 mm		>5.5–6.4 mm
8.0 mm	20, 30 mm		>6.4–7.3 mm
9.0 mm	20, 30 mm		>7.3–8.2 mm
10.0 mm	20, 30 mm		>8.2–9.1 mm
Tapered stents			
6–8 mm taper	30, 40 mm	ICA: 4.8–5.5 mm	CCA: >6.4–7.3 mm
7–9 mm taper	30, 40 mm	ICA: >5.5–6.4 mm	CCA: >7.3–8.2 mm
8–10 mm taper	30, 40 mm	ICA: >6.4–7.3 mm	CCA: >8.2–9.1 mm

equipment now utilized for a standard carotid stent procedure. Many other devices (especially stents and EPDs) are under clinical evaluation, and will soon be approved by the FDA. We hope that future generations of catheters, wires, balloons, stents, and emboli protection devices will further improve the safety and long-term outcome of carotid stenting.

REFERENCES

1. Wholey MH, Al-Mubarek N. Updated review of the global carotid artery stent registry. Catheter Cardiovasc Interv 2003;60:259–266.
2. Ness J, Aronow WS. Prevalence of coexistence of coronary artery disease, ischemic stroke, and peripheral arterial disease in older persons, mean age 80 years, in an academic hospital-based geriatrics practice. J Am Geriatr Soc 1999;47:1255–1256.
3. Ohki T, Marin ML, Lyon RT, Berdejo GL, Soundararajan K, Ohki M, et al. Ex vivo human carotid artery bifurcation stenting: correlation of lesion characteristics with embolic potential. J Vasc Surg 1998;27:463–471.
4. Rapp JII, Pan XM, Sharp FR, et al. Atheroemboli to the brain: size threshold for causing acute neuronal cell death. J Vasc Surg 2000;32:68–76.
5. Topol EJ, Yadav JS. Recognition of the importance of embolization in atherosclerotic vascular disease. Circulation 2000;101:570–580.
6. Mukherjee D, Kalahasti V, Roffi M, et al. Self-expanding stents for carotid interventions: comparison of nitinol versus stainless-steel stents. J Invasive Cardiol 2001;13:732–735.

11 Emboli Protection Devices

Jacqueline Saw, MD

CONTENTS

INTRODUCTION
FILTER EMBOLI PROTECTION DEVICES
DISTAL BALLOON OCCLUSION EMBOLI PROTECTION DEVICE
PROXIMAL BALLOON OCCLUSION EMBOLI PROTECTION DEVICES
CONCLUSIONS
REFERENCES

Summary

Distal embolization occurs routinely during carotid artery stenting (CAS), and some of these debris may result in devastating neurologic complications. The use of an emboli protection device (EPD) is crucial to reduce distal embolization, and has been shown in nonrandomized studies to decrease stroke or death event rates by two to three times during CAS. This chapter reviews both the filter and balloon occlusion EPD.

Key Words: Distal embolization, emboli protection device.

INTRODUCTION

Distal embolization occurs routinely during carotid artery stenting (CAS), and some of these debris may result in devastating neurologic complications *(1)*. The use of an emboli protection device (EPD) is crucial to reduce distal embolization, and has been shown in nonrandomized studies to decrease stroke or death event rates by two to three times during CAS *(2,3)*. In the updated global experience of 12,392 CAS reported by Wholey et al., the 30-d death or stroke event rate was 2.23% with EPD use, and 5.29% without EPD use ($p < 0.0001$) *(2)*. In a meta-analysis of 3196 CAS by Kastrup et al., the combined 30-d death and stroke rate was 1.8% with EPD use compared to 5.5% without EPD use *(3)*.

In the original *ex vivo* model of 24 carotid angioplasty and stent procedures by Ohki et al. *(1)*, distal embolization was demonstrated in all cases and correlated with echolucency and stenosis severity. Further, the occurrence of distal embolization may be higher with percutaneous CAS than with surgical carotid endarterectomy, when an EPD is not used. In a retrospective analysis by Jordan et al., transcranial Doppler detected eight times higher microembolization rate with CAS when no EPD was used, compared with carotid endarterectomy *(4)*. In fact, only 7.5% of patients who underwent

From: *Contemporary Cardiology: Handbook of Complex Percutaneous Carotid Intervention*
Edited by: J. Saw, J. E. Exaire, D. S. Lee, and S. Yadav © Humana Press Inc., Totowa, NJ

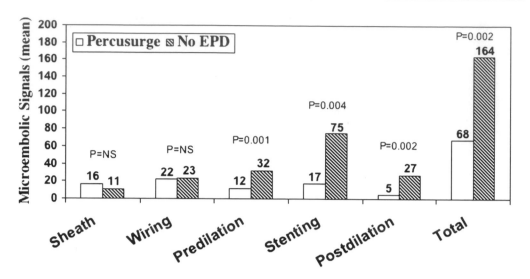

Fig. 1. Mean microembolic signals with or without the use of the Percusurge GuardWire™ emboli protection device (EPD) during each step of carotid stenting (sheath placement, wiring, balloon predilation, stent deployment, postdilation, and total for procedure). (Adapted from ref. 5.)

CAS without EPD did not have distal emboli *(4)*. Fortunately, clinical studies using transcranial Doppler have shown that the use of an EPD can dramatically reduce microembolic signals with CAS. Al-Mubarak compared a series of 76 patients, 37 of whom underwent CAS with the Percusurge® GuardWire™ (Medtronic, Minneapolis, MN) and 39 underwent CAS without EPD *(5)*. The use of the balloon occlusion EPD significantly reduced microembolic signals during the critical phases of CAS: predilation, stent deployment, and postdilation (Fig. 1) *(5)*.

As transcranial Doppler is not readily available or routinely used during CAS, clinicians often assess for the presence of visible embolic debris in the filters of EPD (or in the aspirated blood of balloon occlusion EPD) to gage the success of distal protection. In clinical studies using EPD for CAS, visible embolic debris were aspirated in all patients when the Percusurge® device is used (size range 56–2652 µm) *(6)*, and in approx 50% of patients with filter EPD *(7)*. Although these devices do reduce distal embolization, they do not completely prevent all events *(5)*. Fortunately, not all distal emboli cause clinically relevant ischemic events, which depend on the size, quantity, and location of embolization. The minimum particle size capable of producing clinical ischemic events has not been established. A few magnetic resonance imaging (MRI) studies have shown that silent cerebral infarctions do occur during CAS *(8,9)*, however, the long-term clinical significance is unknown. In one study of unprotected CAS, of 20/69 (29%) of patients who had ipsilateral cerebral infarcts on MRI, only one patient (1.4%) was symptomatic *(8)*. In another study on CAS with EPD, 2/16 (1.2%) of patients had new cerebral infarcts on MRI, but none had permanent neurologic deficits *(9)*. Nevertheless, there is no reliable predictive characteristics that can predict occurrence of visible debris *(10)*, and thus routine EPD use is recommended for all CAS procedures. In fact, all modern CAS trials require the adjunctive use of an EPD. To date, no randomized trials comparing CAS with EPD vs without EPD have been done, and for ethical reasons likely never will be done.

Table 1
Filter vs Balloon Occlusion Emboli Protection Devices

	Filter devices	Balloon occlusion devices
Crossing profile	More bulky and larger crossing profile, may require predilatation for very tight lesions	Smaller crossing profile and better flexibility
Embolic potential	Potentially higher risk of embolization during wire crossing	Potentially lower risk of embolization during wire crossing
Vessel visualization	Unhindered visualization of vessel, allow accurate stent placement	Difficulty visualizing vessel when balloon is inflated
Perfusion	Permit antegrade blood flow to distal bed, well tolerated by patients	Blood flow to distal bed occluded, may cause ischemia if collateral flow is poor
Ease of use	Easy to use	More cumbersome, requires aspiration and fast operation
Emboli protection	Captures emboli that are larger than the pore size of the filter	Theoretically traps and captures all emboli with occlusion balloon and aspiration catheter
Apposition to vessel wall	May have incomplete apposition if inappropriate size or eccentric placement	Usually good apposition if balloon size is appropriate
Retrieval profile	May have difficulty collapsing filters full of embolic debris, and extruding debris through pores	Low profile

EPD can be divided into filter and balloon occlusion devices. The balloon occlusion devices can be further subdivided into proximal and distal occlusion types. The potential advantages and disadvantages of these devices are described in Table 1.

FILTER EMBOLI PROTECTION DEVICES

The prototypical filter EPD consists of a guidewire with an integrated filter basket, although some devices are designed to have a separate guidewire and filter basket system. They are packaged with their delivery and retrieval catheters. When these EPD are deployed, they allow antegrade blood flow through the filter pores, but trap embolic debris that are larger than the pore size. Because these devices do not interrupt distal blood flow, angiography can be performed when filters are deployed to allow visualization of balloon and stent placement. Ideally, anticoagulation with unfractionated heparin is recommended with ACT >250 ms, and the filter should be deployed at least 2 cm beyond the stenosis, and situated in the straight portion of the cervical internal carotid artery (ICA) before the petrous portion. Once deployed, the filter guidewire functions as a conventional angioplasty guidewire accommodating balloons and stents with filter protection. These devices are simple to use and are the most commonly utilized EPD during CAS. However, their main disadvantages are their high crossing profiles and

Table 2
Filter Emboli Protection Devices

Device	Pore size (μm)	Filter diameter (mm)	Delivery profile (Fr)
AngioGuard XP™	100	4–8	3.2–3.9
AccuNet™	120	4.5–7.5	3.5–3.7
EmboShield™	140	3–6	3.9
FilterWire EZ™	110	3.5–5.5	3.2
SPIDER™	50–200	3–7	3.2
Interceptor™	100	4.5–6.5	2.9
Rubicon Filter	100	4–6	2.1–2.7

Table 3
Examples of High-Risk Carotid Stent Registries

High-risk registries	Company	EPD	Stent	N
ARCHER 1	Guidant	None	AccuLink OTW	158
ARCHER 2	Guidant	AccuNet	AccuLink OTW	278
ARCHER 3	Guidant	AccuNet	AccuLink MR	145
BEACH	Boston Scientific	FilterWire	Wallstent	747
CABERNET	EndoTex	FilterWire	NexStent	443
CASES	Cordis	AngioGuard	Precise	1500
MAVErIC II	Medtronic	Percusurge	Exponent	399
MAVErIC III	Medtronic	Interceptor PLUS	Exponent	413
MO.MA	Invatec	MO.MA	Any stent	157
PASCAL	Medtronic	Any	Exponent	115
SECURITY	Abbott	EmboShield	Xact	398

dependency on their predetermined pore size to capture emboli (missing particles smaller than the pore size).

There are two carotid stents and filter EPD that are currently FDA approved, the AccuLink™ and AccuNet™ system (Guidant, Santa Clara, CA) [approved August 2004], and the Xact® and EmboShield™ system (Abbott Vascular Devices, Redwood City, CA) [approved in September 2005]. The FDA's Circulatory System Devices Panel also had recommended approval of the Cordis Carotid System (Precise™ stent and AngioGuard™ EPD), although this system has not received final FDA approval. Several other filter EPD have been developed and are available under clinical trials of coronary, carotid, and peripheral interventions. Table 2 compares the filter size diameters, pore sizes, and delivery profiles of these EPD. Examples of high-risk CAS registries utilizing these EPD are listed in Table 3.

AngioGuard XP™

The AngioGuard XP™ (Cordis Corporation, Warren, NJ) guidewire-filter system consists of a polytetrafluoroethylene (PTFE)-coated stainless steel 0.014-in. guidewire with a 3.5-cm shapeable floppy tip. This guidewire is integrated with a filter basket

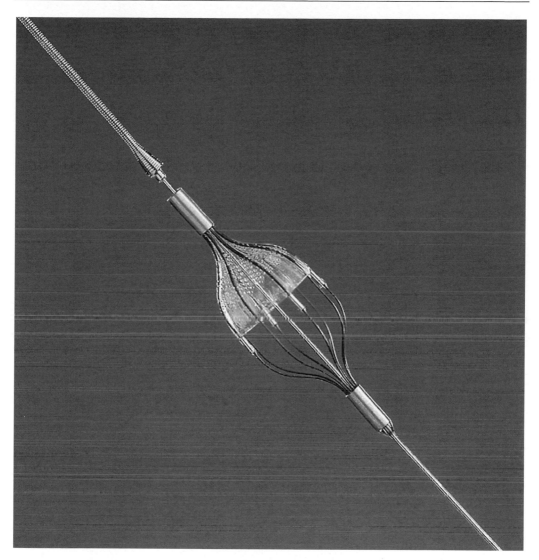

Fig. 2. AngioGuard™ device.

that is constructed of thin, porous polyurethane membrane (100 μm pore size) supported by an eight-wire nitinol system (four with radiopaque markers) (Fig. 2). The system comes with different basket sizes, with diameters from 4 to 8 mm (in 1-mm increment). In general, the filter basket should be oversized by 0.5–1.0 mm compared with the vessel diameter. The current over-the-wire delivery system has a crossing profile of 3.2–3.9 Fr depending on the filter size. The retrieval sheath has a larger crossing profile of 5.1 Fr. The length of the filter varies from 4.11 mm to 6.91 mm, depending on the filter diameter. This system is compatible with a 6 Fr sheath or an 8 Fr guide catheter. This device was evaluated in the SAPPHIRE (Stenting and Angioplasty with Protection in Patients at High Risk for Endarterectomy) study. As well, the GUARD (Saphenous Vein Graft Intervention Using AngioGuard™ for Reduction of Distal Embolization) study is randomizing patients undergoing SVG intervention to the AngioGuard™ device or no EPD.

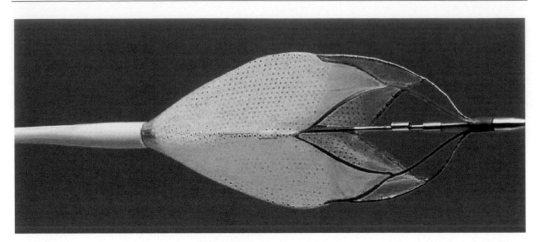

Fig. 3. AccuNet™ device.

Table 4
AccuNet™ Filter Sizes and Recommended
Reference Vessel Diameters

Filter size	Reference vessel diameters	Delivery profile (Fr)
4.5 mm	3.25–4.0 mm	3.5
5.5 mm	4.0–5.0 mm	3.5
6.5 mm	5.0–6.0 mm	3.7
7.5 mm	6.0–7.0 mm	3.7

AccuNet™

The RX AccuNet™ Embolic Protection System (EPS) (Guidant Corporation, Indianapolis, IN) is a guidewire-filter system that has a similar design to the AngioGuard™ device. It has a PTFE-coated stainless steel 0.014-in. guidewire (ACS Hi-Torque Balance Heavyweight) with a 3-cm shapeable floppy tip, available in 190-cm and 300-cm lengths. The filter basket is integrated on the guidewire, and is constructed of thin, porous polyurethane (pore size ≤150 μm) supported by a four-wire nitinol system (four radiopaque markers to guide wall apposition) (Fig. 3). The baskets come in different sizes with 1-mm diameter increment, from 4.5 to 7.5 mm in diameter. The reference vessel diameter ranges recommended for this device is listed in Table 4. The length of the filter basket cone ranges from 10 mm to 12 mm (according to filter size). This system is compatible with a 6 Fr sheath or an 8 Fr guide catheter. The packaged delivery sheath has a profile of 3.5–3.7 Fr, and has a peel-away design for rapid exchange. The packaged retrieval catheter has a shapeable tip, which allows easier access to retrieve the filter in the setting of tortuous vessels. This device was evaluated in the ARCHeR (ACCULINK for Revascularization of Carotids in High-Risk Patients) studies.

EmboShield™

The MedNova NeuroShield™ was renamed EmboShield™ after the acquisition by Abbott Laboratories (Abbott Park, IL). This device consists of a separate guidewire

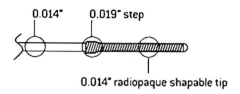

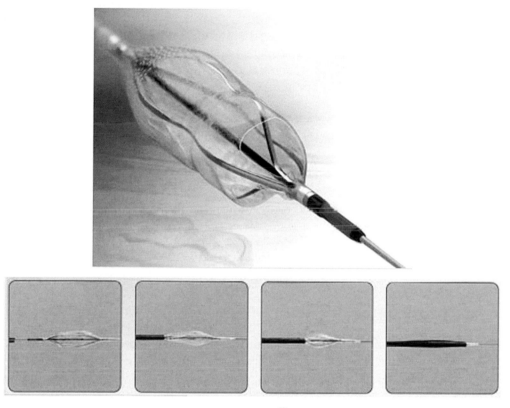

Fig. 4. EmboShield™ device.

(BareWire™) and filter system, thus allowing lesion crossing with a bare guidewire, prior to delivering the filter. There are five types of 0.0140-in. BareWire™ that can be chosen (each available in 190-cm or 315-cm lengths): soft, medium, extra, super, and maximum. These proprietary guidewires are PTFE-coated and have a 3-cm platinum shapeable radiopaque tip, followed by a 0.019-in. "step" for filter retrieval (Fig. 3). After the BareWire™ has crossed the lesion, the filter delivery catheter is advanced over the BareWire™ to the intended deployment site, proximal to the 0.019-in. step. The filter is then deployed and the deliver sheath removed. The design of the retrieval catheter allows full capture of the entire filter during retrieval (Fig. 4). The filter basket is constructed of polyurethane membrane (with pore size 140 μm) with an internal nitinol support frame. The filter diameters come in sizes from 3 to 6 mm, in 1-mm increments. The delivery catheter profile is 3.9 Fr and the retrieval catheter is 5.7 Fr. This device was studied in the SECURITY (Registry Study to Evaluate the Neuroshield Bare Wire Cerebral Protection System and X-Act Stent in Patients at High Risk for Carotid Endarterectomy) trial.

FilterWire EZ™

The FilterWire EZ™ (Boston Scientific, Natick, MA) guidewire-filter system consists of a stainless steel 0.014-in. guidewire, with a 3-cm long shapeable floppy tip, available in 190-cm and 300-cm lengths. The guidewire is integrated with the filter basket, which is constructed of thin, porous polyurethane (with 110-μm pores) mounted on a nitinol wire loop. This nitinol loop has a 360° apposition to the vessel wall and accommodates vessel diameters from 3.5 to 5.5 mm. The earlier EX™ version has an off-center design with the guidewire attached to the side of the nitinol basket. The newer generation EZ™ version has a suspension loop, to allow good apposition of the filter in curved vessels. The EZ™ version also has the delivery sheath preloaded, and has a peel-away design to allow for rapid exchange. The nitinol loop has a "fish-mouth" opening that closes during retrieval for efficient particle retention. This system is compatible with a 6 Fr guide catheter, and has a crossing profile of 3.2 Fr with the delivery sheath (Fig. 5). The retrieval sheath has a 4 Fr crossing profile. This device is simple to use, and comes in only one size (fitting 3.5- to 5.5-mm vessels). However, vessels >5.5 mm will not be adequately protected by this filter. The FilterWire has been studied in the BEACH (Boston Scientific/EPI: A Carotid Stenting Trial for High-Risk Surgical Patients) and CABERNET (Carotid Artery Revascularization Using the Boston Scientific EPI FilterWire EX™ and the EndoTex NexStent) trials.

SPIDER™ Embolic Protection Device

EV3 acquired Microvena's Trap™ filter device, and has since introduced the new SPIDER™ (EV3, Plymouth, MN), which has received CE mark approval to prevent distal embolization during general vascular interventions (including peripheral, coronary, and carotid interventions). The advantage of this system includes the ability to use any guidewire of choice to initially cross the lesion. A short 0.014-in. coronary guidewire is first inserted into a supplied stylet, and as a unit, the guidewire within the stylet is then inserted into the delivery catheter. The low profile delivery catheter (3.2 Fr) is compatible with a 6 Fr guide catheter. After the lesion is crossed with the guidewire, the delivery catheter is advanced over the guidewire, followed by removal of the guidewire and stylet. The filter basket is then introduced into the delivery sheath and positioned at the distal end of the delivery sheath. The filter basket is attached to a 0.014-in. capture wire, which comes in 190-cm or 320-cm lengths. The delivery sheath is then retracted to deploy the filter basket (Fig. 6). This nitinol filter is coated with HEPROTEC™, which maintains patency for up to 60 min. The pore sizes vary, being smaller distally at the tip of the basket and larger at the proximal end (varying from 50 to 200 μm). Five filter sizes are available (3–7 mm diameter, in 1-mm increments) to match the appropriate vessel size. The retrieval sheath has a crossing profile of 4.2 Fr. This device is currently being studied in the CREATE (Carotid Revascularization with ev3 Arterial Technology Evolution) trial.

Interceptor® PLUS Carotid Filter System

The Interceptor® plus Carotid Filter System (Medtronic, Minneapolis, MN) is a guidewire-filter device that recently received CE Mark approval in 2004. This low profile (2.9 Fr) filter is mounted on a guidewire, and is constructed of a spring-loaded braided nitinol filter, with pore size of 100 μm (Fig. 7). The filter sizes are available to fit vessel diameter from 4.25 to 6.25 mm. The system is compatible with a 6 Fr guiding

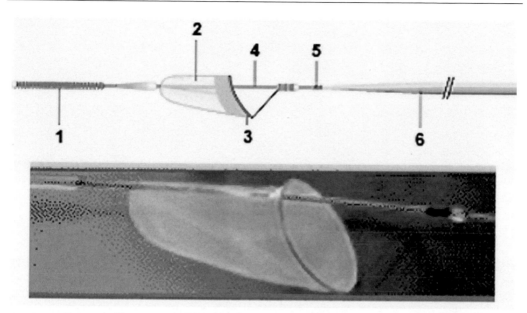

Fig. 5. FilterWire EZ™ device: *1*, radiopaque 3-cm tip; *2*, polyurethane filter; *3*, radiopaque nitinol loop; *4*, spinner tube; *5*, proximal stop; *6*, 0.014-in. PTFE-coated wire.

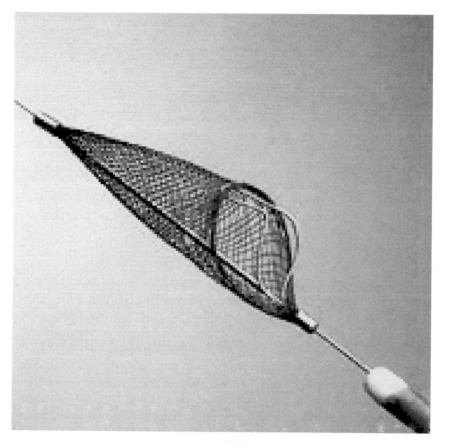

Fig. 6. SPIDER™ device.

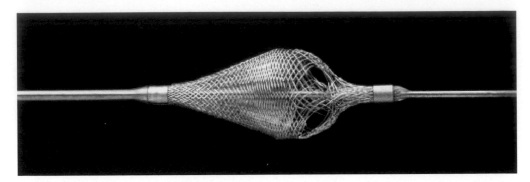

Fig. 7. Interceptor® PLUS device.

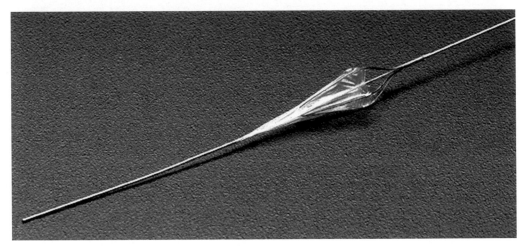

Fig. 8. Rubicon Filter.

catheter. This device is currently being evaluated in the MAVErIC III (Evaluation of the Medtronic AVE Self-Expanding Carotid Stent System in the Treatment of Carotid Stenosis) study.

Rubicon Embolic Filter

The Rubicon Embolic Filter (Rubicon Medical, Salt Lake City, UT) is the lowest profile guidewire-filter device that has been developed, which is unique in that a delivery catheter is not required. This device received CE Mark approval in April 2005. The filter is mounted on a 0.014-in. guidewire. A unique coaxial actuating wire design at the proximal end of the wire deploys the filter, thus eliminating the need for a delivery catheter. The filter basket has 100-μm pores, and is supported by floating nitinol struts for superior apposition to vessel wall (Fig. 8). This device is compatible with 6 Fr guide catheters, and is available in three filter sizes: 4, 5, and 6 mm diameters (with crossing profile of 2.1 Fr, 2.4 Fr, and 2.7 Fr, respectively). At the completion of the procedure, the filter is retrieved by a large-bore capture catheter, which is telescoped over the filter and trapped debris.

DISTAL BALLOON OCCLUSION EMBOLI PROTECTION DEVICE

The Percusurge® GuardWire™ (Medtronic, Minneapolis, MN) was the first balloon-occlusive EPD that was commercially available. It was also the first EPD used during carotid angioplasty. It has a simple design and concept, but is more cumbersome technically compared to the filter EPD, and may not be tolerated by all patients. It is recommended that four-vessel cerebral angiography be performed prior to contemplating use of this device, to evaluate collateral circulation (assess Circle of Willis, external to internal carotid artery collaterals, and external to vertebral artery collaterals) and contralateral stenosis.

The guidewire is a 0.014-in. specially constructed hollow nitinol hypotube, with an inflatable compliant balloon incorporated near the distal end of the guidewire. The tip of this guidewire has a 3.5-cm shapeable segment, and it comes in total lengths of 200 cm or 300 cm. There are two choices of balloon diameters, either 2.5–5 mm or 3–6 mm. To inflate the balloon, the GuardWire™ is attached to the EZ Adapter, and through a turn of the knob, opens the Microseal. The EZ Flator inflation device is then dialed up to inflate the balloon to the desired pressure. The Microseal can then be sealed off with the EZ Adapter to keep the balloon inflated. This device comes with the Export® catheter to aspirate debris while the balloon is inflated (Fig. 9).

During CAS, the GuardWire™ is advanced across the carotid stenosis to at least 2–3 cm distal to the lesion, ideally at the prepetrous cervical ICA, particularly if the vessel is large. The GuardWire™ balloon is then inflated to the desired diameter to occlude the internal carotid artery. Contrast is then injected to confirm complete occlusion of blood flow. The EZ Adapter is sealed to keep the balloon inflated, and then disconnected to allow angioplasty balloon predilation and stent placement. After postdilation, the Export® catheter is advanced to the GuardWire™ balloon, and blood is suctioned to retrieve liberated debris that are suspended throughout the stagnant blood column. The EZ Adapter is then reattached to open up the Microseal, and the GuardWire™ balloon is then deflated and removed.

Alterations to the aforementioned technique may be required if the patient is intolerant (e.g., decrease level of consciousness, complete loss of consciousness, seizure, neurologic deficit) to the GuardWire™ balloon occlusion. This may occur in about 5% of patients, particularly those with contralateral carotid occlusion or poor collateral circulation (6). In these patients, the GuardWire™ balloon has to be deflated more than once (with aspiration prior to each deflation) during CAS (usually between predilation and stenting). In about 1% of cases, patients are completely intolerant of the GuardWire™ balloon occlusion, in which case this EPD would be abandoned in favor of filter EPD.

Flushing of the carotid artery prior to aspiration is generally not recommended, as this will divert suspended emboli toward the external carotid artery (ECA). This can be detrimental when there are external to internal carotid artery collaterals via the ophthalmic artery, ascending pharyngeal, or internal maxillary arteries, which would then result in cerebral and/or retinal embolization (5,11). Similarly, embolization may be diverted to the posterior circulation if there are collaterals between the ECA and the vertebral artery. Therefore, it is important that four-vessel cerebral angiography be performed before the use of the GuardWire™, and operators should favor filter EPD if these collaterals are noted.

PROXIMAL BALLOON OCCLUSION EMBOLI PROTECTION DEVICES

The proximal balloon occlusion EPD was designed with the intention of preventing emboli during all stages of CAS. With the filter and distal balloon occlusion EPD, the

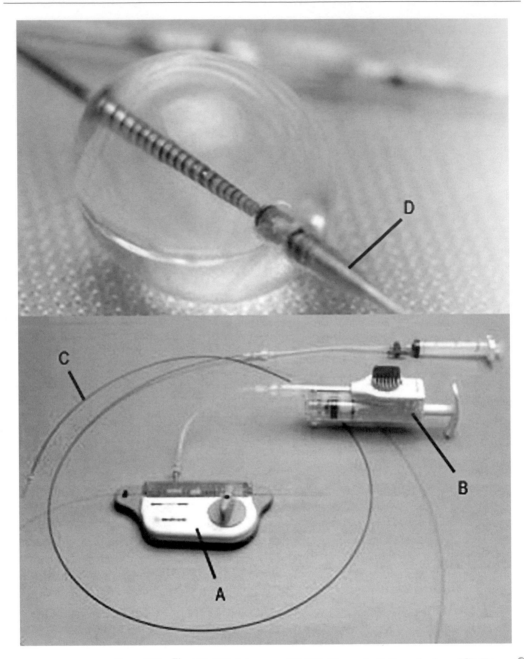

Fig. 9. Percusurge GuardWire™: (**A**) EZ Adapter, (**B**) EZ Flator inflation device, (**C**) Export®
catheter, (**D**) GuardWire™ with inflated occlusion balloon.

stenotic lesions have to be crossed with these devices prior to protection, whereas the
proximal balloon occlusion EPD allows cerebral protection prior to lesion crossing.
There are two commercially available systems in Europe, the Parodi Anti-Embolic
System (Gore, Flagstaff, AZ) [who acquired this device from ArteriA Medical Science]
and the MO.MA system (Invatec, Roncadelle, Italy). Both devices are investigational
only in the United States.

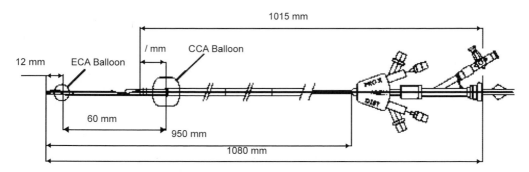

Fig. 10. MO.MA device.

Both devices have a similar designs, with a large compliant balloon attached to the end of the guiding sheath to be inflated in the common carotid artery (CCA), and a smaller compliant balloon delivered through the sheath to be inflated in the ECA. With both balloons inflated in the CCA and ECA, forward blood flow through the ICA is prevented. In fact, reversal of flow may be achieved in the ICA by establishing a "fistula" with the lower pressure femoral venous system (the Parodi device). However, up to 10% of patients do not tolerate this flow reversal, especially those with contralateral stenosis or poor cerebral collateral circulation. With the MO.MA device (Fig. 10), blood and debris are aspirated from the guiding sheath from the ICA (which can also be done with the Parodi device). Once the CCA and ECA balloons are inflated, operators can proceed with protected CAS using guidewire, balloon, and stents of their choice (Fig. 11).

Preliminary data with these devices are promising. In a nine-patient experience with the Parodi device, no microembolic signals were detected with transcranial Doppler during CAS *(12)*. In a small 42-patient comparative study of FilterWire EX™ vs MO.MA, there were significantly lower numbers of microembolic signals with the MO.MA device (Table 5) *(13)*. In the initial 42-patient experience with the MO.MA device, 12% were intolerant to the transient clamping, and there were two minor stroke events post-CAS. However, there were no major stroke or death at 3 mo *(14)*. In the large PRIAMUS prospective registry, 416 patients underwent CAS with the MO.MA device *(15)*. Technical success was achieved in 99%. Twenty-four (5.8%) patients had transient intolerance to the device, 12 of whom still completed the study with the MO.MA device, 7 required intermittent balloon deflation, and 5 required conversion to filter EPD. The incidence of in-hospital stroke or death complication was 4.6% (0.7% TIA, 3.8% minor stroke, 0.2% major stroke, 0.5% death). In 59% of cases, there were visible debris after filtration of the aspirated blood *(15)*.

The disadvantages of the proximal balloon EPD are that they are cumbersome to use, technically challenging, and require large arterial access with 10 Fr guiding sheaths. They are unlikely to surpass the filter EPD as the protection device of choice with their ease of use, although they may have a niche market for patients with tortuous ICA, where filter EPDs are inaccessible.

CONCLUSIONS

The use of an EPD is indispensable for carotid artery stenting. Numerous devices are now available, which could be classified into filter or balloon occlusion devices. They

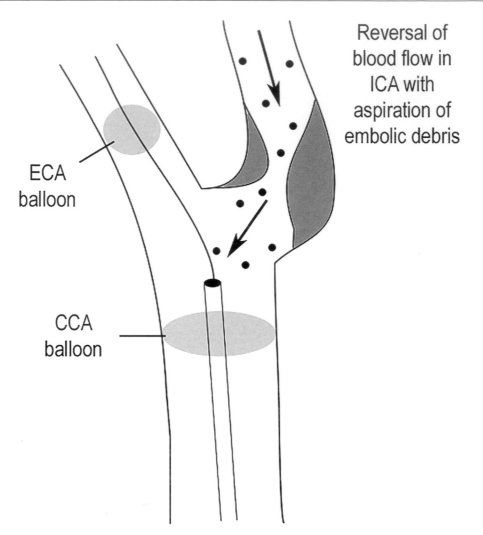

Fig. 11. Proximal balloon occlusion device with compliant balloon occlusions of the common carotid artery (CCA) and external carotid artery (ECA). Embolic debris can be aspirated through the guiding sheath.

Table 5
Comparison of Microembolic Signals (Means ± SD) During Carotid Artery Stenting with the MO.MA vs the FilterWire EX™ Devices

Procedural step	MO.MA	FilterWire EX™	p value
Sheath and EPD placement	18 ± 10	20 ± 15	NS
Crossing lesion with guidewire	2 ± 3	25 ± 22	<0.0001
Deploying stent	11 ± 19	73 ± 49	<0.0001
Balloon postdilation	12 ± 21	70 ± 31	<0.0001
Retrieval of EPD	19 ± 15	14 ± 15	NS
Total	57 ± 41	196 ± 84	<0.0001

Adapted from ref. *13*.
EPD, Emboli protection device; NS, not significant; SD, standard deviation.

have been shown to reduce distal embolization and clinical neurologic events. The filter EPD are the most popular devices used at present, and several devices are currently available or are being investigated in clinical trials. With further technological development, we could anticipate lower profile devices and easier delivery.

REFERENCES

1. Ohki T, Marin ML, Lyon RT, et al. Ex vivo human carotid artery bifurcation stenting: correlation of lesion characteristics with embolic potential. J Vasc Surg 1998;27:463–471.
2. Wholey MH, Al-Mubarek N. Updated review of the global carotid artery stent registry. Catheter Cardiovasc Interv 2003;60:259–266.
3. Kastrup A, Groschel K, Kraph H, Brehm B, Dichgans J, Schulz J. Early outcome of carotid angioplasty and stenting with and without cerebral protection devices. A systematic review of the literature. Stroke 2003;34:813–819.
4. Jordan WD, Jr., Voellinger DC, Doblar DD, Plyushcheva NP, Fisher WS, McDowell HA. Microemboli detected by transcranial Doppler monitoring in patients during carotid angioplasty versus carotid endarterectomy. Cardiovasc Surg 1999;7:33–38.
5. Al-Mubarak N, Roubin G, Vitek J, Iyer S, New G, Leon M. Effect of the distal-balloon protection system on microembolization during carotid stenting. Circulation 2001;104:1999–2002.
6. Henry M, Polydorou A, Henry I, Hugel M. Carotid angioplasty under cerebral protection with the PercuSurge GuardWire System. Catheter Cardiovasc Interv 2004;61:293–305.
7. Reimers B, Corvaja N, Moshiri S, et al. Cerebral protection with filter devices during carotid artery stenting. Circulation 2001;104:12–15.
8. Jaeger HJ, Mathias KD, Hauth E, et al. Cerebral ischemia detected with diffusion-weighted MR imaging after stent implantation in the carotid artery. AJNR Am J Neuroradiol 2002;23:200–207.
9. Jaeger H, Mathias K, Drescher R, et al. Clinical results of cerebral protection with a filter device during stent implantation of the carotid artery. Cardiovasc Intervent Radiol 2001;24:249–256.
10. Sprouse LR, 2nd, Peeters P, Bosiers M. The capture of visible debris by distal cerebral protection filters during carotid artery stenting: Is it predictable? J Vasc Surg 2005;41:950–955.
11. Wilentz JR, Chati Z, Krafft V, Amor M. Retinal embolization during carotid angioplasty and stenting: mechanisms and role of cerebral protection systems. Catheter Cardiovasc Interv 2002;56:320–327.
12. Parodi JC, La Mura R, Ferreira LM, et al. Initial evaluation of carotid angioplasty and stenting with three different cerebral protection devices. J Vasc Surg 2000;32:1127–1136.
13. Schmidt A, Diederich KW, Scheinert S, et al. Effect of two different neuroprotection systems on microembolization during carotid artery stenting. J Am Coll Cardiol 2004;44:1966–1969.
14. Diederich KW, Scheinert D, Schmidt A, et al. First clinical experiences with an endovascular clamping system for neuroprotection during carotid stenting. Eur J Vasc Endovasc Surg 2004;28:629–633.
15. Coppi G, Moratto R, Silingardi R, et al. PRIAMUS - Proximal flow blockage cerebral protection during carotid stenting: results from a Multicenter Italian registry. J Cardiovasc Surg (Torino) 2005;46: 219–227.

12 Complications of Carotid Artery Stenting

Jacqueline Saw, MD

CONTENTS

Summary

It is important for operators of carotid artery stenting (CAS) to have a thorough understanding of potential complications associated with CAS, and strategies to prevent and manage these complications. With improvements in technology and equipments, periprocedural complications related to CAS has progressively diminished, especially since the introduction of emboli protection devices. The most devastating complications of CAS are stroke and death. In this chapter, potential complications associated with each step of CAS are reviewed, including delayed postprocedural complications.

Key Words: Carotid artery stenting, cerebral ischemia, distal embolization, hyperperfusion syndrome, in-stent restenosis, procedural complications, stroke.

INTRODUCTION

It is important for operators of carotid artery stenting (CAS) to have a thorough understanding of potential complications associated with CAS, and strategies to prevent and manage these complications. With improvements in technology and equipment, periprocedural complications related to CAS has progressively diminished, especially since the introduction of emboli protection devices (EPDs). The most devastating complications of CAS are stroke and death. In the updated global experience of 12,392 procedures reported by Wholey et al. the combined procedure-related death and stroke (major and minor) was 3.98% *(1)*. The incidences of individual end points were: transient ischemic attacks (TIAs) 3.07%, minor strokes 2.14%, major strokes 1.2%, and death 0.64% *(1,2)*. In a separate meta-analysis of 3,196 patients by Kastrup et al. the combined 30-d stroke and death rate was 1.8% in those with EPD use compared to 5.5% without EPD use during CAS *(3)*.

From: *Contemporary Cardiology: Handbook of Complex Percutaneous Carotid Intervention*
Edited by: J. Saw, J. E. Exaire, D. S. Lee, and S. Yadav © Humana Press Inc., Totowa, NJ

Patients with symptomatic carotid stenosis have approx 2.5 times more likelihood of developing stroke during CAS compared to asymptomatic patients *(4)*. Other clinical predictors of strokes during CAS are advanced age and the presence of long (>10 mm) or multiple stenoses *(5)*. Although involving a different vascular bed, patients undergoing CAS may suffer periprocedural myocardial infarction (MI), with reported incidence of 0.9 to 2.6% *(6–8)*. Nonetheless, in the SAPPHIRE trial of high-risk patients, CAS was not inferior to endarterectomy at 1 yr, with a trend to reduction in 30-d death, stroke, or MI event rate with CAS (4.8% vs 9.8%, $p = 0.09$) *(9)*.

Although the majority of ischemic complications tend to occur during the procedure, late postprocedural complications do occur. The incidence of neurologic events and deaths after the initial 30 d was 1.39% in 3924 patients at up to 1-yr follow-up *(10)*. In this chapter, potential complications associated with each step of CAS are reviewed, including delayed postprocedural complications (Tables 1 and 2).

PROCEDURAL COMPLICATIONS

Arterial Access Complications

The most common arterial access for CAS is via the femoral artery. Brachial and radial accesses are feasible for contralateral carotid interventions; however, these approaches render CAS more challenging because of difficult guide or sheath access and support. Direct carotid puncture is no longer used because of complication risks (carotid dissection, thrombosis, or hematoma that may compromise airway). With advances in equipment (guides, sheaths, balloons, and stents), access via the retrograde femoral artery has been simplified and can be performed with small arteriotomies (for 6 Fr sheaths or 8 Fr guides). Complications associated with femoral, brachial, and radial arterial access sites and their management are well described in standard catheterization textbooks, and are not discussed here. Briefly stated, femoral complication rate varies from 0.7% to 9% *(11)*, and encompasses bleeding, hematoma, pseudoaneurysm, retroperitoneal hemorrhage, arteriovenous fistula, dissection, thrombosis, and embolism. The majority of these complications can be treated successfully without surgery.

Carotid Artery Catheterization Complications

Operators may encounter difficulties with catheter access of common carotid arteries, especially with type III aortic arches, presence of significant aortic arch atheroma, or presence of stenoses involving the ostial or proximal carotid arteries. In patients in whom the origins of the innominate or left common carotid artery are markedly displaced inferiorly (i.e., type III arch), reverse-curved catheters (e.g., Vitek, Simmons) are often required to selectively engage these vessels. These complex catheters need to be reformed in the descending aorta to redirect the catheter tip to point into the carotid arteries (Fig. 2 in Chapter 9). Despite careful manipulations in the aortic arch, these catheters may dislodge aortic arch atheroma, causing distal embolization to the brain or peripheral organs. In the presence of ostial or proximal carotid artery stenosis, catheter engagement may also cause plaque embolization or dissection of the carotid artery. This risk can be increased with the use of larger guide catheters compared to smaller and softer-tip diagnostic catheters. Thus, many operators favor the use of the telescoping approach (Fig. 3 in Chapter 9) to lower the risk of plaque scraping and dissection. With this technique, a smaller caliber 5 Fr diagnostic catheter (e.g., JR4 or Vitek) is

Table 1
Summary of Complications Related to Carotid Artery Stenting

A. Procedural complications
    1. Arterial access complications
    2. Carotid artery access complications during guide or sheath placement
    3. Complications with emboli protection devices
    4. Cerebral ischemia
    5. Distal cerebral embolization
    6. Retinal embolization
    7. Reflex bradycardia and hypotension
    8. Acute vessel closure

B. Early postprocedural complications
    1. Cerebral hyperperfusion syndrome
    2. Stent thrombosis
    3. Late distal embolization

C. Late postprocedural complications
    1. Stent deformation
    2. In-stent restenosis

Table 2
Prevalence Estimates of Carotid Artery Stenting Complications

Complications	Estimated prevalence (%)
Death	0–1
Major stroke	0–1
Minor stroke	1–2
Transient ischemic attack	1–3
Death or stroke (30 d)	2–4
Myocardial infarction	0–3
Retinal embolization	1–2
Slow flow	10
Reflex bradycardia and hypotension	20–30
Hyperperfusion syndrome	1
Intracranial hemorrhage	0–1
Acute stent thrombosis	0.5
In-stent restenosis (late)	2–5

telescoped within an 8 Fr guide catheter, and is advanced ahead of the guide catheter along a guidewire within the diagnostic catheter. Alternatively, the use of a sheath with its packaged dilator introducer to track into the carotid artery may also reduce embolic/dissection risks, because of the smoother transition between the dilator and sheath tip (Fig. 1).

Complications with Emboli Protection Devices

Microembolization to the brain during carotid angioplasty occurs frequently as measured with transcranial Doppler *(12)*, and thus EPDs have been developed to reduce

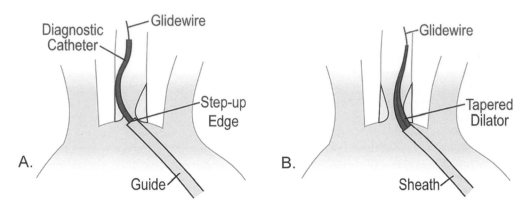

Fig. 1. (A) Use of a telescoping setup with a 5 Fr diagnostic catheter within an 8 Fr guide, with a step-up edge crossing an ostial common carotid artery lesion. **(B)** Use of a sheath with its packaged dilator introducer, showing smoother transition when traversing an ostial common carotid artery lesion.

distal embolization. Although these devices reduce stroke event rates by at least 50% *(1,3)* and are now considered mandatory during CAS, there are potential risks associated with the use of such devices. Further, complex lesions (such as critical stenosis, heavily calcified, or tortuous vessel) may preclude successful delivery and deployment of EPDs.

Numerous EPDs have been developed and can be divided into occlusive (distal or proximal balloon occlusions) and nonocclusive devices (see Chapter 11). Although currently available filter EPD (see Chapter 11) are of relatively small profile (about 3–4 Fr diameter), they are still considered somewhat bulky, especially while crossing critical lesions. Crossing with an EPD may roughen up the intimal surface of the carotid atheroma, and shear off embolic debris distally. When the EPD is deployed in the desired location, depending on the size of the carotid artery and tortuosity of the vessel, the filter basket may not be well opposed to the arterial wall. This would allow atheroemboli to escape cephalad around the device, especially for filters with an eccentric guidewire location. Even if the filter EPD is adequately opposed to the vessel wall, the smallest pore sizes in current filters are approx 80 μm in diameter, and thus smaller-sized embolic particles may still escape through these pores. The deployed EPD could also injure the vessel wall if it is inadvertently displaced aggressively (especially with balloon occlusive devices), causing dissection and embolization. Moreover, prolonged balloon inflation with occlusive EPD or complete filling of filter baskets can protract cerebral ischemia. Therefore, like all steps in the CAS procedure, operators need to be vigilant about placement and retrieval of EPD to reduce complications.

Cerebral Ischemia

There are numerous steps during CAS in which transient obstructions of cerebral blood flow occur, such as during balloon inflation, inflation of balloon occlusive EPD, and when filter EPD baskets are clogged. Most patients tolerate short ischemic episodes relatively well, unless the collateral circulation is compromised (e.g., incomplete Circle of Willis with hypoplastic anterior communicating or posterior communicating arteries), or if the contralateral carotid artery has a severe stenosis. Thus, symptom presentations vary among patients, from none to loss of consciousness, seizures, or TIA. In a report by Yadav et al. the 4 patients (of 107 CAS patients) who transiently lost

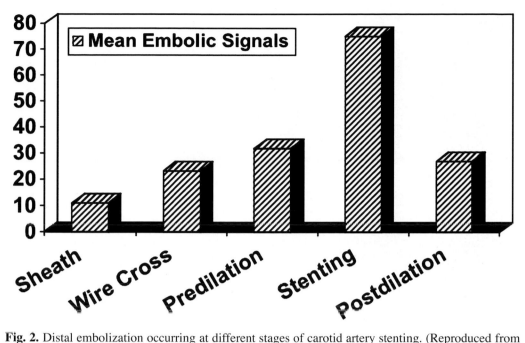

Fig. 2. Distal embolization occurring at different stages of carotid artery stenting. (Reproduced from ref. *15*.)

consciousness during angioplasty balloon inflation had contralateral carotid occlusions *(4)*. TIAs can occur in up to 3% of CAS procedures, manifesting as either amaurosis fugax or transient motor–sensory deficits *(10)*. There are no long-term sequelae from these transient ischemic episodes. Prevention and management includes short angioplasty balloon inflation, and expeditious but meticulous techniques to limit occlusive EPD balloon inflation times.

Distal Cerebral Embolization

Microembolization occurs in virtually all stages of CAS as documented on transcranial Doppler during carotid angioplasty *(13,14)*, with the majority occurring during stent deployment and balloon dilatation (Fig. 2) *(13–15)*. In a more recent retrospective analysis of 414 patients who underwent CAS, 10.1% developed slow flow due to distal embolization, with higher risks associated with increasing age, larger stent diameters, and among those with symptomatic carotid stenosis *(16)*. Remarkably, 71.4% of these slow flow events occurred after postdilatation of the deployed self-expanding stent *(16)*. And the risk of 30-d stroke event rate was much higher in these patients with slow flow (9.5% vs 1.7%) despite the use of EPDs *(16)*. Fortunately, the majority of patients with distal embolization do not manifest significant neurologic deficits, because of the amazing tolerance of the brain to smaller-sized particles. This is further exemplified by a CEA study involving 301 patients, whereby the adverse clinical event rate was only 5.7% despite the occurrence of detected embolization in the majority of patients *(17)*. Nevertheless, the quantity and size of embolic particles do correlate with the incidence of neurologic deficits and infarcts after CEA *(17–19)*.

The use of an EPD is crucial to prevent distal embolization (Fig. 3), and has been shown to reduce stroke or death event rates by two to three times during CAS *(1,3)*. In

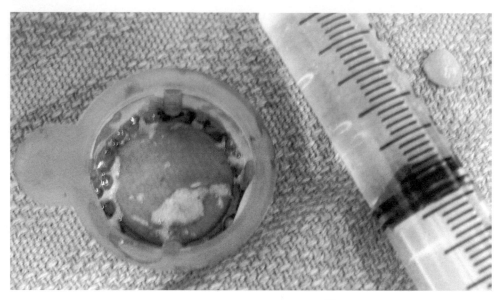

Fig. 3. Large emboli debris retrieved from an AngioGuard XP™ emboli protection device during carotid stenting.

fact, all modern CAS trials necessitate the adjunctive use of EPD. There is no lesion or procedural characteristics that can reliably predict the occurrence of visible distal debris *(20)*, and thus routine EPD use is recommended for all CAS procedures. However, slow flow and distal embolization may still occur despite the use of EPD. With non-occlusive EPDs, if the filters are coated with debris leading to slow flow, it is crucial to prevent embolization by suctioning the stagnant column of blood proximal to the filter basket with either a 5 Fr multipurpose catheter or an Export catheter of the PercuSurge® GuardWire™ (Medtronic, Minneapolis, MN) device before retrieval of the filter. The stagnant column of blood contains suspended debris, which will go to the brain if the filter is collapsed and retrieved without aspiration of the internal carotid artery.

In the event that neurologic symptoms develop despite EPD use and suctioning, further management depends on the significance of the intracranial arterial occlusion. If no occlusion is identified on intracerebral angiography, medical management with fluid resuscitation and maintenance of blood pressure is recommended. However, if the M1 or M2 segment of the middle cerebral artery is occluded, a mechanical approach is recommended. This can include using a hydrophilic wire to cross the blockage and dislodge the embolus, inflation of a small coronary angioplasty balloon, or a small snare to capture the embolus *(21)*. Although adjunctive intraarterial tissue plasminogen activator (tPA) or glycoprotein (GP) IIb/IIIa antagonists (specifically abciximab) may be administered, it is important to weigh the benefits against the risk of intracranial hemorrhage *(22)*. Occlusions beyond the M2 segment of the middle cerebral artery are generally associated with good prognosis and do not require mechanical interventions.

Retinal Embolization

This specific form of distal embolization is worth separate discussion. It has been described with CAS, occurring in 1.3% of patients with the use of PercuSurge® system *(23)*. The occurrence was much higher (13.2%) with the use of the Theron system, which is an EPD that requires balloon occlusion in the distal internal carotid artery and routine flushing toward the external carotid artery *(23)*. It is postulated that these embolizations occur through external to internal carotid artery anastomotic pathways via the ophthalmic artery. Embolization can also occur as the occlusion balloon of the PercuSurge® device is deflated, allowing the stagnant column of blood and remnant suspended debris that was not suctioned by the aspiration catheter to flow downstream.

It is foreseeable that retinal embolization may also occur with filter EPD via these two mechanisms (especially if slow flow occurs with the use of filter EPD), and we have seen this in clinical practice. Although fewer than half of retinal embolizations are symptomatic *(23)* and some may have only transient deficits, unfortunately others may develop permanent visual field defects (especially if the emboli are large and cause central retinal artery occlusion). Thus, when patients complain of visual field defects after CAS, prompt referral to an ophthalmologist for retinal examination is necessary. Although the treatment of central retinal artery occlusion is often unsatisfactory, various treatment trials may be attempted (e.g., ocular massage to dislodge emboli to smaller arterioles, decrease intraocular pressure with acetazolamide or anterior chamber paracentesis, hyperbaric oxygen, intravenous heparin or tPA).

Reflex Bradycardia and Hypotension

Balloon dilatation of the carotid bulb stimulates the carotid baroreceptors, which relay signals via the afferent glossopharyngeal nerve to the efferent vagal nerve, decreasing cardiac chronotropy and inotropy (Fig. 4) *(21)*. The efferent reflex arc is also relayed to the spinal cord sympathetic nervous system, causing vasodilatation. These reflex-mediated bradycardia and hypotension are frequently encountered during CAS, 27.5% and 22.4%, respectively, in a study by Qureshi et al. *(24)*. They tend to occur during stent postdilatation, with larger sized diameter balloons. In a study by Yadav et al. 71% of patients developed significant bradycardia during balloon dilatation of the carotid sinus *(4)*. These bradycardic episodes are generally self-limited, resolving with balloon deflation within a few minutes, and do not cause permanent high-grade atrioventricular block *(4)*. More severe cases can be treated with intravenous atropine (0.6 mg–1 mg), but temporary transvenous pacemaker is almost never required.

On the other hand, the vasodilatory component may be more persistent, with a small proportion of patients experiencing prolonged hypotension lasting several hours. This may require fluid boluses (normal saline), with or without temporary vasoconstrictor therapy (e.g., pseudoephedrine, norepinephrine, dopamine) *(21)*. Patients who have persistent hypotension postprocedure on the ward can be treated with oral pseudoephedrine (30–60 mg q4h prn), to keep systolic blood pressure 90–140 mmHg.

Acute Vessel Closure

With the use of current techniques, equipment, and pharmacology, abrupt closure of the carotid artery is now exceedingly rare. This complication was essentially limited to the days of carotid angioplasty alone, whereby dissection and thrombosis were more commonly encountered. The routine use of self-expanding nitinol or elgiloy stents in modern practice allows treatment of dissections created by balloon dilatation. Contemporary antiplatelet and anticoagulant therapies also decrease procedural and postprocedural thrombotic complications (see Chapter 9 for recommendations).

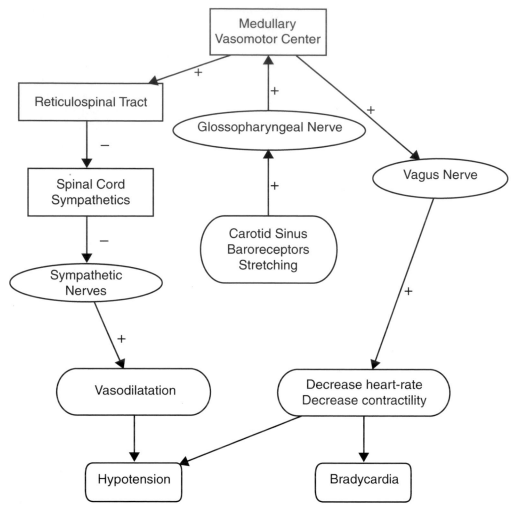

Fig. 4. Pathways of the carotid sinus reflex resulting in bradycardia and hypotension.

EARLY POSTPROCEDURAL COMPLICATIONS

Cerebral Hyperperfusion Syndrome

When a significant high-grade carotid stenosis is rendered widely patent by CAS or CEA, there is often a dramatic and instantaneous increase in ipsilateral cerebral blood flow. This may be particularly problematic in the setting of chronic cerebral ischemia, which is accompanied by impaired cerebrovascular autoregulation. The cerebral hyperperfusion that occurs is often transient, but may provoke severe symptoms (ipsilateral headache, vomiting, altered sensorium, stupor, hypertension, seizures, focal neurologic deficits, and intracranial hemorrhage). In a retrospective analysis from the Cleveland Clinic CAS Registry, 5/450 (1.1%) patients developed hyperperfusion syndrome, with 3/450 (0.67%) progressing to intracranial hemorrhage *(25)*. Patients with high-grade stenosis (>90%), severe contralateral stenosis, severe underlying hypertension, poor collateral circulation, and recent stroke or ischemia are at increased risk for hyperperfusion (Table 3) *(25)*. Treatment is key to prevent intracranial hemorrhage (Fig. 5),

Table 3
Patients at Risk of Developing Hyperperfusion Syndrome
and Subsequent Intracranial Hemorrhage

1. Underlying severe uncontrolled hypertension
2. High-grade carotid artery stenosis (>90%)
3. Severe contralateral carotid artery stenosis
4. Poor collateral cerebral circulation
5. Recent stroke or cerebral ischemia

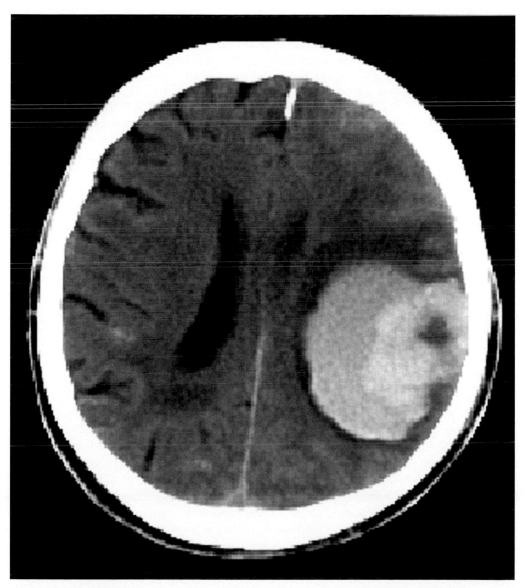

Fig. 5. Hyperperfusion syndrome complicated by intracranial hemorrhage.

which is associated with extremely poor prognosis. Thus, management of hyperperfusion includes early recognition, with careful blood pressure (β-blockers and diuretics) and seizure control. Some authors even recommend withholding antiplatelet therapy until the blood pressure is adequately controlled (25). Prompt imaging should be performed (computed tomography [CT] or magnetic resonance imaging [MRI]) to diagnose cerebral edema or hemorrhage. Transcranial Doppler may also be helpful to demonstrate increase ipsilateral flow velocity and pulsatility index in the middle cerebral artery (26).

Stent Thrombosis

Thrombosis of carotid artery stents is relatively rare. In a CAS study by Yadav et al. (89% received balloon-expandable stents), stent thrombosis occurred in only 0.8% (4). In the modern era with the use of nitinol self-expanding stents, the risk of stent thrombosis is even lower (0.4%) (27). The use of balloon-expandable stents for carotid bifurcation has been abandoned, because of the risk of stent deformation by external compression of this superficial vessel (28). On the contrary, self-expanding stents have superior apposition and conformability to vessel walls, and their innate flexibility allows compression without fracture in the carotid position. The use of dual antiplatelet therapy (aspirin and clopidogrel) is also crucial in reducing stent thrombosis. Pretreatment with both agents is recommended preprocedure. Postprocedure, aspirin is recommended lifelong and clopidogrel for at least 4 wk. Even though longer clopidogrel therapy has been shown to be beneficial for percutaneous coronary interventions (29,30), similar data for CAS are lacking.

Late Distal Embolization

Although the majority of embolization occurs during the procedure, late embolic events may occur hours to days after CAS. These infrequent late events probably arise from detachment of atherosclerotic fragments protruding through stent struts. This is similar to the pathophysiology of the "cheese-grater" effect during coronary stenting (Fig. 6). They often manifest as TIAs that do not require intervention, although some patients may manifest with minor stroke events, including late retinal embolization. Major deficits require CT scanning and cerebral angiography, and possibly mechanical intervention.

LATE POSTPROCEDURAL COMPLICATIONS

Stent Deformation

The use of a balloon-expandable stent in the carotid artery is not optimal because of external compression of this superficial vessel. Stent collapse, defined as the loss of apposition of the stent to the vessel wall, can occur in 0–16% of cases with the Palmaz balloon-expandable stents (28). Bergeron et al. reported no stent compression in 96 patients treated with Palmaz stents at 13-mo follow-up (31). However, Wholey et al. reported 2.5% stent deformation (≥50% compression of stent) rate with 1804 Palmaz stents at 6-mo follow-up (10). Yadav et al. reported a 6% incidence of Palmaz stent deformation at 6-mo follow-up (4). Patients usually remain asymptomatic, but some may require repeat angioplasty, placement of self-expanding stents, or even surgical excision (28). Stent deformation has essentially been eliminated with the use of self-expanding stents.

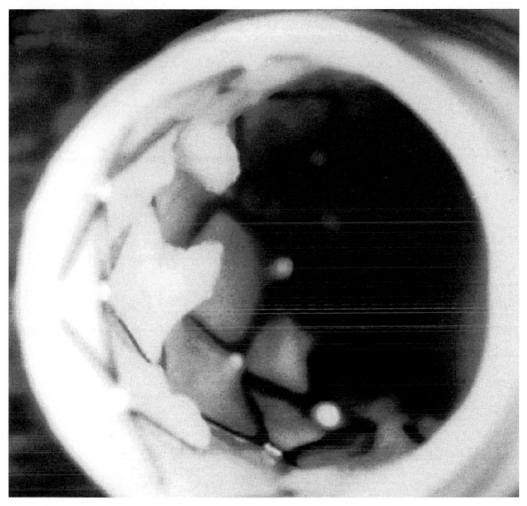

Fig. 6. "Cheese-grater" effect with atherosclerotic plaque protruding through the stent struts.

In-Stent Restenosis

Unlike other arterial beds (peripheral extremities, renals, or coronary arteries), the restenosis rates following stenting of carotid arteries are typically low, approx 2–5% *(1,4,32–34)* (Table 4). This is probably due to the large caliber of the vessel, high arterial blood flow, and low resistance of the cerebral vasculature. In the updated global CAS Registry, Wholey et al. reported a restenosis rate of 2.7% at 1 yr and 5.6% at 4 yr in 12,392 procedures *(1)*. Although not universally accepted, the general definition of in-stent restenosis is an obstruction of at least 50% diameter of the carotid artery. The use of carotid Doppler to diagnose in-stent restenosis has been recognized to be inaccurate *(35)*. In a recent retrospective analysis by Stanziale et al. they correlated 118 carotid Doppler findings to carotid angiography following CAS *(36)*. The standard ultrasound criteria of peak systolic velocity (PSV), and internal carotid artery to common carotid artery ratio (ICA/CCA ratio) were significantly higher in stented carotid arteries vs nonstented arteries. They recommended using the criteria of PSV

Table 4
In-Stent Restenosis Associated with Carotid Artery Stenting

Study	Year published	N	Restenosis (%)
Yadav (4)	1997	107	4.9
Shawl (33)	2002	299	2.7
Wholey (1)	2003	11,243	5.6
Setacci (32)	2005	407	3.6
Levy (34)	2005	138	5.0

Table 5
Higher Carotid Doppler Velocities and Ratios Are Required to Diagnose in-Stent
Restenosis Following Carotid Stenting

Doppler criteria	Sensitivity (%)	Specificity (%)	PPV	NPV
Correlating to ≥70% stenosis on angiography				
PSV ≥350 cm/s	100	96	55	96
ICA/CCA ≥4.75	100	95	50	100
Correlating to ≥50% stenosis on angiography				
PSV ≥225 cm/s	95	99	95	99
and ICA/CCA ≥2.5				

Adapted from ref. 36.
CCA, Common carotid artery; ICA, internal carotid artery; NPV, negative predictive value; PPV, positive predictive value; PSV, peak systolic velocity.

≥350 cm/s or ICA/CCA ratio ≥4.75 to diagnose in-stent restenosis ≥70% and the combined criteria of PSV ≥225 cm/s and ICA/CCA ratio ≥2.5 to diagnose in-stent restenosis ≥50% (Table 5) (36).

Most clinicians would recommend treatment of high-grade restenosis (>70–80%) if patients become symptomatic. The majority of restenosis can be successfully treated with balloon angioplasty alone (32). Although some interventionalists prefer to use cutting balloon for in-stent restenosis, this has not been proven to be superior to regular balloon angioplasty to prevent restenosis. We had previously utilized gamma-brachytherapy for refractory carotid stent restenosis (37); however, this treatment modality is no longer available. CEA may be considered for recurrent in-stent restenosis after failed repeat balloon angioplasty.

CONCLUSIONS

Carotid artery stenting is a rapidly evolving field with novel equipment (catheters, stents, and emboli protection devices) that have effectively reduced periprocedural complications. However, operators still need to be aware of potential complications that are unique to carotid stenting. Meticulous techniques and prompt recognition and management of complications are essential for the continued success of this endovascular therapy.

REFERENCES

1. Wholey MH, Al-Mubarek N. Updated review of the global carotid artery stent registry. Catheter Cardiovasc Interv 2003;60:259–266.
2. Risk of stroke in the distribution of an asymptomatic carotid artery. The European Carotid Surgery Trialists Collaborative Group. Lancet 1995;345:209–212.
3. Kastrup A, Groschel K, Kraph H, Brehm B, Dichgans J, Schulz J. Early outcome of carotid angioplasty and stenting with and without cerebral protection devices. A systematic review of the literature. Stroke 2003;34:813–819.
4. Yadav JS, Roubin GS, Iyer S, et al. Elective stenting of the extracranial carotid arteries. Circulation 1997;95:376–381.
5. Mathur A, Roubin GS, Iyer SS, et al. Predictors of stroke complicating carotid artery stenting. Circulation 1998;97:1239–1245.
6. Yadav J, for The SAPPHIRE Study Investigators. Stenting and angioplasty with protection in patients at high risk for endarterectomy. The American Heart Association Scientific Sessions. Chicago, IL, 2002.
7. Reimers B, Corvaja N, Moshiri S, et al. Cerebral protection with filter devices during carotid artery stenting. Circulation 2001;104:12–15.
8. Wholey MH, Jarmolowski CR, Eles G, Levy D, Buecthel J. Endovascular stents for carotid artery occlusive disease. J Endovasc Surg 1997;4:326–338.
9. Yadav JS, Wholey MH, Kuntz RE, et al. Protected carotid-artery stenting versus endarterectomy in high-risk patients. N Engl J Med 2004;351:1493–1501.
10. Wholey MH, Wholey M, Mathias K, et al. Global experience in cervical carotid artery stent placement. Catheter Cardiovasc Interv 2000;50:160–167.
11. Samal A, White C. Percutaneous management of access site complications. Cathet Cardiovasc Interv 2002;57:12 23.
12. Markus HS, Clifton A, Buckenham T, Brown MM. Carotid angioplasty. Detection of embolic signals during and after the procedure. Stroke 1994;25:2403 2406.
13. Jordan WJ, Voellinger C, Doblar D, Plyushcheva N, Fisher W, McDowell H. Microemboli detected by transcranial Doppler monitoring in patients during carotid angioplasty versus carotid endarterectomy. Cardiol Surg 1999;7:33 38.
14. Rapp J, Pan X, Sharp F, et al. Atheroemboli to the brain: size threshold for causing acute neuronal cell death. J Vasc Surg 2000;32:68–76.
15. Al-Mubarak N, Roubin G, Vitek J, Iyer S, New G, Leon M. Effect of the distal-balloon protection system on microembolization during carotid stenting. Circulation 2001;104:1999–2002.
16. Casserly IP, Abou-Chebl A, Fathi RB, et al. Slow-flow phenomenon during carotid artery intervention with embolic protection devices: predictors and clinical outcome. J Am Coll Cardiol 2005;46: 1466 1472.
17. Ackerstaff RG, Jansen C, Moll FL, Vermeulen FE, Hamerlijnck RP, Mauser HW. The significance of microemboli detection by means of transcranial Doppler ultrasonography monitoring in carotid endarterectomy. J Vasc Surg 1995;21:963–969.
18. Jansen C, Ramos LM, van Heesewijk JP, Moll FL, van Gijn J, Ackerstaff RG. Impact of microembolism and hemodynamic changes in the brain during carotid endarterectomy. Stroke 1994;25:992–997.
19. Tubler T, Schlüter M, Dirsch O, et al. Balloon-protected carotid artery stenting: relationship of periprocedural neurological complications with the size of particulate debris. Circulation 2001;104:2791–2796.
20. Sprouse LR, 2nd, Peeters P, Bosiers M. The capture of visible debris by distal cerebral protection filters during carotid artery stenting: Is it predictable? J Vasc Surg 2005;41:950–955.
21. Yadav JS. Technical aspects of carotid stenting. EuroPCR. Version 3 ed. Paris, 2003:1–18.
22. Qureshi A, Saad M, Zaidat O, et al. Intracerebral hemorrhages associated with neurointerventional procedures using a combination of antithrombotic agents including abciximab. Stroke 2002;33: 1916–1919.
23. Wilentz JR, Chati Z, Krafft V, Amor M. Retinal embolization during carotid angioplasty and stenting: mechanisms and role of cerebral protection systems. Catheter Cardiovasc Interv 2002;56:320–327.
24. Qureshi A, Luft A, Sharma M, et al. Frequency and determinants of postprocedural hemodynamic instability after carotid angioplasty and stenting. Stroke 1999;30:2086–2093.
25. Abou-Chebl A, Yadav JS, Reginelli J, Bajzer CT, Bhatt DL, Krieger DL. Intracranial hemorrhage and hyperperfusion syndrome following carotid artery stenting: risk factors, prevention, and treatment. J Am Coll Cardiol 2004;43:1596–1601.

26. Meyers P, Higashida R, Phatouros C, et al. Cerebral hyperperfusion syndrome after percutaneous transluminal stenting of the craniocervical arteries. Neurosurgery 2000;47:335–345.
27. Ouriel K, Wholey MH, Fayad P, et al. Feasibility trial of carotid stenting with and without an embolus protection device. J Endovasc Ther 2005;12:525–537.
28. Mathur A, Dorros G, Iyer SS, Vitek JJ, Yadav SS, Roubin GS. Palmaz stent compression in patients following carotid artery stenting. Cathet Cardiovasc Diagn 1997;41:137–140.
29. Steinhubl S, Berger P, Mann J, et al. Early and sustained dual oral antiplatelet therapy following percutaneous coronary intervention. JAMA 2002;288:2411–2420.
30. Mehta S, Yusuf S, Peters R, et al. Effects of pretreatment with clopidogrel and aspirin followed by long-term therapy in patients undergoing percutaneous coronary intervention: the PCI-CURE study. Lancet 2001;358:527–533.
31. Bergeron P, Becquemin J, Jausseran J, et al. Percutaneous stenting of the internal carotid artery: the European CAST 1 Study—Carotid Artery Stent Trial. J Endovasc Surg 1999;6:155–159.
32. Setacci C, de Donato G, Setacci F, et al. In-stent restenosis after carotid angioplasty and stenting: a challenge for the vascular surgeon. Eur J Vasc Endovasc Surg 2005;29:601–607.
33. Shawl FA. Carotid artery stenting: acute and long-term results. Curr Opin Cardiol 2002;17:671–676.
34. Levy EI, Hanel RA, Lau T, et al. Frequency and management of recurrent stenosis after carotid artery stent implantation. J Neurosurg 2005;102:29–37.
35. Ringer AJ, German JW, Guterman LR, Hopkins LN. Follow-up of stented carotid arteries by Doppler ultrasound. Neurosurgery 2002;51:639–643; discussion 643.
36. Stanziale SF, Wholey MH, Boules TN, Selzer F, Makaroun MS. Determining in-stent stenosis of carotid arteries by duplex ultrasound criteria. J Endovasc Ther 2005;12:346–353.
37. Chan A, Roffi M, Mukherjee D, et al. Carotid brachytherapy for in-stent restenosis. Cathet Cardiovasc Interv 2003;58:86–92.

13 The Approach to Intracranial Carotid Artery Intervention

Ivan P. Casserly, MD and Jay S. Yadav, MD

Summary

Intracranial large vessel atherosclerosis is believed to account for approx 5–10% of all ischemic strokes in the United States. Compared with extracranial artery atherosclerosis, the natural history of intracranial atherosclerosis, and the effectiveness of medical therapy and revascularization in modifying the natural history of the disease, are poorly defined. This chapter summarizes our current understanding of intracranial atherosclerosis and describes the emerging practice of endovascular revascularization for the treatment of this disease.

Key Words: Intracranial atherosclerosis, intracranial stenting, stroke.

INTRODUCTION

Intracranial large vessel atherosclerosis is believed to account for approx 5–10% of all ischemic strokes in the United States (Fig. 1) *(1–3)*. This figure may actually be an underestimate, given the reliance on invasive angiography to accurately detect the presence of the disease. The mechanism of stroke from intracranial atherosclerosis is thought to be multifactorial: hemodynamic compromise of flow, *in situ* thrombotic occlusion from flow stagnation, and distal embolization as a result of artery-to-artery embolism. Compared with extracranial artery atherosclerosis, the natural history of intracranial atherosclerosis, and the effectiveness of medical therapy and revascularization in modifying the natural history of the disease are poorly defined. This chapter

From: *Contemporary Cardiology: Handbook of Complex Percutaneous Carotid Intervention*
Edited by: J. Saw, J. E. Exaire, D. S. Lee, and S. Yadav © Humana Press Inc., Totowa, NJ

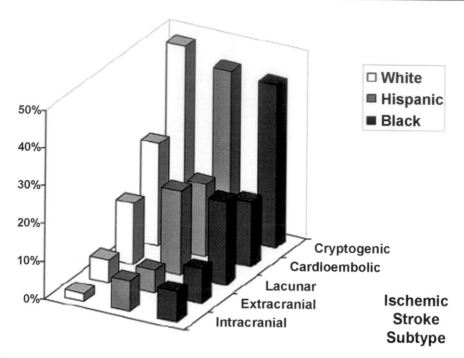

Fig. 1. Proportion of ischemic strokes attributable to various etiologies in different ethnic populations in northern Manhattan. (Reproduced with permission from White et al. Circulation 2005;111: 1327–1331.)

summarizes our current understanding of intracranial atherosclerosis and describes the emerging practice of endovascular revascularization for the treatment of this disease.

EPIDEMIOLOGY

Population-based studies of the incidence of intracranial atherosclerosis have not been performed. However, among symptomatic patients with recent transient ischemic attacks or stroke, several studies have documented the incidence of significant intracranial atherosclerosis and the frequency with which symptoms are ascribed to intracranial disease. For example, among a cohort of 274 patients (60% black, 40% white), Wityk documented a >50% stenosis in an intracranial vessel in 22% of all patients in whom intracranial vascular studies were performed *(4)*. Intracranial disease was determined to be the sole cause of stroke in 8% of all patients. Additional studies have documented an association between intracranial atherosclerosis and traditional risk factors: diabetes, smoking, hyperlipidema, and hypertension. Unique to intracranial atherosclerosis is the propensity for the disease to affect certain ethnic minorities including Asians, Hispanics, and black Americans (Fig. 1) *(5)*.

ANATOMIC DISTRIBUTION

Intracranial atherosclerosis appears to have a predilection for specific sites within the intracranial circulation (Table 1). In the anterior circulation, the most commonly affected sites include (1) the cavernous siphon portion of the intracranial internal carotid artery (ICA), (2) the petrous portion of the ICA, (3) the clinoid portion of the intracranial ICA,

Table 1

Summary of Contemporary Clinical Series of Intracranial Angioplasty for Treatment of Atherosclerotic Disease

Study	Year	N	Lesions	Lesion location		Mean follow-up (mo)	Technical success (%)	In-hospital adverse outcome (%)		
				Anterior	Posterior			Stroke	Hemorrhage	Death
Marks et al. (18)	2005	36	37	16	21	52.9	91	3	0	6
Connors and Wojak (17)	1999	50[a]	N/R	32	18	12	98	0	4	2
Clarke et al. (16)	1995	17	22	6	16	22	82	12	0	0
Mori et al. (19)	1998	42	42	29	13			See Table 2		
Alazzaz et al. (15)	2000	16	17	8	9	24	94	13	0	0

[a]Based on data from interventions performed since 1994.

and (4) the main trunk of the middle cerebral artery (MCA). In the posterior circulation, the distal vertebral artery (VA) (V3 and V4 segments), vertebrobasilar junction, and mid-portion of the basilar artery are typically involved.

NATURAL HISTORY

Knowledge of the natural history of intracranial atherosclerosis is important, as any proposed therapy must compare favorably with the observed event rates that would occur without any intervention. The natural history of asymptomatic intracranial athero-sclerosis is largely unknown. A recent study of 50 patients with mild to moderate asymptomatic MCA disease documented a benign clinical course over a mean follow-up of approx 3 yr, with no patient experiencing an ischemic event in the area of the diseased MCA (6). It is unclear if these results apply to other populations of patients, or to patients with different distributions of intracranial disease. Based on these data or lack thereof, intervention beyond medical therapy for the treatment of asymptomatic intracranial atherosclerosis cannot be recommended.

For patients with symptomatic intracranial disease, there are studies to help define the natural history of patients treated medically. The most contemporary data come from the WASID (Comparison of Warfarin and Aspirin for Symptomatic Intracranial Arterial Stenosis) trial, which studied symptomatic patients with a recent transient ischemic attack (TIA) or stroke caused by an angiographically verified 50–99% stenosis of a major intracranial artery (7). In this trial, the overall 1- and 2-yr risk of an ischemic stroke in the distribution of the stenotic intracranial artery was approx 12% and approx 14%, respectively. Further stratification of risk has been suggested from additional retrospective series (8). Lesion location appears to be an important factor in predicting risk. For example, vertebral and ICA lesions that are proximal to major points of collateral supply have a lower risk than lesions involving the basilar artery or MCA. Patients with basilar and VA lesions also have a high risk of ischemic events compared with patients with posterior cerebral or posterior inferior cerebellar lesions. Recurrent symptoms despite antithrombotic therapy also appear to predict a high risk of adverse outcome. Thijls et al. studied 29 such patients and reported an incidence of recurrent TIA and stroke of 51% in the cohort (9). Finally, increasing severity of steno-sis predicts a worse outcome. This is not surprising, as it is thought that intracranial stenoses most commonly become symptomatic on the basis of compromise of flow and perfusion to the brain, and ultimately, *in situ* thrombosis. These factors highlight the concept of heterogeneity of intracranial atherosclerotic lesions in terms of risk, and argue in favor of an individualized approach to patient management.

MEDICAL THERAPY

Maximal medical therapy for the treatment of patients with intracranial artery steno-sis is poorly defined. One of the major difficulties with prior stroke prevention trials is that they included populations of patients at risk for stroke, of whom an undefined proportion had intracranial artery disease (10). Optimizing the control of vascular risk factors such as hypertension, hyperlipidemia, smoking, and diabetes mellitus should represent the primary goal of therapy in the global management of these patients. More recently, specific trials have been performed that studied patients with well-defined intracranial artery disease and help further refine the medical management of these patients.

Antithrombotic Therapy and the WASID Trial (7)

Before the publication of WASID trial in 2005, retrospective series suggested a benefit of oral anticoagulation with warfarin over antiplatelet therapy with aspirin in patients with significant intracranial atherosclerosis *(11)*. The WASID trial was the first randomized comparison of these two therapies in this patient population. Patients with symptomatic lesions of the intracranial anterior and posterior circulations were included and randomized to treatment with warfarin (target INR of 2.0–3.0) or aspirin (1300 mg/d). Over a mean follow-up of 1.8 yr, there was no significant difference in the incidence of the primary end point of ischemic stroke, brain hemorrhage, or death from vascular causes in both groups (aspirin 22.1% vs warfarin 21.8%). Of concern, however, warfarin was associated with significantly higher rates of adverse events including death (9.7% vs 4.3%, $p = 0.02$), major hemorrhage (8.3% vs 3.2%, $p = 0.01$), and myocardial infarction or sudden death (7.3% vs 2.9%, $p = 0.02$). Therefore, aspirin is now recommended over warfarin in patients with intracranial stenosis.

Cilostazol

Kwon et al. recently reported a randomized comparison of cilostazol (a phosphodiesterase inhibitor) or placebo in 135 patients with symptomatic M1 segment MCA or basilar artery disease on a background of aspirin therapy (100 mg/d) *(12)*. The cilostazol group demonstrated an increased rate of disease regression (24.4% vs 15.4%) and decreased rate of disease progression (6.7% vs 28.8%) as assessed by magnetic resonance (MR) angiography. The study was not powered to detect a difference in clinical outcome between the groups, but the findings suggest that symptomatic intracranial stenosis is a dynamic lesion and may be favorably altered by the combination of aspirin and cilostazol.

REVASCULARIZATION

Surgical Revascularization

Surgical revascularization for the treatment of intracranial disease involving the intracranial ICA and MCA was first performed in 1967, and subsequently tested in a randomized trial, reported in 1985 *(13)*. Nearly 1400 symptomatic patients were randomized to extracranial (EC)-to-intracranial (IC) arterial bypass surgery (by anastomosing the superficial temporal or occipital artery branch of the external carotid artery [ECA] with a cortical branch of the MCA) or medical therapy with aspirin (325 mg four times daily). Over a mean follow-up of 55 mo, the incidence of all strokes in the surgical arm was 31% vs 29% in the medical arm. The difference in event rates was greatest in the first 6 mo because of perioperative events, with a gradual convergence over time. This pattern was repeated for each of the secondary analyses (including the incidence of ipsilateral ischemic strokes) that examined the effect of revascularization. Over the entire duration of the trial, the relative risk of fatal and nonfatal stroke with surgery was 14% higher in the surgical arm. Based on these data, the practice of EC-to-IC bypass for the treatment of intracranial atherosclerosis has been abandoned.

Percutaneous Intervention

The first attempts at percutaneous revascularization of intracranial atherosclerotic lesions were reported in the early 1980s *(14)*. At that time, the only endovascular option was balloon angioplasty. Technical success was limited by the lack of interventional equipment suitable for use in the intracranial vasculature, and also by the lack of operator experience that accompanies any new technique. Complication rates were prohibitively high, causing many to justifiably argue that the treatment was worse than the disease.

By the early to mid-1990s, however, enthusiasm for the technique reemerged based on technological advances and increased operator expertise. The availability of 0.014 in. microwires and low-profile flexible balloon dilation catheters borrowed from coronary intervention improved the technical success of balloon angioplasty from 60% in early series to >90%, with complication rates of <10% (Table 1) *(15–19)*. However, it should be accepted that individual series have reported significantly worse outcomes with the technique. For example, Gupta reported a very high incidence of major complications (50%), intracranial hemorrhage (17%), and disabling stroke (11%) in a series of 21 patients treated at a single institution between 1197 and 2002 *(20)*.

Angiographic outcomes achieved with angioplasty are typically modest: most studies report a mean percent residual stenosis following intracranial angioplasty of approx 40–50%. However, because flow is related to the square of the lumen radius, the modest effect of angioplasty will typically result in a significant improvement in flow and improvement in clinical symptoms. More aggressive dilatation with larger diameter balloons to achieve a lower residual stenosis increases the risk of dissection and abrupt vessel occlusion, and vessel perforation. Intracranial arteries are particularly susceptible to these complications, as the adventitia and elastic layers of the media are sparser compared with extracranial vessels. As perforation in this location will result in subarachnoid or intraparenchymal hemorrhage, which are life-threatening complications, the balance of risk-vs-benefit argues in favor of conservative angioplasty with balloon diameters that are ≥0.5 mm smaller than the reference vessel diameter.

In an effort to identify the intracranial lesions most suitable for angioplasty, Mori et al. classified intracranial lesions as type A, B, or C based on lesion length, severity (stenosis versus occlusion), eccentricity and angulation, the chronicity of occlusive lesions (> or <3 mo old), and the presence of severe tortuosity proximal to the lesion (Table 2) *(19)*. The technical success, complication rate, and angiographic restenosis rates are very favorable for type A lesions, and acceptable for type B lesions. Type C lesions had a low success rate, and prohibitively high complication rate. Based on these findings, it is reasonable to recommend angioplasty of type A lesions, to restrict angioplasty of type B lesions to clinical situations in which there is a strong clinical indication for treatment by an experienced operator, and regard type C lesions as a contraindication for angioplasty.

The availability of balloon-expandable metallic stents in the mid-1990s transformed the field of coronary intervention because stents provided an effective treatment for coronary dissection and elastic recoil following angioplasty *(21,22)*. The incidence of abrupt vessel occlusion fell dramatically, and the acute angiographic result achievable with intervention became highly predictable. In addition, long-term restenosis rates were significantly improved by stenting. Based on this experience, and the known limitations of intracranial angioplasty, stenting of intracranial lesions was attempted. The tortuosity of the intracranial cerebrovascular system, however, represents a greater challenge for stent delivery than the coronary circulation. As a result, significant success with intracranial stenting was not reported until the availability of third- and fourth-generation balloon-expandable coronary stents that had improved flexibility and lower crossing profiles. More recently, balloon-expandable stents with enhanced flexibility have been specifically

Table 2
Rates of Technical Success and Adverse Procedural Outcome Associated with Intracranial
Angioplasty of Different Lesion Types (A, B, and C)

Lesion type	A (n = 12)	B (n = 21)	C (n = 9)
Description			
Length	<5 mm	5–10 mm	>10 mm
Eccentricity	Concentric or moderately eccentric	Extremely eccentric	
Stenosis/occlusion	Stenosis only	Stenosis or occlusion <3 mo old	Occlusion >3 mo
Other	—	—	Angulated lesion, severe tortuosity proximal to lesion
Technical success (%)	92	86	33
Complications (%) (death, stroke or cerebral bypass surgery)	8	26	87
Restenosis (%)	0	33	100

designed for use in the cerebral vasculature (e.g., Neurolink, Guidant Corporation) (Fig. 2) (23). In addition, the use of nitinol self-expanding stents (Wingspan, Boston Scientific/Smart, Fremont, CA) is also being tested for this indication (24).

Although stenting successfully addresses the issues of dissection and elastic recoil, and may improve the rate of restenosis, there is a potential downside to their use in intracranial intervention. Experience in the coronary circulation taught us that adequate stent expansion using high-pressure balloon inflation was important in achieving optimal stent deployment and apposition of the stent struts against the vessel wall (25). This technique is thought critical to minimizing the risk of stent thrombosis and reducing the rate of restenosis. Because of the fragility of intracranial vessels and the risk of perforation, stents are generally undersized in this location and inflated to lower pressures (4–8 atm). The implication of this practice on the risk of stent thrombosis and restenosis in intracranial vessels is largely unknown.

Stenting is also associated with more plaque shift into side branches as compared to angioplasty. Side branches may also be "jailed" by the metal struts of the stent. Although this is generally a benign event in the coronary circulation, compromise of intracranial side branches during intracranial stenting may have catastrophic consequences depending on the particular side branch compromised (e.g., perforating branches of the VA, lenticulostriate branches of the MCA).

Finally, navigation of stents through very tortuous cervicocranial vessels and tight intracranial stenosis may be associated with complications. On occasion, stents have become dislodged from the balloon of the stent delivery system as a result of extreme tortuosity and aggressive maneuvers to deliver the stent. Vessel trauma has also been reported, and embolization of plaque elements from the lesion site may rarely occur.

Despite these potential limitations, the outcomes reported with intracranial stenting have been promising (Table 3) (26–31). It should be stressed that most of these data are

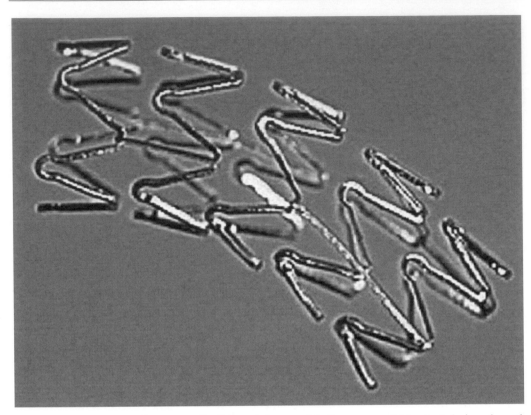

Fig. 2. The NEUROLINK stent—a flexible stainless steel balloon-expandable stent designed specifically for use in the cerebral circulation. (Reproduced with permission from The SSYLVIA Study Investigators. Stroke 2004;35:1388–1392.)

derived from observational case series, and from individual institutions with a small number of highly experienced operators. In most series, procedural success is achieved in 80–90% of cases. Inability to deliver the stent is the most common reason cited for procedural failure, with delivery through the carotid siphon being the most problematic. Mortality rates in different series differ significantly, which strongly relates to the indication for the procedure. In series that include treatment of patients with basilar artery thrombotic occlusions, mortality rates are high. Excluding such patients, mortality rates are generally <5%. Hemorrhagic complications are also uncommon, occurring in 1–5% of cases. The etiology of such hemorrhages is varied and includes wire perforations, vessel rupture, and hemorrhagic transformation of prior infarcts. Procedural stroke rates have been uniformly low, with an incidence of ≤1%.

The true restenosis rates associated with intracranial stenting is not known. The only large prospective study with adequate follow-up angiography was the SSYLVIA study *(23)*. In the subset of 43 patients with treatment of intracranial stenosis treated with the NEUROLINK stent, 37 patients had follow-up angiography. Of these, 12 patients (~32%) had a stenosis of >50% within the stented area. This figure is less than the reported restenosis rates in individual case series, and highlights the bias toward under-reporting of potential issues with the latter observational studies. However, these other series used different coronary balloon-expandable stents, which may explain some of the disparity in restenosis rates between the series.

Table 3
Summary of Contemporary Clinical Series of Intracranial Stenting for Treatment of Atherosclerotic Disease

Study	Year	N	Lesions	Lesion location Anterior	Lesion location Posterior	Mean follow-up (mo)	Technical success	In-hospital adverse outcome Stroke	In-hospital adverse outcome Hem	In-hospital adverse outcome Death	Restenosis	Follow-up stroke rate
Mori (30)	2000	10	12	4	8	12	80	0	0	0	0[a]	0
Levy (28)	2001	11	11	—	11	4	63	1	0	36	14	0
Lylyk (29)	2002	34	34	18	16	5	88	0	1	6	0[b]	0
De Rochemont (26)	2004	18	20	9	11	6	90	0	6	0	—	0
Jiang (27)	2004	40	42	42[c]	—	10	98	0	7.5	2.5	12.5[d]	0
Straube (31)	2005	12	12	6	6	N/R	92	0	0	3	0[e]	0

[a]Based on angiography performed at mean of 4 mo follow-up.
[b]Based on subset of 7 patients that had clinical and angiographic follow-up.
[c]All in MCA MI segment.
[d]Based on angiographic follow-up in eight patients with eight stented vessels.
[e]Based on two patients with angiographic follow-up.

197

While the recurrent stroke rate following intracranial stenting has been reported to be very low in most series (<1%), the more regimented SSYLVIA multicenter trial reported strokes in 7.3% of patients between 30 d and 1 yr following the procedure *(23)*. When added to the periprocedural stroke rate in this study (6.6%), the overall 1-yr stroke rate begins to approach the recurrent stroke rate at 1-yr reported in patients treated with medical therapy alone (12–14%). These data highlight the importance of dedicated trials to closely examine stroke rates following intracranial intervention, and to document the efficacy of this strategy in comparison with medical therapy alone.

PERCUTANEOUS INTRACRANIAL INTERVENTION TECHNIQUES

Patient Preparation: Sedation and Pharmacotherapy

Preprocedural patient preparation centers on two key issues: sedation and anesthesia, and antithrombotic therapy. Most of the published literature on intracranial intervention has reported the use of general anesthesia during the procedure. In contrast, it has been our practice to perform intracranial intervention under conscious sedation, except in circumstances in which patients have an altered level of consciousness and/or cannot protect their airway. While general anesthesia does allow for optimal control of the airway and eliminates patient movement, the ability of the patient to provide feedback during the procedure can be helpful. For example, because the cerebral vessels are richly innervated, excessive stretch of cerebral blood vessels is associated with severe headache, which can warn against excessive dilatation during angioplasty or stenting. In addition, any alteration in neurologic status during the procedure can be detected immediately, which may expedite the recognition of interventional complications and institution of therapeutic maneuvers. We believe that, with greater experience with these procedures, conscious sedation will be used with increased frequency.

The standard preprocedural antithrombotic regimen for intracranial intervention in our practice consists of aspirin (325 mg once daily) and clopidogrel (300-mg load followed by 75 mg once daily) for a minimum of 3 d before the procedure. This regimen is based largely on experience in the coronary interventional literature, in which combined aspirin and clopidogrel therapy is associated with an incidence of acute stent thrombosis of approx 1–2% *(32)*, and preprocedural treatment with clopidogrel appears to obviate the need for glycoprotein (GP) IIb/IIIa inhibitor use in elective interventions *(33)*. The use of anticoagulants (e.g., unfractionated heparin, low molecular weight heparin, coumadin, dextran) before or after coronary intervention has not been shown to add any additional benefit over this combined antiplatelet regimen, but is associated with an increased risk of periprocedural bleeding complications *(34)*.

Procedural Pharmacotherapy

Intracranial intervention is typically performed using unfractionated heparin to achieve an activated clotting time (ACT) of approx 250–300 s. We administer a bolus dose of heparin (50 U/kg) at the beginning of the procedure, and repeat bolus doses as required to maintain therapeutic ACT levels.

The use of GP IIb/IIIa inhibitors during intracranial intervention is controversial. Although some authors use them routinely *(17)*, others reserve their use for situations in which there is abrupt vessel closure. Their use in patients who have rupture of the intracranial vessel can clearly contribute to the mortality associated with the event. For that reason, we do not routinely use these agents during intracranial intervention, limiting their use to patients who do not have adequate pretreatment with antiplatelet agents, or who have atherothrombotic complications associated with the procedure.

Arch Aortography

Before any intracranial intervention, the anatomy of the aortic arch should be defined. In elective situations, this may be done preprocedurally with an MR or computed tomography (CT) angiogram. Alternatively, an arch aortogram may be performed (in 40° LAO view) (Fig. 3a). This helps to define the arch type (i.e., type I, II, or III), and the anatomy of the great vessels. Definition of frequent anomalies of the aortic arch (e.g., bovine origin of left common carotid artery [CCA], anomalous origin of left VA, anomalous origin of right subclavian distal to left subclavian artery) allows for appropriate selection of diagnostic and interventional equipment, and guards against potential confusion created by these anomalies.

Delivery of Sheath and Guide

For anterior and posterior circulation intracranial intervention, the first objective is to deliver a guide or sheath to the distal CCA and proximal subclavian artery, respectively. The inner lumen diameter of an 8 Fr guide or a 6 Fr sheath is usually adequate to allow the delivery of any required interventional equipment for intracranial intervention. Our practice is to use a 6 Fr sheath. The choice of sheath length is important, as choosing a sheath that is too long will limit the ability to treat very distal intracranial lesions due to the limited length of balloon and stent delivery systems. Choosing a sheath length that is too short may compromise the degree of support provided by the sheath. In a normal sized individual, a 70-cm sheath will be adequate.

For anterior circulation intracranial intervention, we typically telescope the diagnostic catheter most suited for engagement of the innominate or left CCA (e.g., JR4 or Berenstein catheter for type I or II arches, Vitek or Simmons catheter for type III arches) through the 6 Fr sheath. With the diagnostic catheter engaged in the appropriate vessel, a stiff angled Glidewire® (Terumo Medical Corporation, Somerset, NJ) is advanced into the ECA using the roadmap function (or into the distal CCA if the ECA is occluded), and the diagnostic catheter is then advanced over the Glidewire®. At this point, the Glidewire® may be exchanged for a stiff Amplatz wire (with 6-cm length soft tip), the catheter removed, and the sheath–dilator combination advanced such that the sheath tip reaches the distal CCA. In patients with a benign anatomy (e.g., type I arch, absence of disease or tortuosity in the CCA), the sheath may be directly advanced over the Glidewire®–catheter combination.

Having successfully delivered the sheath to the distal CCA, a 6 Fr Envoy guide (Cordis Corporation, Miami, FL) is advanced through the sheath over a 0.035-in. wire (e.g., Glidewire®, Wholey wire) to the level of the prepetrous ICA.

For posterior circulation intracranial intervention, a similar strategy is employed to deliver a similar length (i.e., 70 cm) 6 Fr sheath into the proximal subclavian artery. Through this sheath, a 6 Fr Envoy guide is advanced to the level of the distal V2 segment of the VA.

In each case, the platform of a 6 Fr sheath in the CCA or subclavian artery, and the 6 Fr Envoy guide in the prepetrous ICA or V2 segment of the VA, provides the support required for delivery of equipment through the often extremely tortuous intracranial circulation. When additional support is required, more aggressive distal positioning of

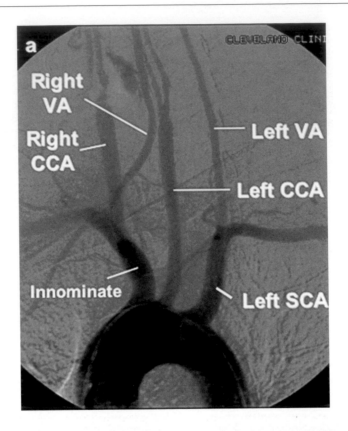

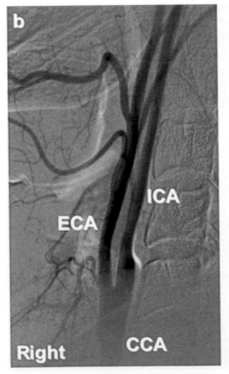

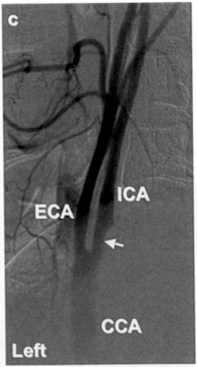

Fig. 3. (*Continued*)

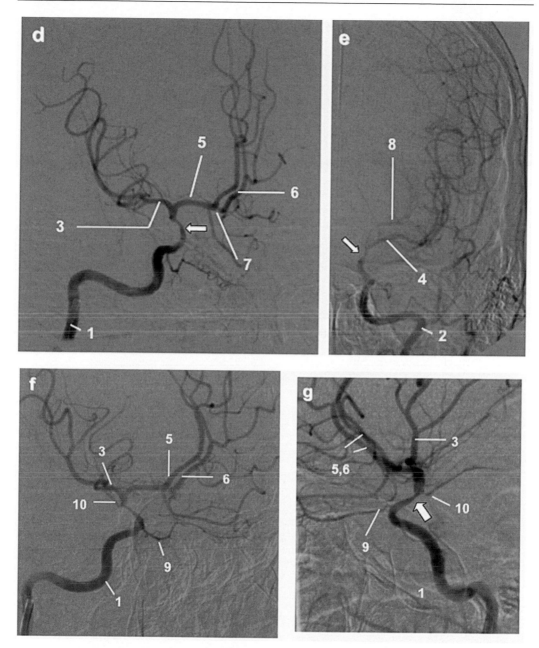

Fig. 3. (*Continued*)

the sheath and/or Envoy guide may be required, accepting that such maneuvers increase the risk of iatrogenic trauma.

Wiring of Lesion

Once a successful platform has been achieved, the lesion may be crossed with a wire. All operators now use 0.010 to 014-in. diameter wires for intracranial intervention. Our wire of choice for initially crossing the lesion is the Synchro™ (Precision Therapeutics, Pittsburgh, PA) wire. This hydrophilic wire is very effective at negotiating

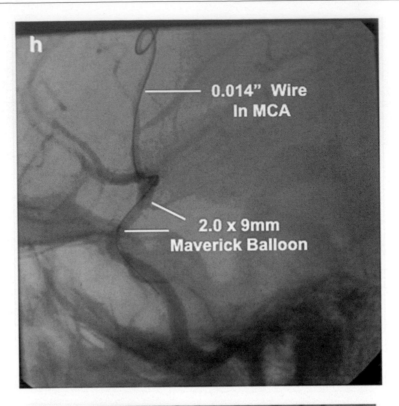

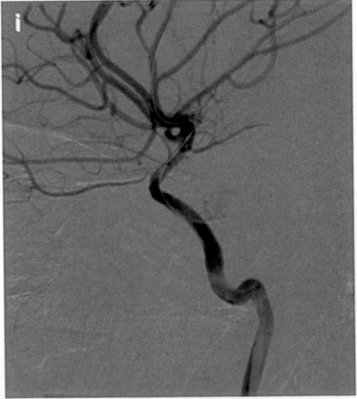

Fig. 3. (*Continued*)

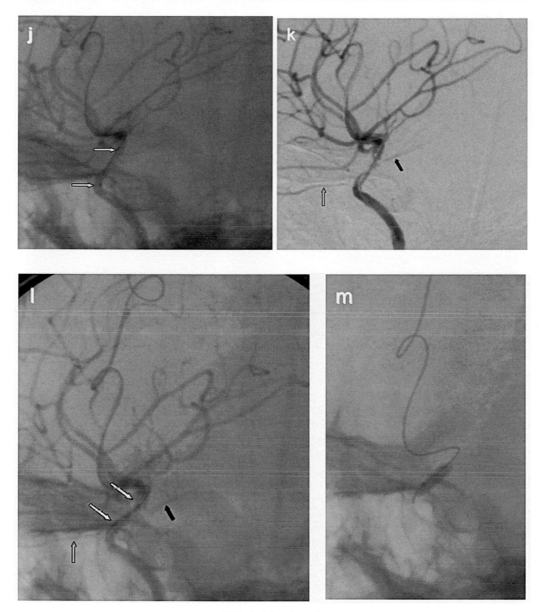

Fig. 3. (*Continued*)

the tortuosity in the intracranial vasculature. To provide sufficient support for delivery of interventional equipment, the distal tip of the wire should be delivered to second- or third-order branches of the middle and posterior cerebral arteries, for anterior and posterior circulation interventions, respectively. Orthogonal views should be performed to ensure correct placement of the wire. The Synchro™ wire is a relatively soft wire, and a more supportive wire is sometimes required to allow delivery of interventional equipment. In this circumstance, an over-the-wire angioplasty balloon e.g., Maverick2™, Boston Scientific) or a hydrophilic microcatheter (Rapid Transit, Cordis) may be used to exchange the Synchro™ wire for a more supportive wire (e.g., Balance Trek/Middle Weight, Guidant, Asahi medium, Abbott Vascular). Because of the

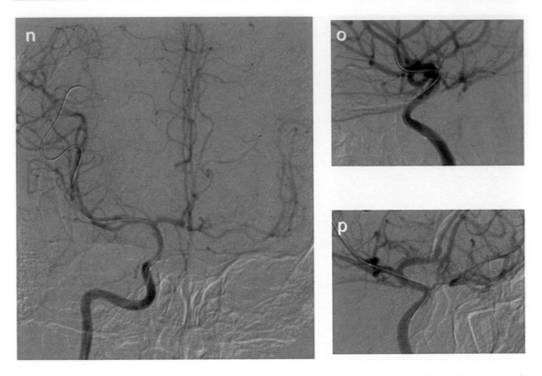

Fig. 3. Angiographic images from intracranial intervention. The patient was a 42-yr-old woman who had a left hemispheric stroke 3 yr previously. She was treated with coumadin and made a complete neurological recovery. While on coumadin therapy, the patient developed severe menorrhagia, which was associated with recurrent right hemispheric stroke-like symptoms. **(a)** Arch aortogram—type I aortic arch with no evidence of atherosclerosis at the origin of the great vessels. **(b,c)** Selective angiography of both common carotid arteries demonstrating mild disease at the origin of the left internal carotid artery (ICA) *(arrow)*. **(d,e)** Right and left PA cerebral angiograms demonstrating a critical eccentric stenosis in the supraclinoid portion of the right ICA and a severe stenosis in the supraclinoid portion of the left ICA extending into the origin of the M1 segment of the left MCA *(white arrows)*. **(f,g)** Oblique PA and lateral view of the supraclinoid portion of the right ICA demonstrating the relationship of the ICA lesion to the origin of the ophthalmic and anterior choroidal branches. **(h)** A 0.014-in. synchro wire was advanced across the lesion into the second-order branches of the right MCA. A 2.0 × 9 mm over-the-wire Maverick balloon was positioned across the lesion and slowly inflated to 6 atm for 60 s. **(i)** Angiographic appearance following angioplasty of the lesion. **(j,k)** A 3.0 × 12 mm Multilink Vision stent was positioned across the lesion (stent markers indicated by *solid white arrows*), but this stent crossed the origins of the ophthalmic *(open arrow)* and anterior choroidal branches *(black arrow)*. This stent was therefore removed. **(l,m)** A 3.0 × 8 mm Multilink Vision stent was then positioned across the lesion and slowly inflated to 8 atm for 30 s. **(n,o,p)** PA, lateral, and lateral oblique angiography following stenting demonstrating excellent angiographic result. There is minimal residual stenosis at the lesion site, and improved cross-filling of the contralateral MCA. *1*, Right internal carotid artery; *2*, left internal carotid artery; *3*, right middle cerebral artery; *4*, left middle cerebral artery; *5*, right anterior cerebral artery; *6*, left anterior cerebral artery; *7*, anterior communicating branch; *8*, lenticulostriate branch; *9*, ophthalmic branch; *10*, anterior choroidal branch.

tortuosity in the cervicocranial vessels, more supportive wires can sometimes create pseudostenoses, which may compromise flow and actually increase the difficulty of stent delivery. One should always confirm antegrade blood flow following placement of more supportive wires.

Angioplasty

With the interventional wire successfully negotiated across the lesion, angioplasty may then be performed. Our practice is to use coronary balloons because of their low profile and compliance, which provides for a very flexible deliverable balloon in the tortuous intracranial circulation (Table 4). Over-the-wire balloons are preferred to monorail balloons because of improved deliverability through tortuous segments.

There is general agreement that, in an effort to minimize the risk of vessel perforation, the choice of angioplasty balloon diameter should be conservative, with a balloon-to-artery ratio of approx 0.7 to 0.8:1. The choice of balloon length needs to be individualized based on lesion location and morphology. In general, the balloon length chosen should be just sufficient to cover the lesion. This minimizes the risk of balloon inflation across adjacent side branches or perforating branches. Many operators have differing opinions as to the optimal method of balloon inflation. Most prefer slow inflation of the balloon to moderate pressures (4–8 atm, i.e., slightly less than nominal pressure) for at least 1 min, followed by slow deflation. Based on observational data, this method is associated with lower rates of dissection and adverse outcomes.

Following angioplasty, an angiogram is performed to assess for: (1) the speed of blood flow across the lesion and into distal circulation; (2) the presence of dissection, recoil, or perforation at the treatment site; (3) compromise of adjacent side branches; and (4) embolization to the distal circulation. It is important to examine the unsubtracted images of the lesion site, as dissections are often masked in the subtracted images. We routinely administer intraarterial nitroglycerin (100- to 200-µg bolus) following angioplasty to eliminate any vasospasm at the treatment site, which might confuse the interpretation of the angiographic outcome. If angioplasty is associated with a significant improvement in lumen diameter, in the absence of significant recoil or dissection, the procedure may be terminated by removing the wire and repeating angiography to confirm a stable angiographic result. Failure to achieve an adequate increase in lumen diameter with angioplasty, or the development of significant recoil or dissection will typically prompt an attempt at stent placement. This strategy of stenting only in the presence of a suboptimal angioplasty result is referred to as "provisional stenting." In cases in which a stent cannot be delivered (~10% of cases), or is contraindicated (e.g., fear of plaque shift into major side branch or perforating branch) repeat prolonged angioplasty may be attempted.

Stenting

As outlined in the preceding text, there are insufficient data to advocate the routine use of stents during intracranial intervention. Despite this lack of data, we have increasingly moved toward a strategy of routine stenting during such procedures. Our practice is to predilate the lesion with a conservatively sized balloon (balloon-to-artery ratio of 0.7:1) to facilitate stent delivery. While some operators have reported performing direct stenting (i.e., stenting without prior angioplasty) in intracranial interventions, we generally avoid this strategy, as aggressive manipulation of stents across an undilated atherosclerotic stenosis may increase the risk of distal embolization of plaque debris. Based on our experience, we have found the newer cobalt-chromium alloy stents (Driver™, Medtronic, and Multilink Vision™, Guidant) to have superior deliverability to the traditional 316L stainless steel stents, and these have become the stents of choice in our practice (Table 4).

Table 4
List of Interventional Equipment that Have Been Reported in Various Series
of Intracranial Intervention

Stents
   Palmaz-Schatz Stent (Cordis) (first-generation coronary stent)
   GR II (Cook) (second generation coronary stent)
   GFX (Advanced Vascular Engineering)
   INX (Advanced Vascular Engineering)
   Multilink (Guidant)
   NIR (NIR Medinol)
   S 660, S 670, S7 (Medtronic AVE)
   Express (Boston Scientific)
   BiodivYsio (Abbott Vascular)
   Multilink Vision (Guidant)
   Driver (Medtronic)

Balloons
   Stealth (Target Therapeutics)
   Valor (Cordis)
   Ranger (Boston Scientific)
   Maverick (Boston Scientific)

Wires
   Dasher-14 (Target Therapeutics)
   0.016-in. GlideGold Wire (Terumo)
   Wizdom-14 (Cordis Neurovascular)
   Prowler-14 (Cordis)
   Transcend-14 (Target Therapeutics, Boston Scientific)
   Choice PT (Boston Scientific)
   High Torque Floppy II (Advanced Cardiovascular Systems)
   Synchro (Precision Therapeutics)

Other
   Transit catheters
   RapidTransit microcatheter (Cordis Endovascular Systems)

As with angioplasty, the stent diameter chosen is at least 0.5 mm smaller than the estimated vessel diameter. Every effort is made to closely match the stent length to the lesion length so as to minimize the effect of plaque shift into adjacent side branches or perforating branches. Stents are generally slowly inflated to moderate pressures (4–8 atm), while the patient is actively questioned for the onset of headache. This is certainly less than the high-pressure inflations that are used to deploy stents in the coronary circulation, based on IVUS studies showing optimal stent expansion at higher pressures. The reason for conservative sizing and inflation pressures in the intracranial circulation is to minimize the risk of vessel rupture. The potential downside of this practice is an increased risk of incomplete stent apposition and stent migration, subacute stent thrombosis, and delayed in-stent restenosis. However, because of the high morbidity and mortality associated with intracranial vessel rupture, this practice seems clinically reasonable.

Following stenting, angiography is performed to examine for the same issues as outlined following angioplasty. Postdilatation of the stent is generally avoided because of the risk of vessel rupture unless the stent is markedly underexpanded.

At the completion of the procedure, orthogonal angiographic views of the lesion site and cerebral circulation with the wire removed are performed to ensure a stable result at the treatment site and document the absence of distal embolization.

Postprocedural Care

Because the majority of our cases are performed under conscious sedation, patients are usually recovered immediately to the neurointensive care unit. Patients have frequent neurologic assessments and particular attention is paid to hemodynamic monitoring. Control of blood pressure should be individualized based on the perceived risk of hyperperfusion syndrome or cerebral ischemia. For example, in patients believed to be at high risk of hyperperfusion syndrome (treatment of critical stenosis, absence of collateral circulation), blood pressure should be managed aggressively with a target systolic blood pressure of 100–120 mmHg. Conversely, in patients at risk of cerebral ischemia (suboptimal angioplasty result, plaque shift into side branches or perforating branches), blood pressure control should be more liberal in an effort to maintain normal cerebral perfusion.

Although some operators continue heparin anticoagulation and/or GP IIb/IIIa inhibition following intracranial procedure, this has not been our practice, unless there has been an ischemic complication.

In the absence of any postprocedural complications, patients are discharged 24–48 h following the procedure. Patients are continued on aspirin therapy for life and clopidogrel for a minimum of 1 mo. At the time of discharge, patients are instructed regarding the importance of meticulous blood pressure control over the next 3–4 wk, and systems should be put in place to provide patients with easy access to healthcare providers to help titrate antihypertensive medications to achieve this goal. There are no guidelines for screening for restenosis in patients following intracranial intervention. CT and MR angiography suffer from artifact created by the metallic stent. Transcranial Doppler is useful for screening for restenosis in patients with stents placed in the ICA siphon, MCA, VA, and the basilar artery, particularly if a baseline measurement was obtained following the procedure for comparison. If the patient develops recurrent symptoms, or if the transcranial Doppler shows significantly increased velocities, repeat angiography is indicated.

CONCLUSIONS

Percutaneous interventional techniques for the treatment of intracranial atherosclerotic lesions have evolved significantly over the last two decades. Our experience to date has shown that these techniques are feasible, and when performed by experienced operators using contemporary interventional equipment and pharmacotherapy, are reasonably safe. The challenges for the future include advancing our understanding of the natural history of the disease in an effort to define those at greatest risk of future events, and performing carefully controlled randomized trials documenting the efficacy of endovascular therapies.

REFERENCES

1. Frey JL, Jahnke HK, Bulfinch EW. Differences in stroke between white, Hispanic, and Native American patients: the Barrow Neurological Institute stroke database. Stroke 1998;29:29–33.
2. Petty GW, Brown RD, Jr., Whisnant JP, Sicks JD, O'Fallon WM, Wiebers DO. Ischemic stroke subtypes: a population-based study of incidence and risk factors. Stroke 1999;30:2513–2516.
3. White H, Boden-Albala B, Wang C, et al. Ischemic stroke subtype incidence among whites, blacks, and Hispanics: the Northern Manhattan Study. Circulation 2005;111:1327–1331.

4. Wityk RJ, Lehman D, Klag M, Coresh J, Ahn H, Litt B. Race and sex differences in the distribution of cerebral atherosclerosis. Stroke 1996;27:1974–1980.

5. Feigin VL, Rodgers A. Ethnic disparities in risk factors for stroke: what are the implications? Stroke 2004;35:1568–1569.

6. Kremer C, Schaettin T, Georgiadis D, Baumgartner RW. Prognosis of asymptomatic stenosis of the middle cerebral artery. J Neurol Neurosurg Psychiatry 2004;75:1300–1303.

7. Chimowitz MI, Lynn MJ, Howlett-Smith H, et al. Comparison of warfarin and aspirin for symptomatic intracranial arterial stenosis. N Engl J Med 2005;352:1305–1316.

8. Gomez CR, Orr SC. Angioplasty and stenting for primary treatment of intracranial arterial stenoses. Arch Neurol 2001;58:1687–1690.

9. Thijs VN, Albers GW. Symptomatic intracranial atherosclerosis: outcome of patients who fail antithrombotic therapy. Neurology 2000;55:490–497.

10. Mohr JP, Thompson JL, Lazar RM, et al. A comparison of warfarin and aspirin for the prevention of recurrent ischemic stroke. N Engl J Med 2001;345:1444–1451.

11. Chimowitz MI, Kokkinos J, Strong J, et al. The Warfarin-Aspirin Symptomatic Intracranial Disease Study. Neurology 1995;45:1488–1493.

12. Kwon SU, Cho YJ, Koo JS, et al. Cilostazol prevents the progression of the symptomatic intracranial arterial stenosis: the multicenter double-blind placebo-controlled trial of cilostazol in symptomatic intracranial arterial stenosis. Stroke 2005;36:782–786.

13. Failure of extracranial-intracranial arterial bypass to reduce the risk of ischemic stroke. Results of an international randomized trial. The EC/IC Bypass Study Group. N Engl J Med 1985;313:1191–1200.

14. Sundt TM, Jr., Smith HC, Campbell JK, Vlietstra RE, Cucchiara RF, Stanson AW. Transluminal angioplasty for basilar artery stenosis. Mayo Clin Proc 1980;55:673–680.

15. Alazzaz A, Thornton J, Aletich VA, Debrun GM, Ausman JI, Charbel F. Intracranial percutaneous transluminal angioplasty for arteriosclerotic stenosis. Arch Neurol 2000;57:1625–1630.

16. Clark WM, Barnwell SL, Nesbit G, O'Neill OR, Wynn ML, Coull BM. Safety and efficacy of percutaneous transluminal angioplasty for intracranial atherosclerotic stenosis. Stroke 1995;26:1200–1204.

17. Connors JJ, 3rd, Wojak JC. Percutaneous transluminal angioplasty for intracranial atherosclerotic lesions: evolution of technique and short-term results. J Neurosurg 1999;91:415–423.

18. Marks MP, Marcellus ML, Do HM, et al. Intracranial angioplasty without stenting for symptomatic atherosclerotic stenosis: long-term follow-up. AJNR Am J Neuroradiol 2005;26:525–530.

19. Mori T, Fukuoka M, Kazita K, Mori K. Follow-up study after intracranial percutaneous transluminal cerebral balloon angioplasty. AJNR Am J Neuroradiol 1998;19:1525–1533.

20. Gupta R, Schumacher HC, Mangla S, et al. Urgent endovascular revascularization for symptomatic intracranial atherosclerotic stenosis. Neurology 2003;61:1729–1735.

21. Fischman DL, Leon MB, Baim DS, et al. A randomized comparison of coronary-stent placement and balloon angioplasty in the treatment of coronary artery disease. Stent Restenosis Study Investigators. N Engl J Med 1994;331:496–501.

22. Serruys PW, de Jaegere P, Kiemeneij F, et al. A comparison of balloon-expandable-stent implantation with balloon angioplasty in patients with coronary artery disease. Benestent Study Group. N Engl J Med 1994;331:489–495.

23. Stenting of Symptomatic Atherosclerotic Lesions in the Vertebral or Intracranial Arteries (SSYLVIA): study results. Stroke 2004;35:1388–1392.

24. Hartmann M, Jansen O. Angioplasty and stenting of intracranial stenosis. Curr Opin Neurol 2005;18:39–45.

25. Nakamura S, Hall P, Gaglione A, et al. High pressure assisted coronary stent implantation accomplished without intravascular ultrasound guidance and subsequent anticoagulation. J Am Coll Cardiol 1997;29:21–27.

26. de Rochemont Rdu M, Turowski B, Buchkremer M, Sitzer M, Zanella FE, Berkefeld J. Recurrent symptomatic high-grade intracranial stenoses: safety and efficacy of undersized stents—initial experience. Radiology 2004;231:45–49.

27. Jiang WJ, Wang YJ, Du B, et al. Stenting of symptomatic M1 stenosis of middle cerebral artery: an initial experience of 40 patients. Stroke 2004;35:1375–1380.

28. Levy EI, Horowitz MB, Koebbe CJ, et al. Transluminal stent-assisted angiplasty of the intracranial vertebrobasilar system for medically refractory, posterior circulation ischemia: early results. Neurosurgery 2001;48:1215–1221; discussion 1221–1223.

29. Lylyk P, Cohen JE, Ceratto R, Ferrario A, Miranda C. Angioplasty and stent placement in intracranial atherosclerotic stenoses and dissections. AJNR Am J Neuroradiol 2002;23:430–436.

30. Mori T, Kazita K, Chokyu K, Mima T, Mori K. Short-term arteriographic and clinical outcome after cerebral angioplasty and stenting for intracranial vertebrobasilar and carotid atherosclerotic occlusive disease. AJNR Am J Neuroradiol 2000;21:249–254.
31. Straube T, Stingele R, Jansen O. Primary Stenting of Intracranial Atherosclerotic Stenoses. Cardiovasc Intervent Radiol 2005;28:289–295.
32. Bhatt DL, Bertrand ME, Berger PB, et al. Meta-analysis of randomized and registry comparisons of ticlopidine with clopidogrel after stenting. J Am Coll Cardiol 2002;39:9–14.
33. Schomig A, Schmitt C, Dibra A, et al. One year outcomes with abciximab vs. placebo during percutaneous coronary intervention after pre-treatment with clopidogrel. Eur Heart J 2005;261:1379–1384.
34. Rabah M, Mason D, Muller DW, et al. Heparin after percutaneous intervention (HAPI): a prospective multicenter randomized trial of three heparin regimens after successful coronary intervention. J Am Coll Cardiol 1999;34:461–467.

14

The Approach to Intracranial and Extracranial Vertebral Artery Stenting

J. Emilio Exaire, MD
and Jacqueline Saw, MD

CONTENTS

Summary

Approximately 25% of ischemic strokes involve the posterior or vertebrobasilar circulation, which is associated with a mortality of 20–30%. Posterior circulation strokes are predominantly due to embolism and large artery disease. This chapter focuses on the percutaneous management of patients with significant atherosclerotic stenosis of the extracranial and intracranial vertebral artery.

Key Words: Vertebral artery stenosis, vertebral artery stenting, vertebrobasilar stroke.

INTRODUCTION

Approximately 25% of ischemic strokes involve the posterior or vertebrobasilar circulation, which is associated with a mortality of 20–30% *(1)*. The posterior circulation perfuses the medulla, cerebellum, pons, midbrain, thalamus, and occipital cortex. Posterior circulation strokes are predominantly due to embolism (40%) and large artery disease (32%) *(2)*. Less common etiologies include penetrating artery disease (14%) and migraine (3%) *(2)*.

Posterior circulation embolism may arise from the heart, aorta, innominate artery, subclavian artery, or the vertebral artery (VA) *(2,3)*. The terminal site of embolization typically involves the posterior inferior cerebellar artery (PICA), superior cerebellar artery (SCA), and posterior cerebral artery (PCA). An acute occlusion of a large vessel (e.g., basilar artery) with an embolism typically results in a catastrophic stroke with major disability or death (mortality as high as 80%).

From: *Contemporary Cardiology: Handbook of Complex Percutaneous Carotid Intervention*
Edited by: J. Saw, J. E. Exaire, D. S. Lee, and S. Yadav © Humana Press Inc., Totowa, NJ

Table 1
Common Posterior Circulation Syndromes

Syndrome	Artery	Symptoms	Clinical signs
Wallenberg	PICA or vertebral	Nausea, vomit, vertigo	Ipsilateral ataxia, dysmetria, Horner syndrome[a]
Locked-in	Basilar	Quadriplegia, intact consciousness	Vertical gaze preserved
Top of the basilar	Basilar (rostral branch)	Confusion, amnesia, and visual symptoms	Hemianopsia, cortical blindness, cranial nerve III palsy
AICA	Anterior inferior cerebellar	Vertigo, unilateral deafness	Ipsilateral facial weakness and ataxia
SCA	Superior cerebellar	Nausea, vomiting, slurred speech	Ataxia, contralateral loss of pain and temperature
Internuclear ophthalmoplegia	Basilar or paramedian	Horizontal gaze palsy	No adduction away from the involved eye

[a]Horner syndrome: ptosis, miosis, hypohidrosis or anhidrosis, enophthalmos. AICA, Anterior inferior cerebellar artery; PICA, posterior inferior cerebellar artery; SCA, superior cerebellar artery.

Large artery disease describes severe stenosis or occlusion of extracranial or intracranial arteries in which a hemodynamic mechanism causes low perfusion. The most common etiology is atherosclerosis. In a series of 260 patients, the most frequent site of stenosis or occlusion in the posterior circulation is the extracranial VA (43.5%), involving primarily the origin off the subclavian artery. Other common sites of involvement are the intracranial VA (41.5%) and basilar artery (41.8%). Less common sites are the PCA (15%), subclavian artery (1.9%) and innominate artery (0.7%) (2). This chapter focuses on the percutaneous management of patients with significant atherosclerotic stenosis of the extracranial and intracranial VA.

POSTERIOR CIRCULATION SYMPTOMS

Patients with disease of the VA often have an asymptomatic course (even despite occlusion of one extracranial VA). Among the symptomatic patients with vertebrobasilar disease, 50% present initially with a stroke, and 26% present with a transient ischemic attack (TIA) followed by a stroke (with a 20–35% stroke risk over 5 yr) (4–6). Vertebrobasilar insufficiency due to low-flow state secondary to hemodynamically critical stenosis is often positional, and may be associated with neck extension or rotational head movements. The clinical symptoms of posterior circulation TIA or stroke are often nonspecific, and thus a high index of suspicion is necessary for diagnosis and prompt management. These symptoms may include nausea, vomiting, nystagmus, vertigo, dysarthria, dysphagia, dysmetria, ataxia, and unilateral Horner's syndrome (with brainstem lesions). Involvement of ipsilateral cranial nerves will result in contralateral corticospinal signs. If the occipital lobe is involved, visual field loss or spatial deficits are common. However, hemispheric symptoms of cortical deficits (e.g., aphasia) are absent. Table 1 summarizes the common posterior circulation ischemic symptoms and syndromes.

ANATOMY OF THE VERTEBROBASILAR SYSTEM

The VA arises from the superior and posterior aspect of the first part of the subclavian artery. In approx 6% of cases, the left VA arises directly from the aortic arch between the left common carotid artery (CCA) and the left subclavian artery (Fig. 1). In rare occasions, the right VA may arise distal to the left subclavian artery *(7)* or from the right CCA (0.18%) *(8,9)*. Usually, one of the VA is considered "dominant" (e.g., larger caliber), with 50–60% of individuals having the left VA as dominant *(10)*. On the other hand, a hypoplastic VA is seen in about 10–40% of cases on angiography *(11)*. The VA is divided into three extracranial and one intracranial segments (Fig. 2):

1. Extracranial V1 segment (usual diameter 3.0–5.0 mm) starts from the origin of the VA to where it enters the transverse foramina at the fifth or sixth cervical vertebra.
2. The extracranial V2 segment (diameter 3.0–5.0 mm) is within the intervertebral foramina and ends when the VA courses behind the atlas.
3. The extracranial V3 segment is between the C2 transverse process and the base of the skull where it enters the foramen magnum.
4. The intracranial V4 segment (diameter 2.5–3.5 mm) starts where the VA pierces the dura and arachnoid mater at the base of the skull, and ends where it joins the contralateral VA form the basilar artery at the base of the medulla oblongata.

The branches of the VA are divided into cervical branches and cranial branches. There are spinal and muscular branches off the cervical VA. The cranial branches are the meningeal, posterior spinal, anterior spinal, PICA, and medullary arteries. The PICA is the largest branch of the VA, and courses backward to the under surface of the cerebellum. It divides into medial and lateral branches, and may anastomose with the anterior inferior cerebellar artery (AICA) and the SCA of the basilar artery. The PICA may be absent unilaterally in approx 20% of cases, and bilaterally in approx 2% of cases *(11)*. In 1% of cases, the VA terminates in the PICA. The VA ends when it joins the contralateral VA to form the basilar artery (so named as it is located at the base of the skull).

The basilar artery gives off several important branches on both sides (Figs. 3, 4a, 4b). The pontine branches are small vessels that arise at right angles on both sides of the basilar artery, supplying the pons and adjacent brain. The bilateral AICAs passes backward to the under surface of the cerebellum to supply the anterior portion, and anastomose with the ipsilateral PICA. The bilateral SCAs come off distally near the termination of the basilar artery, and travel to the upper surface of the cerebellum, and anastomose with the inferior cerebellar arteries. The basilar artery ends when it divides into both PCAs, which travel laterally and each are joined by the ipsilateral posterior communicating artery (PCOM) from the distal internal carotid artery (ICA) as part of the Circle of Willis. The PCA supplies the temporal and occipital lobes.

The PCOM tends to diminish in size with age, with large diameter PCOMs found with higher incidence in children (39–75%) than in adults (8–29%) *(12)*. And in about 30% of cases, the PCOM is of the same caliber or larger than the PCA, in which case the P1 segment may be hypoplastic (fetal-type PCOM) with predominant supply of the PCA via the anterior circulation *(13)*. The PCOM varies in length and diameter, and is absent unilaterally in about one third of cases on autopsy *(14)*. On magnetic resonance angiography (MRA), 40% of patients were found to have absent PCOM *(15)*. In older series with conventional angiographically, however, only 30–40% of PCOM may be visualized on anteroposterior projection *(12)*.

DIAGNOSIS OF VERTEBRAL ARTERY STENOSIS

Duplex Ultrasound

The overall sensitivity of duplex ultrasound in detecting extracranial VA stenosis is 70–80% *(16,17)*. Specificity and negative predictive value >95% have been reported

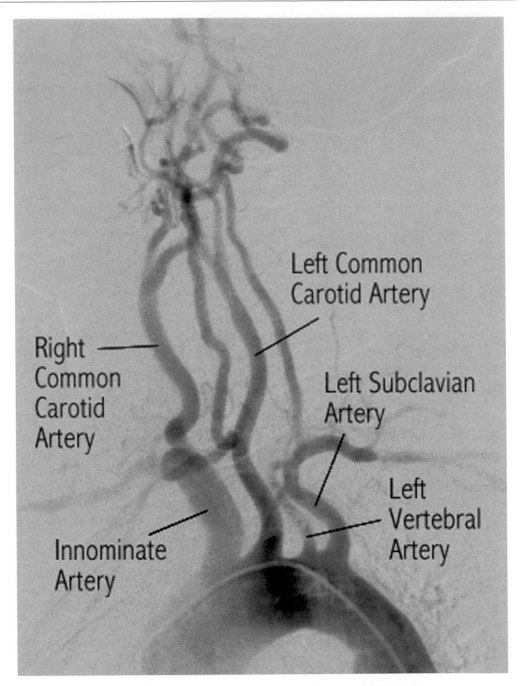

Fig. 1. Aortic arch angiogram demonstrating a normal variant of separate left vertebral artery origin from the aorta.

(16,17). The extracranial V1–3 segments can be visualized with duplex ultrasound. The VA ostium, the most common site of atherosclerotic stenosis in the VA, can be imaged in 80–90% of patients with duplex ultrasound *(18,19).* For intracranial VA stenosis, transcranial Doppler can be used, with a sensitivity of approx 80% and specificity of 80–97% *(20).* However, transcranial Doppler may underestimate stenosis and occlusion.

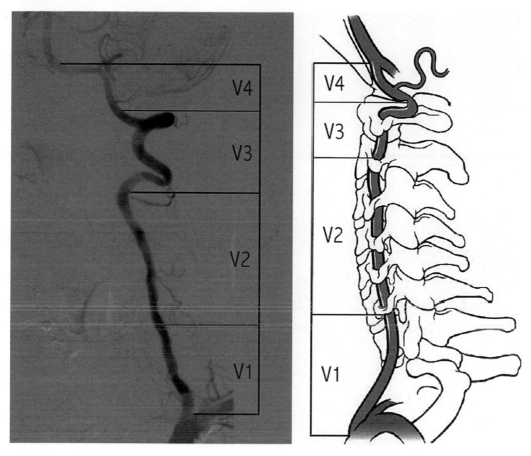

Fig. 2. Angiographic and schematic diagrams showing the three extracranial vertebral artery segments (V1–3) and one intracranial segment (V4). (Adapted from ref. *41*.)

Magnetic Resonance Angiography

MRA is increasingly used to evaluate the extracranial and intracranial cerebrovasculature. The VA can be assessed by gadolinium-enhanced MRA with high sensitivity (97–100%) and specificity (85–99%) *(21,22)*. Sometimes the degree of stenosis may be overestimated by MRA because this is a flow-related image technique. Therefore, severe stenosis with significant flow compromise may result in poor visualization of the vessel and thus resemble an occlusion. It appears that the extracranial portion of the VA is more accurately visualized than the intracranial portion with MRA *(23)*.

Computed Tomography Angiography

CT angiography is a helpful tool to identify posterior circulation anomalies in the acute stroke setting, especially in lesions involving the basilar artery. However, the role of CT angiography for VA imaging is limited because of the proximity of bone, due to the course of the VA within the transverse foramina and through the skull base. In a small study involving 103 patients, the specificity of diagnosing VA stenosis was only 50% *(24)*. Introduction of multidetector CT and modern image processing techniques appear promising in improving visualization of the VA.

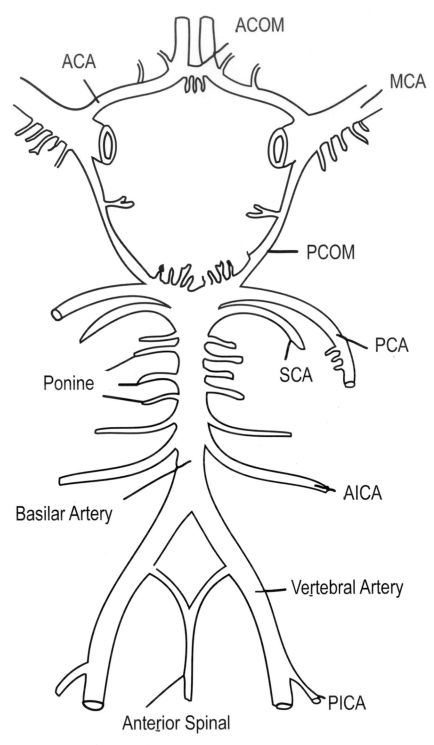

Fig. 3. Schematic diagram of the vertebrobasilar system and the Circle of Willis. ACA, Anterior cerebral artery; ACOM, anterior communicating artery; AICA, anterior inferior cerebellar artery; PCA, posterior cerebral artery; PCOM, posterior communicating artery; PICA, posterior inferior cerebellar artery; SCA, superior cerebellar artery.

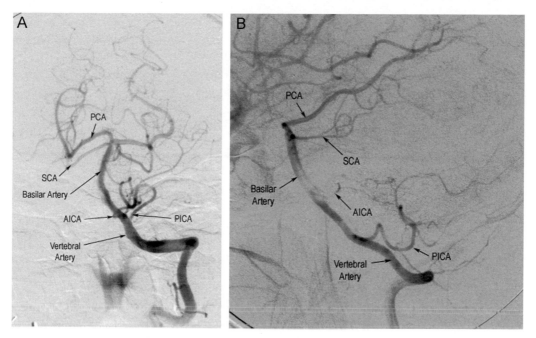

Fig. 4. Angiographic diagrams of the intracranial vertebrobasilar system in the (**A**) PA projection, (**B**) Lateral projection. See Fig. 3 for abbreviations.

Digital Subtraction Angiography

Digital subtraction angiography remains the gold standard to diagnose VA disease. We typically begin with an aortic arch angiogram (45° LAO) to view the great vessels and arch classification. It is important to assess the origin of the great vessels for stenosis, and the great vessel branching morphology for normal variants. An adequate field of view to visualize the origin and proximal portions of the VA is necessary. A longer cine run may be necessary if there is VA or subclavian occlusion with retrograde vertebral flow into the subclavian artery (i.e., subclavian steal syndrome).

A full four-vessel angiogram (including both carotid and both vertebral arteries with intracerebral runoff) is then performed to assess the morphology of the VA stenosis and the intracerebral collateral circulation (Circle of Willis). A very meticulous technique is necessary to prevent embolization and dissection. A 5 Fr JR4 catheter is typically used to perform the diagnostic angiography, and the catheter is placed in close proximity to the ostium of the VA without selectively engaging. This is a precaution to avoid dissection of the VA. Occasionally, a reverse-curved catheter (e.g., VTK) may be necessary to engage the subclavian arteries with type III aortic arch. An ipsilateral blood pressure cuff is then inflated above the systolic pressure to maximize contrast filling of the vertebral system. To visualize the origin of the VA, a 20°–30° contralateral angulation is often used to separate the ostium of the VA from the subclavian artery. At times, additional PA and/or ipsilateral angulation (with or without cranial 20° angulation) views are helpful to visualize the ostium. For the rest of the extracranial VA, a PA or shallow ipsilateral 20° angulation (with or without cranial 20° angulation) is adequate for proper visualization. For the intracranial segments, a PA view with steep cranial angulation (usually ~40°) (Townes view) and cross-table lateral views with digital subtraction are performed. In addition, a PA caudal view with the patient's mouth wide open may be useful, as this avoids the overlying bony structures.

With meticulous techniques, the risks associated with VA diagnostic angiography are low, but may include embolization and dissection *(25)*.

TREATMENT OF VERTEBRAL ARTERY STENOSIS

Medical Treatment

There is a general lack of randomized data on medical therapy specifically for VA stenosis. Empirically, patients with VA stenosis should be on aspirin, a statin, and an angiotensin converting enzyme inhibitor (ACE inhibitor). Aggressive management of atherosclerotic risk factors is also recommended.

There had been some controversy regarding the use of anticoagulant for patients with symptomatic intracranial vertebral disease, until the recent publication of the WASID (Warfarin-Aspirin Symptomatic Intracranial Disease) trial *(26)*. In this study, 551 patients with symptomatic intracranial stenosis (TIA or stroke within last 6 mo) were randomized to aspirin 1300 mg/d or warfarin (to achieve INR 2–3). Of these patients, 39.7% had intracranial vertebral or basilar artery disease. This study was halted prematurely because of higher adverse events in the warfarin group at mean follow-up of 1.8 yr: mortality 9.7% warfarin vs 4.3% aspirin ($p = 0.02$), major hemorrhage 8.3% warfarin vs 3.2% aspirin ($p = 0.01$), and myocardial infarction or sudden death 7.3% warfarin vs 2.9% aspirin ($p = 0.02$). The primary composite end point of ischemic stroke, hemorrhagic stroke, and cardiovascular death was similar in both treatment groups, 21.8% warfarin vs 22.1% aspirin ($p = 0.83$). Thus, warfarin had no benefit over high-dose aspirin in patients with symptomatic intracranial stenosis, and is associated with higher adverse event rate. One of the major criticisms of this study is that in the warfarin group, patients were in the therapeutic INR range only 63% of the time. Further, a high daily dose of aspirin was used (1300 mg/d) in this study; it is unknown if lower doses will provide similar efficacy.

Surgical Treatment

Surgery for VA stenosis is challenging because of difficult access of the VA origin. The two approaches are endarterectomy and reconstruction procedures. For disease involving the V1 segment, especially the ostium, endarterectomy may be performed via a supraclavicular incision. Reconstruction may also be performed by transposing the VA to the CCA or ICA, and less frequently, to the subclavian artery or thyrocervical trunk. Sometimes, a bypass graft (saphenous or polytetrafluoroethylene) may be used *(27)*. The V2 segment, because it travels within the transverse foramina, is prone to external compression by osteophytes or intervertebral joints; rarely, a ligation at C1–C2 level and bypass to the V3 segment may be indicated. The V3 segment can be reconstructed with a saphenous vein bypass from the common carotid, subclavian, proximal vertebral arteries, or transposition of the external carotid onto the distal vertebral, or transposition of the distal VA onto the distal ICA *(27)*. The vertebro–basilar junction can be accessed surgically above the level of the transverse process of C1. Reconstruction may be achieved with saphenous vein bypass from the distal ICA.

The complication rates with these procedures are not trivial. Berguer had reported a series of 369 extracranial VA reconstructions, showing a stroke and death rate of <2%

for proximal and 6% for distal extracranial VA reconstruction *(28)*. Patency rate at 5 yr was 80%, and survival at 5 yr was 70% *(28)*. Other surgical complications include Horner's syndrome (10%), lymphoceles (10%), thrombosis of transposed vessel (11%), vocal cord paralysis, and phrenic nerve injury *(20)*. Given the technical challenges and complication rates, a percutaneous approach with VA stenting is considered the first-line treatment for patients requiring revascularization.

PERCUTANEOUS INTERVENTION

Percutaneous intervention of the VA can be done safely and with good technical feasibility. It is much less challenging than the surgical approaches. Technical success has been reported at 97–100% (defined as ability to deliver the stent, and residual stenosis <20–50%) *(29–31)*. There is a lack of appropriate randomized trials comparing surgery, medical treatment, and percutaneous intervention of the VA. In fact, in a literature review, only one completed randomized trial of VA percutaneous intervention versus medical treatment in 16 patients within the CAVATAS (Carotid and Vertebral Artery Transluminal Angioplasty Study) had been published *(32)*. However, data from small case series have demonstrated safety and acceptable long-term patency. The long-term clinical efficacy, especially the reduction of posterior circulation strokes, is still unknown and would require randomized comparison to best medical therapy.

Early experience with VA intervention with angioplasty alone was associated with high restenosis rates, especially for ostial lesions *(33,34)*. Extending the experience from coronary interventions (where stent has been shown to reduce restenosis, acute and sub-acute thrombosis, and treat intimal dissection), modern extracranial and intracranial VA interventions now include routine stenting. In the case series by Chastain et al., 55 extracranial VA stents were performed without any periprocedural complications, and the restenosis (>50% diameter) rate was 10% at 25-mo follow-up *(29)*. In a smaller case series by Albuquerque et al., the restenosis rate was 43% among 33 patients who underwent extracranial VA ostium stenting *(30)*. In the study by Jenkins et al., of 32 patients who underwent VA stenting, there was one procedural TIA and one in-stent restenosis (3%) at 3.5 mo *(31)*. In the SSYLVIA (Stenting of Symptomatic Atherosclerotic Lesions in the Vertebral or Intracranial Arteries) study, which enrolled 61 symptomatic patients with intracranial disease (22/43 were posterior circulation) or extracranial VA stenosis (*n* = 18, with 6 involving ostia), the 6-mo restenosis (>50% diameter) rate was 32.4% for intracranial vessels and 42.9% for extracranial VA lesions *(35)*.

Indications for Vertebral Artery Stenting

ACUTE STROKE

This is the least controversial indication of vertebrobasilar intervention, especially for patients with acute occlusion or critical stenosis of a major arterial branch. It has been proposed that patients with extensive acute posterior circulation stroke should undergo percutaneous intervention *(36,37)*. It has been reported that a combined approach with intraarterial thrombolysis (9 mg r-pro-urokinase locally) *(36)* and stent placement can achieve improvement of symptoms in up to 70% of the patients *(37,38)*. Symptomatic brain hemorrhage, however, can occur in 10–15% of patients with the use of thrombolysis *(36,39)*. The use of glycoprotein (GP) IIb/IIIa inhibitors may be used in the setting of refractory intraarterial thrombolysis or unsuccessful intervention. In a small series of 21 patients presenting with acute ischemic stroke due to large-vessel occlusion, GP IIb/IIIa inhibitors was administered to patients who failed rtPA with or without mechanical thrombolysis. Seventeen of 21 patients achieved complete or partial recanalization of the culprit artery *(39)*.

SYMPTOMATIC PATIENTS WITH TIA

Patients with posterior circulation TIA should undergo noninvasive tests including MRI and MRA. MRI may rule out parenchymal hemorrhage, edema, or the presence of arteriovenous malformations. If any of these lesions are present, the risk of procedural hemorrhagic complications may be increased and risk–benefit should be weighed. MRA helps to identify the presence of significant arterial lesions. Although some experts advocate percutaneous intervention only after failed initial medical therapy (e.g., antiplatelet agent), others proceed directly to percutaneous intervention if MRA reveals significant atherosclerotic disease (≥50% stenosis) attributing to the symptoms *(40,41)*.

ASYMPTOMATIC PATIENTS

The vast majority of asymptomatic patients do not require revascularization. Asymptomatic patients with elevated risk of stroke may benefit from prophylactic percutaneous intervention, although this remains highly controversial, and expert opinion varies with respect to such high-risk indications. It has to be emphasized that the efficacy in stroke prevention and long-term outcome of such strategy have not been studied. However, given the high mortality associated with posterior circulation stroke *(1)*, it is our practice to consider percutaneous intervention of severe VA stenosis ≥70% if any of the following is present: (a) contralateral VA occlusion, (b) bilateral severe VA stenosis ≥70%, or (c) hypoplastic contralateral VA. Percutaneous intervention of a high-grade unilateral VA stenosis is even more controversial (even of the "dominant" VA), and we do not advocate routine revascularization for such lesions until more data are available.

Patient Preparation

MEDICAL PRETREATMENT

Conscious sedation is not used routinely because it may mimic some of the posterior circulation stroke symptoms. Thus, patients are kept awake during the procedure, which allows prompt assessment of neurologic symptoms.

1. Aspirin (325 mg daily) should be started at least 3 d before the procedure, and continued indefinitely *(42)*.
2. Clopidogrel (75 mg/d) should be administered 5–7 d before the procedure; a suitable alternative is to give 600-mg loading dose at least 2 h before the intervention. It should be continued for 30 d postprocedure. If drug-eluting stents are used, it should be continued for 6 mo–1 yr based on coronary intervention data.
3. Unfractionated heparin (50–100 U/kg to maintain an activated clotting time (ACT) of 250–300 s) is given intravenously after the sheath is inserted and before the angiography. Alternatively, low molecular weight heparin (enoxaparin 1 mg/kg SQ) may be used, but no published data are available. Bivalirudin may also be used in place of heparin (bolus of 0.75 mg/kg followed by an infusion of 1.75 mg/kg per hour for the duration of the procedure), although this has also not been evaluated for vertebral interventions.
4. GP IIb/IIIa inhibitors are not routinely used for elective VA intervention, unless procedural slow flow or embolization occurs, or patient presented initially with acute stroke.

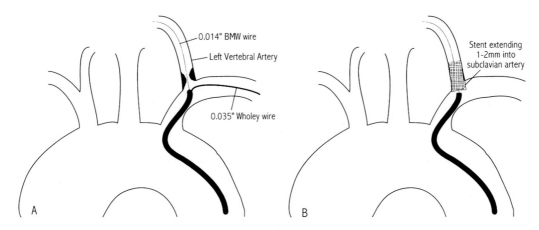

Fig. 5. Schematic diagrams of extracranial vertebral artery stenting showing (**A**) A 0.035-in. Wholey® wire in the subclavian artery for catheter stabilization, and a 0.014-in. Balance Middle Weight (BMW) wire in the vertebral artery. (**B**) Balloon-expandable stent in the ostium of the left vertebral artery, with proximal edge extending into the left subclavian artery.

VASCULAR ACCESS

Most of the interventions are performed via the femoral artery approach. A 5 Fr system is usually sufficient to perform the diagnostic angiography. Most of the interventions can be performed with a 6–8 Fr sheath. If bilateral occlusive iliac disease is present, the access may be obtained via the ipsilateral brachial artery (e.g., right vertebral, right brachial artery) or radial artery *(43,44).*

Approach to Extracranial Vertebral Stenting

Either a guide or sheath approach is suitable for treatment of V1–V3 segment stenosis. A sheath approach requires a 6 Fr system, such as a 70–90 cm length Raabe sheath (Cook, Bloomington, IN) or Shuttle sheath (Cook, Bloomington, IN). A guide approach would require typically an 8 Fr system (although a 6–7 Fr system may suffice if a coronary balloon-expandable stent is used), and guides such as JR4 or multipurpose catheters are suitable. The telescoping technique can be used to deliver either the guide or the sheath into the subclavian artery in close proximity to the VA ostium. We favor the use of a 5 Fr JR4 125 cm length catheter telescoped within the guide or sheath, to engage the subclavian artery and advanced beyond the VA ostium. The guide or sheath is then tracked over the 5 Fr JR4 close to the VA ostium. For tortuous subclavian artery, a 0.035-in. wire (e.g., Wholey®) may be left in place in the subclavian artery for support (Fig. 5a). We purposely do not selectively engage the guide or sheath into the VA, to avoid trauma or dissection of the vessel.

A 0.014-in. coronary wire (e.g., Balance Middle Weight [BMW, Guidant, Indianapolis, IN]) is then advanced into the VA and positioned distal to the stenosis. Operators may decide to use an emboli protection device (EPD) instead (see below). Predilatation is almost always done, using a monorail coronary balloon 3–4 mm in diameter. The stent diameter used is usually 3.0–6.0 mm, in a 1:1 stent-to-artery ratio to the vessel diameter.

For stenosis involving the VA ostium, a balloon-expandable stent with good radial strength is used. We favor using peripheral 0.014-in. platform stents, e.g., Genesis

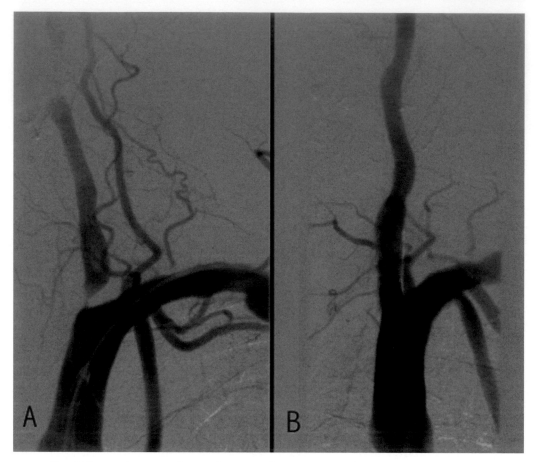

Fig. 6. Pre- and poststenting angiograms of severe ostial left vertebral artery stenosis.

(Cordis Corporation, Warren, NJ) or Herculink (Guidant, Indianapolis, IN), which has better radial force than coronary stents. It should be noted that peripheral stents are less flexible, and thus more difficult to deliver. Therefore, in patients with severe tortuosity of the vessel in whom support may be an issue, a coronary stent may be preferred. To ensure that the ostium of the artery is covered (to reduce restenosis), the stent should prolapse 1–2 mm into the subclavian artery (Fig. 5b). The balloon is then partially withdrawn into the subclavian artery, and an additional inflation done to flare the proximal edge of the stent (Fig. 6). For stenosis involving the V2 segment, a coronary balloon-expandable stent (e.g., Ultra™ [Guidant, Indianapolis, IN]) is chosen for this fixed extracranial bony location. For stenosis involving the V3 segment, a nitinol self-expanding stent (e.g., Radius stent [Boston Scientific, Natick, MA]) is recommended because of vessel tortuosity.

Approach to Intracranial Vertebral Stenting

To treat intracranial lesions, a 7 Fr 70-cm Raabe™ (Cook, Bloomington, IN) is advanced into the subclavian artery using the same telescoping approach as above. Then a 100-cm 6 Fr soft tip guide catheter (Envoy™ [Cordis, Warren, NJ]) is telescoped within the sheath and engage the VA ostium. A stiff angle tip Glidewire® (Terumo

Medical, Somerset, NJ) is then advanced into the V3 segment, and the Envoy™ tracked into the distal V2 segment. Careful flushing of the manifold is done to avoid air embolism.

A 300-cm 0.014-in. soft hydrophilic wire (Synchro™ [Boston Scientific, Natick, MA]) or Whisper® ([Guidant, Indianapolis, IN]) is advanced across the lesion and parked sufficiently distal to the lesion for support (in the proximal PCA). Because of tortuosity of the intracranial vessels, over-the-wire balloon and stent systems are preferred for better profile and trackability. We generally predilate intracranial VA lesions with small 2.0- to 3.0-mm coronary balloons (e.g., Maverick2™ [Boston Scientific, Natick, MA]), which helps with stent delivery. Stent size is chosen to match a 1:1 stent-to artery ratio. Most coronary stents can be used for the intracranial VA lesion, although we do prefer the cobalt-chromium stents (e.g., Multilink Vision™ [Guidant, Indianapolis, IN]), Driver™ ([Medtronic, Minneapolis, MN]), which have thinner struts and are more flexible and deliverable. Coronary drug eluting stents have been used to treat VA stenosis (45); however, long-term outcome data are not available.

Emboli Protection Devices

The use of EPD for extracranial ostial or proximal VA stenting is controversial and not commonly done. There are no randomized data to guide treatment; only anecdotal cases of EPD use in the vertebral circulation have been reported (46). Further, the need for EPD in the setting where there is retrograde flow in the VA (i.e., subclavian steal syndrome) (Fig. 7) has been questioned. In the classic study by Ringelstein et al., 12 patients with subclavian stenosis or occlusion with subclavian steal syndrome underwent angioplasty. Continuous ultrasound monitoring of the ipsilateral VA flow pattern showed a delay in normalization (i.e., antegrade flow) of the VA flow up to several minutes after sufficient recanalization of the subclavian artery (47). This delay of flow reversal may serve as a protective mechanism against cerebral embolization during and shortly after angioplasty of the subclavian artery. Whether this phenomenon of delayed flow reversal occurs in patients with critical proximal VA stenosis is unknown; mechanistically, the VA stenosis would have to be severe enough to have baseline retrograde flow, unless there is concomitant subclavian artery disease.

Using EPD does add additional time and challenges to the VA stenting procedure. It may be difficult to direct and advance an EPD into the VA when the guide catheter is not engaged in the VA ostium (particularly so for stenosis involving the ostium). Further, the vessel diameter at the V2 segment needs to be large enough to accommodate an EPD (e.g., FilterWire EZ device requires a minimum vessel diameter of 3.5 mm). Therefore, with the lack of evidence and the technical challenges associated with EPD use for VA stenting, it is currently not advocated unless the operator is concerned that the risk of embolization is very high (e.g., bulky, ulcerated lesions).

Complications of Vertebral Artery Stenting

SPASM AND SLOW OR NO REFLOW

Occasionally spasm develops within the VA after placement of the wire, especially if there is tortuosity of the V1 segment. The spasm usually subsides after the removal of the wire or after injection of 100–200 µg of intraarterial nitroglycerin. Slow flow may result from distal spasm, dissection, or distal embolization. If a dissection flap is clearly identified, and spasm is ruled out, an additional stent should be deployed to cover the

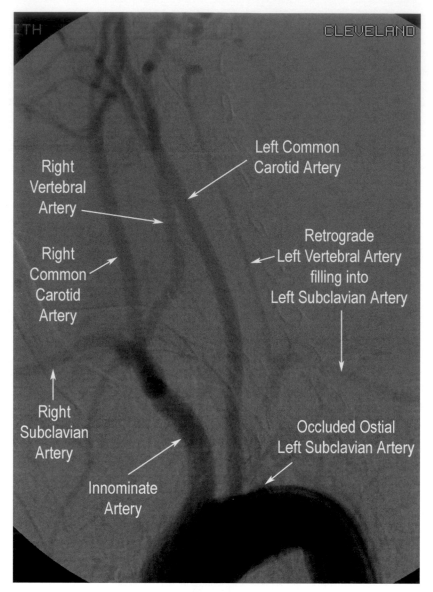

Fig. 7. Aortic arch angiogram showing occluded ostial left vertebral artery with retrograde filling of the left vertebral artery into the left subclavian artery (subclavian steal syndrome).

dissection. In the setting of distal embolization, intraarterial abciximab may be administered through an over-the-wire balloon to improve the flow.

DISTAL EMBOLIZATION

As in other angioplasty and stenting procedure, some degree of distal embolization is anticipated to occur during VA intervention. However, symptomatic cerebral embolization during VA intervention is thought to be uncommon. In a small study by Sawada et al., 12 patients undergoing VA angioplasty (no stenting) were monitored with transcranial Doppler. Intraprocedurally, only one patient had a microembolic signal during balloon deflation. There were several microembolic signals immediately postprocedure in a few patients, and this continued until 3 d postprocedure. None of these microembolic signals were associated with neurologic symptoms, and brain CT did not show any silent infarction (48). Thus, the clinical consequence of this distal cerebral embolization during VA intervention is not known.

STROKES AND TIA

Complications of TIA or stroke during VA stenting is low, reported at 0–3% (29,31). In the SSYLVIA trial whereby patients underwent intracranial or VA interventions (41/61 patients had posterior circulation lesions), procedural strokes occurred in 3% of patients, and 30-d stroke event was 6.6% (49).

IN-STENT RESTENOSIS

In-stent restenosis has been reported to range widely from 3% to 67% (30,31,35,50). Drug-eluting stents have been used in this vascular territory, as they may reduce restenosis (45,51). However, randomized trials comparing long-term patency and clinical efficacy (e.g., reducing TIA or stroke) of drug-eluting stents vs bare-metal stents are lacking. Small retrospective series suggest that restenosis in this vascular territory may not necessarily result in recurrent neurologic symptoms (29,30,35).

HYPERPERFUSION SYNDROME

This is an infrequent complication seen in patients undergoing carotid stenting or endarterectomy. There is a recent case report of hyperperfusion with bilateral thalamic hemorrhage in a patient who underwent intracranial VA stenting (52). Therefore, similar precaution with aggressive blood pressure control, as with carotid stenting, is important.

Postprocedural Care

Aggressive management of the blood pressure is mandatory. If needed, intravenous β-blockers such as metoprolol are carefully used to keep the systolic blood pressure below 140 mmHg. The use of IV nitrates is discouraged, especially in patients undergoing intracerebral intervention, as the nitrates may cause headache that may obscure the diagnosis of cerebral hemorrhage, a rare (52) but potentially catastrophic complication.

Patients should be discharged with clopidogrel (75 mg daily) for at least 1 mo with bare-metal stents, and 1 yr with drug-eluting stents (following the coronary artery intervention guidelines) (53). Aspirin (81 mg–325 mg daily) should be administered indefinitely. The use of statins in high doses (atorvastatin 80 mg daily) (as recommended for coronary artery disease) is suggested to decrease the progression of atherosclerosis (54). The use of an ACE inhibitor is also recommended.

Patients should undergo routine follow-up Doppler ultrasound for vertebral stents involving the ostial or proximal region, in the V1 or V2 segments. This should be performed every 6 mo for the first year and yearly thereafter. If the stent was deployed within the V3 or V4 segments, a transcranial Doppler may be performed. If the clinical suspicion of restenosis is high (e.g., recurrence of symptoms or a positive noninvasive test), however, repeat angiography is recommended.

CONCLUSIONS

Posterior circulation stroke and TIA are often misdiagnosed. A high index of clinical suspicion along with noninvasive tests such as MRA and Doppler ultrasound are necessary to identify patients with posterior circulation atherosclerosis. The current

interventional equipment allows treatment of most extracranial and intracranial vertebral artery lesions with great success and few complications. Studies evaluating the
long-term outcomes of percutaneous vertebral intervention are limited. Further studies
are necessary to address the clinical indications for treatment and the utility of drug-
eluting stents in this vascular territory.

REFERENCES

1. Patrick BK, Ramirez-Lassepas M, Synder BD. Temporal profile of vertebrobasilar territory infarction. Prognostic implications. Stroke 1980;11:643–648.
2. Caplan L. Posterior circulation ischemia: then, now, and tomorrow. The Thomas Willis Lecture— 2000. Stroke 2000;31:2011–2023.
3. Caplan LR, Wityk RJ, Glass TA, et al. New England Medical Center Posterior Circulation registry. Ann Neurol 2004;56:389–398.
4. Wityk RJ, Chang HM, Rosengart A, et al. Proximal extracranial vertebral artery disease in the New England Medical Center Posterior Circulation Registry. Arch Neurol 1998;55:470–478.
5. Cartlidge NE, Whisnant JP, Elveback LR. Carotid and vertebral-basilar transient cerebral ischemic attacks. A community study, Rochester, Minnesota. Mayo Clin Proc 1977;52:117–120.
6. Whisnant JP, Cartlidge NE, Elveback LR. Carotid and vertebral-basilar transient ischemic attacks: effect of anticoagulants, hypertension, and cardiac disorders on survival and stroke occurrence—a population study. Ann Neurol 1978;3:107–115.
7. Lemke AJ, Benndorf G, Liebig T, Felix R. Anomalous origin of the right vertebral artery: review of the literature and case report of right vertebral artery origin distal to the left subclavian artery. AJNR Am J Neuroradiol 1999;20:1318–1321.
8. Gluncic V, Ivkic G, Marin D, Percac S. Anomalous origin of both vertebral arteries. Clin Anat 1999;12:281–284.
9. Palmer FJ. Origin of the right vertebral artery from the right common carotid artery: angiographic demonstration of three cases. Br J Radiol 1977;50:185–187.
10. Shrontz C, Dujovny M, Ausman JI, et al. Surgical anatomy of the arteries of the posterior fossa. J Neurosurg 1986;65:540–544.
11. Wollschlaeger G, Wollschlaeger PB, Lucas FV, Lopez VF. Experience and result with postmortem cerebral angiography performed as routine procedure of the autopsy. Am J Roentgenol Radium Ther Nucl Med 1967;101:68–87.
12. Baskaya M, Coscarella E, Gomez F, Morcos J. Surgical and angiographic anatomy of the posterior communicating and anterior choroidal arteries. Neuroanatomy 2004;3:38–42.
13. Bisaria KK. Anomalies of the posterior communicating artery and their potential clinical significance. J Neurosurg 1984;60:572–576.
14. Wells CE. The cerebral circulation. The clinical significance of current concepts. Arch Neurol 1960;3:319–331.
15. Schomer DF, Marks MP, Steinberg GK, et al. The anatomy of the posterior communicating artery as a risk factor for ischemic cerebral infarction. N Engl J Med 1994;330:1565–1570.
16. Ackerstaff RG, Hoeneveld H, Slowikowski JM, Moll FL, Eikelboom BC, Ludwig JW. Ultrasonic duplex scanning in atherosclerotic disease of the innominate, subclavian and vertebral arteries. A comparative study with angiography. Ultrasound Med Biol 1984;10:409–418.
17. de Bray JM, Pasco A, Tranquart F, et al. Accuracy of color-Doppler in the quantification of proximal vertebral artery stenoses. Cerebrovasc Dis 2001;11:335–340.
18. Cloud GC, Markus HS. Vertebral artery stenosis. Curr Treat Options Cardiovasc Med 2004;6: 121–127.
19. Kuhl V, Tettenborn B, Eicke BM, Visbeck A, Meckes S. Color-coded duplex ultrasonography of the origin of the vertebral artery: normal values of flow velocities. J Neuroimaging 2000;10:17–21.
20. Cloud GC, Markus HS. Diagnosis and management of vertebral artery stenosis. Qjm 2003;96:27–54.
21. Clifton AG. MR angiography. Br Med Bull 2000;56:367–377.
22. Randoux B, Marro B, Koskas F, Chiras J, Dormont D, Marsault C. Proximal great vessels of aortic arch: comparison of three-dimensional gadolinium-enhanced MR angiography and digital subtraction angiography. Radiology 2003;229:697–702.
23. Bhadelia RA, Bengoa F, Gesner L, et al. Efficacy of MR angiography in the detection and characterization of occlusive disease in the vertebrobasilar system. J Comput Assist Tomogr 2001;25:458–465.

24. Graf J, Skutta B, Kuhn FP, Ferbert A. Computed tomographic angiography findings in 103 patients following vascular events in the posterior circulation: potential and clinical relevance. J Neurol 2000;247:760–766.

25. Fayed AM, White CJ, Ramee SR, Jenkins JS, Collins TJ. Carotid and cerebral angiography performed by cardiologists: cerebrovascular complications. Catheter Cardiovasc Interv 2002;55:277–280.

26. Chimowitz MI, Lynn MJ, Howlett-Smith H, et al. Comparison of warfarin and aspirin for symptomatic intracranial arterial stenosis. N Engl J Med 2005;352:1305–1316.

27. Carney AL, Anderson EM, Martinez DM. Advances in vertebral artery surgery at the skull base. Tex Heart Inst J 1986;13:83–90.

28. Berguer R, Flynn LM, Kline RA, Caplan L. Surgical reconstruction of the extracranial vertebral artery: management and outcome. J Vasc Surg 2000;31:9–18.

29. Chastain HD, 2nd, Campbell MS, Iyer S, et al. Extracranial vertebral artery stent placement: in-hospital and follow-up results. J Neurosurg 1999;91:547–552.

30. Albuquerque FC, Fiorella D, Han P, Spetzler RF, McDougall CG. A reappraisal of angioplasty and stenting for the treatment of vertebral origin stenosis. Neurosurgery 2003;53:607–614; discussion 614–616.

31. Jenkins JS, White CJ, Ramee SR, et al. Vertebral artery stenting. Catheter Cardiovasc Interv 2001;54:1–5.

32. Hankey GJ, Coward LJ, Featherstone RL, Brown MM. Percutaneous transluminal angioplasty and stenting for vertebral artery stenosis. Stroke 2005;36:2047–2048.

33. Crawley F, Brown MM, Clifton AG. Angioplasty and stenting in the carotid and vertebral arteries. Postgrad Med J 1998;74:7–10.

34. Storey GS, Marks MP, Dake M, Norbash AM, Steinberg GK. Vertebral artery stenting following percutaneous transluminal angioplasty. Technical note. J Neurosurg 1996;84:883–887.

35. Stenting of Symptomatic Atherosclerotic Lesions in the Vertebral or Intracranial Arteries (SSYLVIA): study results. Stroke 2004;35:1388–1392.

36. Higashida RT, Furlan AJ, Roberts H, et al. Trial design and reporting standards for intra-arterial cerebral thrombolysis for acute ischemic stroke. Stroke 2003;34:e109–e137.

37. Lin DD, Gailloud P, Beauchamp NJ, Aldrich EM, Wityk RJ, Murphy KJ. Combined stent placement and thrombolysis in acute vertebrobasilar ischemic stroke. AJNR Am J Neuroradiol 2003;24:1827–1833.

38. Nomura M, Hashimoto N, Nishi S, Akiyama Y. Percutaneous transluminal angioplasty for intracranial vertebral and/or basilar artery stenosis. Clin Radiol 1999;54:521–527.

39. Deshmukh VR, Fiorella DJ, Albuquerque FC, et al. Intra-arterial thrombolysis for acute ischemic stroke: preliminary experience with platelet glycoprotein IIb/IIIa inhibitors as adjunctive therapy. Neurosurgery 2005;56:46–54; discussion 54–55.

40. Barakate MS, Snook KL, Harrington TJ, Sorby W, Pik J, Morgan MK. Angioplasty and stenting in the posterior cerebral circulation. J Endovasc Ther 2001;8:558–565.

41. Wehman JC, Hanel RA, Guidot CA, Guterman LR, Hopkins LN. Atherosclerotic occlusive extracranial vertebral artery disease: indications for intervention, endovascular techniques, short-term and long-term results. J Interv Cardiol 2004;17:219–232.

42. Bhatt DL, Kapadia SR, Bajzer CT, et al. Dual antiplatelet therapy with clopidogrel and aspirin after carotid artery stenting. J Invasive Cardiol 2001;13:767–771.

43. Fessler RD, Wakhloo AK, Lanzino G, Guterman LR, Hopkins LN. Transradial approach for vertebral artery stenting: technical case report. Neurosurgery 2000;46:1524–1527; discussion 1527–1528.

44. Bendok BR, Przybylo JH, Parkinson R, Hu Y, Awad IA, Batjer HH. Neuroendovascular interventions for intracranial posterior circulation disease via the transradial approach: technical case report. Neurosurgery 2005;56:E626; discussion E626.

45. Abou-Chebl A, Bashir Q, Yadav JS. Drug-eluting stents for the treatment of intracranial atherosclerosis: initial experience and midterm angiographic follow-up. Stroke 2005;36:e165–e168.

46. Mintz EP, Gruberg L, Kouperberg E, Beyar R. Vertebral artery stenting using distal emboli protection and transcranial Doppler. Catheter Cardiovasc Interv 2004;61:12–15.

47. Ringelstein EB, Zeumer H. Delayed reversal of vertebral artery blood flow following percutaneous transluminal angioplasty for subclavian steal syndrome. Neuroradiology 1984;26:189–198.

48. Sawada M, Hashimoto N, Nishi S, Akiyama Y. Detection of embolic signals during and after percutaneous transluminal angioplasty of subclavian and vertebral arteries using transcranial Doppler ultrasonography. Neurosurgery 1997;41:535–540; discussion 540–541.

49. Wiviott SD, Antman EM. Clopidogrel resistance: a new chapter in a fast-moving story. Circulation 2004;109:3064–3067.

50. Cloud GC, Crawley F, Clifton A, McCabe DJ, Brown MM, Markus HS. Vertebral artery origin angio-plasty and primary stenting: safety and restenosis rates in a prospective series. J Neurol Neurosurg Psychiatry 2003;74:586–590.
51. Levy EI, Hanel RA, Howington JU, et al. Sirolimus-eluting stents in the canine cerebral vasculature: a prospective, randomized, blinded assessment of safety and vessel response. J Neurosurg 2004;100:688–694.
52. Rezende MT, Spelle L, Mounayer C, Piotin M, Abud DG, Moret J. Hyperperfusion syndrome after stenting for intracranial vertebral stenosis. Stroke 2006;37:e12–e14.
53. Steinhubl SR, Berger PB, Mann JT, 3rd, et al. Early and sustained dual oral antiplatelet therapy fol-lowing percutaneous coronary intervention: a randomized controlled trial. Jama 2002;288:2411–2420.
54. Nissen SE. Effect of intensive lipid lowering on progression of coronary atherosclerosis: evidence for an early benefit from the Reversal of Atherosclerosis with Aggressive Lipid Lowering (REVERSAL) trial. Am J Cardiol 2005;96:61F–68F.

15 Endovascular Treatment of Acute Ischemic Stroke

Mikhael Mazighi, MD, Qasim Bashir, MD, and Alex Abou-Chebl, MD

CONTENTS

Summary

Acute ischemic stroke is caused by a variety of mechanisms including cardiac embolism, atherosclerosis/thrombosis, intracranial atherosclerosis, or penetrating artery disease. The highly complex clinical manifestations of ischemia, which are often unique to the individual patient, the wide variety of medical conditions that often accompany stroke, and diverse anatomical and technical factors all combine to make each patient unique in terms of the endovascular approach to treatment.

Key Words: Endovascular treatment, intraarterial thrombolytic, intravenous thrombolytic, ischemic stroke, mechanical embolectomy.

INTRODUCTION

Morbidity and mortality from stroke remain a major public health problem, as stroke represents the leading cause of disability and the third leading cause of death. There are approx 700,000 new cases of stroke in the United States each year (1), but unlike an acute coronary artery syndrome, which in the vast majority of patients is the result of an atherosclerotic plaque rupture, acute ischemic stroke (IS) is caused by a variety of mechanisms including cardiac embolism, atherosclerosis/thrombosis, intracranial atherosclerosis or penetrating artery disease (i.e., lipohyalinosis). The highly complex clinical manifestations of ischemia, which are often unique to the individual patient, the wide variety of medical conditions that often accompany stroke, and diverse anatomical and technical factors all combine to make each patient unique in terms of the endovascular approach to treatment (2).

From: *Contemporary Cardiology: Handbook of Complex Percutaneous Carotid Intervention*
Edited by: J. Saw, J. E. Exaire, D. S. Lee, and S. Yadav © Humana Press Inc., Totowa, NJ

Each patient problem must be tempered by the unique qualities of the intracranial cerebral vasculature, which make cerebrovascular interventions very complex and dangerous in ways that are different from cardiac and peripheral vascular interventions. Unlike coronary arteries, which consist of thickly muscular vessels that have an adventitia and are surrounded by the myocardium, the cerebral arteries are very thin and have no external elastic lamina or adventitia and course in the subarachnoid space. Combined with the great deal of tortuosity in their proximal segments, the fragility of the cerebral arteries greatly increases the risk of vessel injury and perforation during attempted endovascular interventions. The consequences of even a mild vessel injury can produce catastrophic results because intracerebral hemorrhage (subarachnoid or intraparenchymal) can result in a rapid increase in the intracranial pressure because of the noncompliant skull. Although all tissues can potentially be affected by embolization, the brain is uniquely sensitive even at the nearly microscopic artery and arteriolar level. The production of embolic debris during endovascular therapy, even if microscopic, can occlude the smaller vessels, which are less likely to have collateral flow than the more proximal larger vessels, and can lead to clinically apparent ischemia. These qualities should be considered in every case and appropriate measures taken to decrease the risk of complications.

CEREBROVASCULAR CIRCULATION

The major cerebral vessels most commonly involved in the pathogenesis of IS include the intracranial internal carotid artery (ICA), the middle cerebral artery (MCA), the anterior cerebral artery (ACA), the intracranial vertebral artery (VA), the basilar artery (BA), and the posterior cerebral artery (PCA) (Fig. 1). These vessels are connected at the base of the brain with three anastomotic channels, the paired posterior communicating arteries (PCom) and the single anterior communicating artery (ACom), that complete the Circle of Willis, a major source of potential collateral blood supply. The cerebral arteries lose their adventitia and external elastic lamina within 1 cm of entering the skull base, and follow their course on the surface of the brain within the subarachnoid space; most muscular arteries elsewhere in the body have dual elastic lamina and substantial adventitia. As a result, perforation or rupture of an artery often results in intracranial hemorrhage (ICH). Intracranial hemorrhage can lead to a rapid and marked elevation of intracranial pressure (ICP), which in turn can lead to the cessation of cerebral blood flow when the ICP approaches mean arterial pressure (MAP), or to herniation and brainstem compression leading to immediate tissue injury and death *(3,4)*. Another important and unique characteristic of the brain and cerebral circulation is that the brain is extremely sensitive to embolization. In the peripheral tissues, except for massive embolization in a patient with poor collaterals, embolization is not often of clinical consequence.

With the preceding in mind, the following principles should guide all interventional procedures on the cerebral vasculature:

- Meticulous technique must be used in every aspect of the procedure to minimize the risk of embolization—all air, dried blood and contrast must be removed from all equipment, all flushes and contrast should be heparinized unless the patient has a heparin allergy, endovascular equipment should not be kept in the cerebrovascular circulation any longer than absolutely necessary, and catheter and wire exchanges should be minimized.
- Finesse and gentle technique rather than brute force should be used and stents and balloons should be sized accurately to the vessel being treated and should never be oversized.

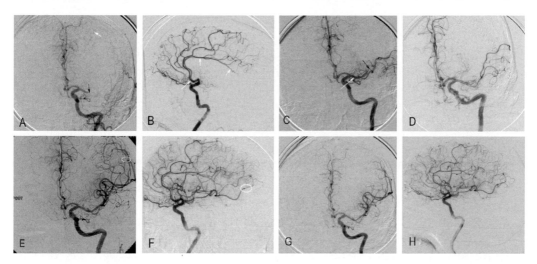

Fig. 1. Intraarterial thrombolysis. A 58-yr-old man presented 3 h after onset with a severe left middle cerebral artery (MCA) syndrome. Computed tomography of the brain was negative for hemorrhage or acute ischemic changes. An urgent angiogram revealed a left MCA occlusion (*black arrow* in **A** [AP angiogram]) with some pial collaterals from the anterior cerebral artery (*white arrow* in **A**). In **B** (lateral angiogram) note the absence of MCA branches and filling of only the anterior cerebral artery territory (*arrows*). Internal carotid artery access was obtained as described in the text and a microcatheter was placed within the MCA thrombus. One unit of reteplase and 1/4 bolus of abciximab were injected into the thrombus. Within 15 min there was recanalization of the MCA trunk (*white arrow* in **C**) but a persistent thrombus in the inferior division (*black arrow* in **C**). The microcatheter was then repositioned within the inferior division (**D**) and an additional 1 U of reteplase and 1/4 U of abciximab were injected. Within 10 min there was complete recanalization of all of the proximal branches (**E** [AP image] and **F** [lateral image]). There was, however, a single, small, distal thrombus in an angular artery branch (*white circle* in **E** and **F**). No more interventions were performed and within another 10 min there was complete recanalization of all branches (**G** and **H**). The patient began to improve immediately and returned to normal within 2 d.

ACUTE ISCHEMIC STROKE TREATMENT

Unlike patients with acute myocardial ischemia, there has been only one randomized study of an endovascular acute stroke treatment *(5)* and only one successful trial of intravenous thrombolysis *(6)*. Most of the data on the endovascular approaches to acute stroke treatment are from small case series or nonrandomized safety studies, all of which have differed greatly in their methodologies and patient populations studied. As a consequence there are no standardized or widely accepted endovascular techniques for the treatment of acute IS. These difficulties are all attributable not only to the risk of ICH but also to the heterogeneous nature of stroke. In contrast with the most common cause of the acute coronary artery syndrome, that is, atherosclerotic plaque rupture and thrombosis, acute strokes have a number of potential causes. Eighty-five percent of strokes are ischemic and the remainder are hemorrhagic. The cause is due to cardiogenic embolism in 20%, atherosclerosis/thrombosis (i.e., artery to artery embolism from cervical atherosclerosis or intracranial stenosis leading to occlusion or embolism) in 20%, and penetrating artery disease, otherwise known as small-vessel disease, in 25%. Thirty percent of strokes have no identifiable cause. Therefore no single approach or pharmacologic agent will be effective in all cases and treatment must be individualized based on the needs of each patient and on the probable mechanism of ischemia.

To date there has been only one FDA-approved treatment for acute IS (intravenous [IV] administration of recombinant tissue plasminogen activator [rt-PA]), and only one randomized trial of endovascular treatment for acute IS (PROACT II [Prolyse in Acute Cerebral Thromboembolism II]) *(5)*. PROACT II is the only placebo-controlled, randomized trial that evaluated the safety and efficacy of intraarterial (IA) thrombolysis. PROACT II studied the effects of recombinant pro-urokinase (r-pro-UK) in 180 patients with MCA occlusion. Despite showing a 66% TIMI II or III recanalization rate and a 15% absolute benefit (58% relative benefit) for the treatment group over placebo, the symptomatic hemorrhage rate was only 10% (for comparison the ICH rate in the definitive IV rt-PA study that led to FDA approval was 6%) *(6)*. Although the PROACT II trial was positive, IA thrombolysis is not yet FDA approved treatment despite the fact that IA thrombolysis has superior recanalization efficacy (~70%, compared to ~34% with IV thrombolysis) *(7)*. There have been no randomized or direct studies of the clinical efficacy of IA compared with IV thrombolysis; it is generally accepted, however, that larger vessels and greater clot burdens (e.g., occlusions of the ICA, MCA, or BA) are more resistant to thrombolysis, particularly IV thrombolysis and that IA thrombolysis is the best option for those patients *(8,9)*. Most clinicians accept the PROACT II results as a proof of the safety and efficacy of IA thrombolysis for strokes of less than 6 h duration, and many have adopted the "PROACT protocol" for IA thrombolysis (of course, other thrombolytic agents are used in place of r-pro-UK).

The PROACT protocol was remarkable for its stringent inclusion criteria and standardized protocol. All patients received the same dose of periprocedural heparin, which consisted of a 2000 U bolus at the start of the procedure and was then followed by a 500 U/h infusion for 4 h only. The r-pro-UK dose was 9 mg infused over 2 h in all patients irrespective of the clot burden, and mechanical disruption of the thrombus was not permitted. As a result, although there was nearly 70% recanalization at 2 h, the complete, TIMI 3 recanalization rate was only 19% *(5)*.

In addition to the longer time window for treatment (6 h for IA and 3 h for IV) and the higher recanalization rates, IA thrombolysis is useful in circumstances where IV thrombolysis is contraindicated (such as for patients with recent noncerebral hemorrhage, major organ surgery or arterial puncture, and patients on systemic anticoagulation). Although the risk of hemorrhage exists with IA thrombolysis in these circumstances, in general smaller doses of thrombolytics are needed so the risks are minimized *(10)*.

Patient Selection

All patients should be evaluated clinically and with laboratory tests and cerebral imaging before an intervention is contemplated. Clinical assessments of stroke severity are typically performed using the National Institutes of Health Stroke Scale (NIHSS) *(11)*, which has been validated as a reliable tool for this task. This scale, which ranges from 0 (normal) to 42 (no neurologic function), is based on a 12-item focused neurologic examination. In general, strokes in the 0–3 range are considered minor, those between 4 and 7 are considered mild, those between 8 and 15 are moderate, and strokes with scores of >15 are severe. The NIHSS value can also suggest the size of the vessel involved and has a prognostic value. Deficits with a score of <4 are more likely to resolve completely (these patients should not be considered for IA thrombolysis because their the prognosis for recovery is usually good and the probability of finding a large artery occlusion that would be amenable to IA thrombolysis is small), whereas patients with a score >20 are less likely to derive benefit from any treatment, including IV and IA thrombolysis *(5)*. Patients with a score of 8–20 are the most likely to benefit from intervention and are also less likely to have hemorrhagic transformation, so they are the ideal group of patients to select for IA thrombolysis.

The time of stroke onset must be known with certainty before an intervention can be performed because the duration of ischemia is a predictor of prognosis and the risk of ICH *(12,13)*. In most circumstances 6 h appears to be the upper limit for safe intervention. Despite the 6-h window the earlier the treatment can be started, the better the prognosis.

It is of great value to determine the likely etiology of the stroke before beginning the intervention, to allow as much planning as possible. This is because the approach to the patient with a fresh cardioembolic stroke may be different than that for a patient with a long atherosclerotic ICA occlusion. Although there is no completely reliable means of determining etiology, particularly without angiography, there may be historical or clinical clues that may be of value. The presence of atrial fibrillation or a history of it in someone who is not anticoagulated greatly increases the likelihood that this arrhythmia is the cause. Similarly a history of vasculopathy (e.g., known coronary artery disease, peripheral vascular disease), especially if there is known carotid artery disease, should raise the possibility of atherothrombosis as the mechanism of stroke. In African Americans and Asians who have no cardiac history but have vascular risk factors (particularly diabetes and renal failure), there is a high likelihood that intracranial atherosclerosis and thrombosis will be the mechanism of stroke. Therefore, as much clinical history as possible should be obtained before, but without delaying the intervention.

A computerized tomographic (CT) scan of the brain is mandatory in all patients presenting with acute IS. CT is currently the standard means of evaluating the brain in the setting of acute IS primarily because of its high sensitivity and specificity for ICH. Magnetic resonance imaging (MRI) is a more sensitive and specific tool for the assessment of cerebral ischemia and can also provide data on the viability of brain tissue as well as the area of brain at risk. The major limitation of MRI is the prolonged imaging and processing time (up to 15–30 min or longer) compared with CT, which can be performed within seconds on the latest generation of multidetector spiral scanners. A full discussion of the merits of one imaging modality over another is beyond the scope of this chapter. The interventionist should therefore work in concert with a colleague in neurology who is familiar with the evaluation of stroke patients to determine the best imaging study and to determine which patients are candidates for intervention.

Indications and Contraindications for Intraarterial Thrombolysis

Table 1 lists the indications and contraindications to IA thrombolytics. The contraindications to IA thrombolysis are all based on the need to decrease the risk of ICH. A history of ICH at any time in the recent or remote past should be considered an absolute contraindication in most cases. Similarly, patients with Alzheimer's disease who are predisposed to ICH because of amyloid angiopathy should be considered as very high risk for IA thrombolysis. Other factors such as patient age >80 yr old; elevated serum glucose level; active treatment with heparin or a heparinoid; or therapy with high-dose aspirin, clopidogrel, or platelet glycoprotein (GP) IIb/IIIa receptor antagonists should be considered as potential contraindications for intraarterial thrombolysis. The clinician deciding on whether to treat an individual patient or not should weigh all of these factors

Table 1
Indications and Contraindications for Intraarterial Thrombolysis

Indications

- Acute, ischemic stroke <6 h in duration
- Significant stroke (i.e., disabling or life-threatening)
- Suspected occlusion of a large artery (i.e., nonlacunar stroke syndrome)
- No hemorrhage on screening CT scan

Contraindications

- Intracerebral hemorrhage is suspected or evident on CT
- Initial CT scan shows evidence of acute ischemia in a large portion of the affected territory (i.e., more than one third of the middle cerebral artery territory)
- History of intracranial or subarachnoid hemorrhage
- Presence of an arteriovenous malformation or large thrombosed aneurysm (non-thrombosed or unruptured aneurysms are not absolute contraindications to thrombolysis)
- Uncontrolled hypertension >185/110 mm Hg
- History of Alzheimer's dementia
- Stroke duration unknown or >6 h
- Recent stroke within 3 mo
- Bleeding diathesis, INR >1.7, or thrombocytopenia <100,000 cells/mm^3

together. For example, an octogenarian with no other risk factors and stroke duration of 3 h may be a better candidate than a 55-yr-old who is receiving dual antiplatelet therapy with aspirin and clopidogrel who also has profound hyperglycemia and elevated blood pressure who presents at 5.5 h after stroke onset with some evidence of ischemia on CT scan.

INTERVENTIONAL APPROACH

Diagnostic Angiography

Access is obtained rapidly via the femoral artery and a 5 Fr diagnostic catheter is used for diagnostic angiography. If time permits, an arch angiogram should be performed to assess the tortuosity of the vessels and the complexity to engage the symptomatic vessel. This step will determine the equipment used for access. If the ICA or MCA are the symptomatic vessels, ipsilateral common carotid artery (CCA) angiography should be performed, as well as angiography of the carotid bifurcation and ICA origin. The intracranial ICA and MCA are best visualized with both an antero–posterior (AP) image (with slight, 10–15°, of cranial angulation) and a true lateral image. For suspected ischemia in the vertebrobasilar (VB) circulation, the subclavian artery should be cannulated first and the ostium of the VA visualized. The left subclavian and VA are usually more easily cannulated than the right VA. If the left VA cannot be found arising from the subclavian artery, the right subclavian artery should be cannulated and angiography of the right VA then performed. Of note, the left VA rarely can arise from the aorta, usually in between the left common carotid and left subclavian artery origins. In addition, many individuals have a dominant VA on one side, with the other smaller VA ending in the posterior inferior cerebellar artery (PICA), which does not contribute significant flow to the BA and the brainstem. Lastly, the VA supplies small arterial feeders, which arise medially from its cervical portion, to the anterior spinal artery; therefore the wire tip should be pointed laterally when possible to avoid precipitation of a spinal cord infarct.

When performing digital subtraction angiography, image capture should be continued until the end of the venous phase. Branch occlusions may be indicated only angiographically by delayed arterial filling and emptying, which at times can be subtle. Following angiography of the symptomatic vessel, cannulation of the contralateral carotid artery and at least one vertebral artery, whichever is appropriate, should be performed to search for evidence of collateral blood flow from either the ACom, the PCom, or pial collaterals from the PCA to the MCA or ACA, or vice versa. The presence of collaterals is a positive prognostic sign and their presence suggests a high probability of recanalization success with a lower risk of ICH. Conversely, their absence suggests a high likelihood of infarction of the affected territory even if rapid recanalization is achieved (14). In addition, angiography is performed to exclude the presence of large, thrombosed aneurysms or arteriovenous malformations or vascular brain tumors, all of which should be considered as contraindications to thrombolysis because of the risk of ICH. Spontaneous dissections of the extracranial or intracranial vessels do not represent contraindications to thrombolysis; however, these are conditions that do increase the risk of subarachnoid hemorrhage (even without the use of thrombolytics and anticoagulants) and can make access to the intracranial vessels difficult and risky and should be handled with extreme caution.

Access

Because of the tortuosity and sharp angles of the cervicocranial vessels the most critical technical factor that determines procedural failure or success is stable access to the site of occlusion or stenosis. In patients who have straight vessels both proximally and distally, a 6 Fr guide catheter in the distal cervical ICA or distal cervical VA provides sufficient support to allow equipment access to the most distal intracranial vessels. Roadmapping or trace subtraction should be considered, as they greatly increase the margin of safety. In patients with tortuous vessels the approach may be different. Proximal tortuosity prevents the effective transmission of kinetic energy to the tips of wires and catheters, which when combined with distal tortuosity makes delivery very difficult, particularly for stiff equipment such as balloon-mounted stents. In addition to the tortuosity, the vessels in the elderly are stiff and noncompliant, which makes equipment navigation that much more difficult. For this reason a long sheath should be preferentially used: 7 Fr or 8 Fr for enough support, considering a 55-cm-length sheath if there is extreme iliac tortuosity or abdominal aortic dilatation (but with straight cerebral vessels), or a 70- to 80-cm length sheath if the tortuosity is in the great vessels (90 cm sheaths are too long and will not permit sufficiently high guide-catheter placement since most guide catheters are only 100 cm in length).

For ICA and MCA interventions, the sheath should be placed in the distal CCA. Sheath placement that high within the CCA carries risk of vessel injury and the approach we have found to be most effective and safest is to place in the external carotid artery (ECA) a stiff, angled 0.035-in. hydrophilic wire. Roadmapping makes this procedure very simple. After the wire is placed in the ECA, a 5 Fr diagnostic catheter is inserted into the ECA and the hydrophilic wire is exchanged for a super-stiff 0.035-in. wire; this wire will straighten out most tortuous segments and will give sufficient support even for cannulation of a right CCA that is arising from a very low-lying innominate artery. The diagnostic catheter is then removed. The sheath exchange is carried out over the super-stiff wire, keeping it securely within the ECA. The sheath should be inserted with its introducer securely in place rather than over the diagnostic or guide catheters to avoid dissection of the CCA. The introducers are quite stiff and caution should be used not to dissect the ICA as the tip approaches the CCA bifurcation. With back traction maintained on the sheath to prevent it from "jumping" into the ICA, the stiff wire and introducer are carefully removed after the sheath is placed just below the carotid bifurcation.

For VB interventions a variation of the procedure described above can be used but since the sheath is needed only within the proximal subclavian, if there is no severe innominate or subclavian tortuosity, there is no need for exchange of the hydrophilic wire for a super-stiff wire. This wire is placed in the axillary artery and unless a super-stiff wire is needed, the sheath can be inserted over it. If a super-stiff wire is needed, then as was described for CCA placement, a 5 Fr diagnostic catheter is placed distally in the axillary or distal subclavian artery and the wires exchanged. VB access can be quite difficult if there is severe tortuosity as even a rigid sheath may have a tendency to fall out of the subclavian, particularly the right subclavian. In those cases there are two options. The first is to place a 0.018-in. stiff wire or 0.035-in. nonhydrophilic wire distally within the axillary or brachial arteries for sheath support. If that is not adequate and stable access cannot be obtained via a femoral approach then the second option is to obtain brachial access with insertion of a 6 Fr sheath into the subclavian just distal to the VA origin.

Following the sheath exchange, a 2000 U bolus of heparin is given and is followed by a 500 U/h infusion for 4 h. This was the heparin regimen that was validated in the PROACT II trial (5). This regimen is the most commonly used, but in our experience higher doses of heparin with an activated clotting time (ACT) of one to two times baseline or a value of 250–300 s is often needed, particularly if mechanical interventions are attempted. Lower doses of heparin are used if the patient was treated with GP IIb/IIIa inhibitors and/or thrombolytics, if there is no underlying endothelial injury, if the patient has had recalcitrant hypertension or if a large infarct is suspected. The heparin is reversed with protamine sulfate at the end of the procedure.

A 6 Fr soft-tipped and curved guide catheter is then placed within the distal cervical ICA or VA. This is typically performed over a soft, hydrophilic 0.035-in. wire or over a small coronary balloon, which was been advanced over a 0.014-in. wire. If resistance is felt, force should not be used to advance the guide; rather, a very gentle injection of contrast can be performed to look for spasm or dissection. These vessels have a high propensity for spasm, particularly in younger patients. If spasm is found, then nitroglycerin 200–400 μg should be given directly into the vessel or the guide catheter can be withdrawn slightly to alleviate the spasm. With the availability of embolectomy devices designed specifically for the neurovascular tree, placement of a balloon occlusion guide catheter rather than a conventional neuroguide may be prudent in cases of cardioembolism. Doing so will facilitate embolectomy and obviate the need to exchange guide catheters in the middle of the case.

Following proximal access, a 0.014-in. hydrophilic, soft-tipped wire should be passed through the stenotic or occluded segment and placed distally. Crossing an occluded segment should be performed very carefully, remembering that the intracranial vessels have no adventitia and are easily perforated. The wire tip should always be free and mobile: any buckling or loss of ability to torque the wire tip should raise the possibility of subintimal migration. In advancing the wire through an occluded segment the operator must also be aware of the normal branches arising from the occluded segment and their usual course so that the wire is not directed inadvertently into one of the small branches which can easily be perforated. The essential branches to be aware of are the ophthalmic artery arising anteriorly from the ICA, the PCom arising posteriorly from the carotid siphon, and the smaller anterior choroidal also arising posteriorly just above the PCom. The MCA has multiple perforators that arise superiorly (dorsally) along the length of the main trunk; the wire tip should be kept pointing downward in the AP view when it is being passed through the MCA trunk. The MCA bifurcation can be variable in its location: it can bifurcate normally with a long trunk and two main branches arising just as the MCA enters the Sylvian fissure and takes an upward (dorsal) course or the bifurcation can be early or even be a tri- or quadrifurcation. Often the anterior temporal artery can arise anteroinferiorly (ventrally) from the mid to distal MCA trunk.

The VA has several muscular branches in its distal cervical segments and the PICA can often arise extracranially at the C1 level and should not be cannulated inadvertently. Intracranially the VA gives off the PICA dorsally and just before the VB junction each VA gives off a very small vessel, the anterior spinal artery to the spinal cord, dorsomedially. The BA has multiple nearly microscopic perforating branches posteriorly (dorsal) that supply the pons and midbrain, as well as the large paired anterior inferior cerebellar arteries (AICA) arising laterally at the juncture of the proximal and middle thirds and the paired superior cerebellar arteries (SCA) arising laterally at the BA terminus just before the BA bifurcation into the PCA. The wire tip should be carefully maneuvered into the third-order MCA and PCA branches for adequate support. If roadmapping is available and sufficient flow, either antegrade or retrograde, is present, the wire should be placed into the largest possible branch. Careful shaping of the wire tip is essential; not enough of a tip can lead to perforation and the inability to navigate very tortuous vessels and too much of a curve on the tip can make manipulation of the wire difficult in the smaller distal branches. A two-component curve on the wire tip, a very small and short (1–2 mm) distal curve with a slightly longer secondary curve 1–2 mm more proximally, is highly effective.

Wire placement can be greatly facilitated by loading the wire through a microcatheter or small balloon angioplasty catheter, which are then advanced with the wire leading. If there is a low likelihood of underlying atherosclerotic plaque as the cause of the vessel occlusion and thrombolysis is the first planned treatment, then a microcatheter may be more appropriate so that thrombolysis can be immediately begun. However if there is a high likelihood of underlying stenosis then loading the wire through a small 1.5- to 2.5-mm diameter, flexible balloon catheter will allow for more rapid angioplasty. In almost all intracranial interventions, an over-the-wire balloon catheter is preferred to a rapid-exchange or monorail system because it permits wire exchanges and is generally more deliverable to tortuous segments. Also, if needed, angiography can be performed through the central lumen of the balloon catheter just as with a microcatheter. Regardless of whether a microcatheter or balloon is used, the device should be advanced into the occluded segment and thrombus.

Recanalization Technique

Several approaches to achieve recanalization have been described. Most of the published series have reported on the use of thrombolytics alone, similar to the PROACT II protocol, but using a different agent *(15)*. More recently some have reported on the use of a combination of pharmacological agents, while a few series have described a purely mechanical approach (16). A multimodal approach combining multiple pharmacological agents and mechanical disruption may be superior to a single modality approach because IS is heterogeneous (Fig. 1) (17); not all thrombi are composed of the same platelet and fibrin components, and not all emboli are thrombi. Therefore, the treatment should be adapted to the needs of each patient. For example, in cases with a high likelihood of cardioembolism as the cause of the stroke, higher doses of thrombolytics may be preferred, whereas in patients with an atherothrombotic lesion GP IIb/IIIa inhibitors may be combined with thrombolytics and angioplasty or even stenting. However, in clinical practice, the first-line treatment remains the infusion of a single thrombolytic agent. This approach may be performed with significant differences in the technique. Some interventionists do advance the microcatheter distally to the occluded segment with the goal to define the distal most extent of the occlusion or to permit infusion of thrombolytic agent distally. This approach carries a risk of distal embolization, so another approach is to place the microcatheter within the thrombus and to infuse the pharmacologic agents directly into the thrombus. Other aspects of IA thrombolysis that vary from one center to another include the choice of pharmacological agent as well as the dose, the rate of infusion, and the duration of the infusion.

The most widely used thrombolytic agent is rt-PA (18,19), but other agents are also used including streptokinase, urokinase, reteplase, and TNK-ase (16,20,21). The only agent whose efficacy and safety were validated in a controlled trial, r-pro-UK, is unfortunately not commercially available. One agent in particular, streptokinase, is no longer used and should be avoided, because in early studies it was associated with excessive risks of ICH (4). Although rt-PA is the most commonly used, there is a suggestion that it may not be ideal because it has some neurotoxic effects, and it may be associated with higher risks of ICH (22). The optimal dose of each agent is unknown because of the significant variation in the doses used in the various reported series: 5–50 mg of rt-PA, 250,000–1,000,000 U of urokinase, and 1–8 U of reteplase. In general lower doses are preferred and excessive dosing may not only increase the risk of ICH, it may lead to a paradoxical increase in thrombosis. The doses of each agent should be adjusted to the needs of each patient based on the presence or absence of several patient characteristics that are associated with higher risks of ICH or poor prognosis: increasing patient age (especially >80 yr), hypertension (especially if >185/110 mmHg and if difficult to control), elevated serum glucose, duration of ischemia >4 h, the absence of collateral blood flow, underlying large brain infarct >1/3 of the MCA territory, large clot burden (e.g., complete ICA occlusion from bulb to MCA), other extenuating circumstances (e.g., anticoagulant use or coagulopathy, thrombocytopenia, etc.), or the intended use of other agents or aggressive mechanical manipulation during the intervention (23). The presence of several of these factors may best be handled by avoiding thrombolytics all together or by using a purely mechanical approach, whereas the absence of all of the factors would favor an aggressive approach, particularly if the clinical deficit is severe. No systematic study of IA thrombolysis has yet been done and no approach has been proven to be superior to another.

In regard to the dosing frequency and infusion rate, the rule remains "the more rapid the recanalization the better the chance of a good neurologic outcome." Therefore, two to three boluses of thrombolytic given over 30 min may be better than the 2-h infusion used in the PROACT II trial. As with practically all aspects of the procedure, clinical data are lacking on the best approach.

Adjunctive Pharmacotherapy

In the setting of acute IS, platelet GP IIb/IIIa receptor antagonists have been used in combination with thrombolytics quite successfully without significantly increasing the risk of ICH *(3,16,17)*. These agents may have a facilitatory effect on thrombolysis when combined with a thrombolytic agent because thrombi are often composed of a combination of aggregated platelets bound with fibrin strands *(24)*. In addition the administration of a GP IIb/IIIa receptor antagonist is typically performed if a balloon angioplasty is planned, as there is a risk of endothelial injury *(17)*. The two most commonly used agents are abciximab and eptifibatide. The typical doses are similar to those used to treat the acute coronary syndrome, although it is preferable to start slowly and give more as needed, that is, abciximab in bolus increments. The GP IIb/IIIa inhibitor doses are alternated with boluses of thrombolytic agent. These agents are typically infused IV but IA administration directly into the thrombus through the microcatheter may facilitate thrombolysis by saturating the platelets within the thrombus *(17)*. A continuous (12-h) infusion should be considered following successful thrombolysis if a stent is placed or if there is an underlying atherosclerotic plaque and small doses of thrombolytics were used. The risk of ICH appears to be low with this approach but this has not been studied in a randomized fashion; therefore, it should not be considered for centers without much experience.

Clot Disruption

Manipulation of the thrombus with the wire is of benefit for fresh thrombi as in those complicating endovascular procedures, for example, coronary catheterization or cerebral angiography, or for small clot burdens, for example, an MCA branch occlusion. Mechanical clot disruption can be performed with repeated passes of the microwire or microcatheter through the thrombus. Larger occlusions or those due to an atherosclerotic plaque are unlikely to be disrupted sufficiently with wire manipulation; in these cases a more elaborate approach, such as angioplasty, is warranted. In particular, individuals in whom a thrombotic occlusion due to an underlying stenosis is the cause of the stroke may benefit greatly from angioplasty. These patients often have poorly controlled diabetes mellitus or are of African or Asian descent *(25)*.

Mechanical manipulation increases the risk of the procedure, so great care should be taken to not traumatize the underlying vasculature. Wire passes must be performed without letting the wire tip get "caught" or entering a small perforator. Adjunct balloon angioplasty for acute stroke has been reported both in combination with other techniques or as the sole treatment *(17,26–28)*. We perform gentle balloon angioplasty with undersized coronary balloons in most patients who do not respond quickly to thrombolysis. Because thrombi often have a gelatinous consistency, the inflations should be somewhat prolonged, typically 1–2 min in duration and multiple inflations may be required. Adjunctive GP IIb/IIIa antagonists can be considered in patients treated with angioplasty because of the likelihood of underlying endothelial injury, either iatrogenic or preexisting due to plaque rupture (similar to the approach that interventional cardiologists use to treat acute coronary syndrome). After each infusion, sufficient time should be given for thrombolysis (5–15 min) before repeating the angiogram to see if more drugs should be given.

In some circumstances, not only is angioplasty warranted and effective, but stenting of the occluded vessel may also be needed. At our institution, we have treated several acute stroke patients with stenting, most of whom we have treated with stenting alone, that is, without thrombolysis (unpublished data) (Fig. 2). All of our patients and the

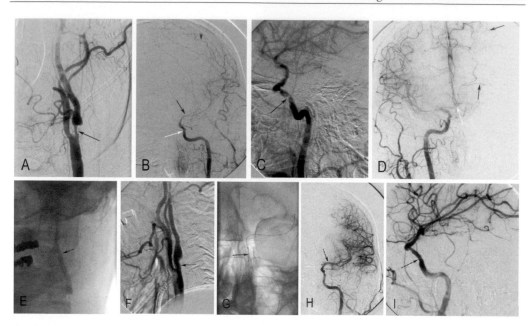

Fig. 2. Stenting for acute ischemic stroke. A 54-yr-old man developed progressive right hemiplegia and aphasia 12 h after coronary bypass graft surgery. Computerized tomography of the brain did not show any evidence of acute injury. Because of the recent surgery, intravenous thrombolysis was contraindicated and an urgent cerebral angiogram was performed. The left internal carotid artery (ICA) had an 80% stenosis at it origin (*arrow* in **A**). There was decreased and markedly delayed filling of the left middle cerebral artery (MCA) and its branches. In **B** compare the filling of the MCA *(black arrow)* and branches of the external carotid artery *(short arrow)*. The latter should fill latter than the MCA but in this case filled earlier consistent with the presence of a critical, flow-limiting stenosis within the cavernous ICA (*white arrow* in **B** and black arrow in **C**). An angiogram of the right ICA (**D**) revealed the presence of collateral flow to the left anterior cerebral artery (ACA) via the anterior communicating artery *(white arrow)* as well as pial (surface) collateral from the left ACA to the left MCA *(black arrows)*. Using the vessel access technique described in the text an 8 Fr sheath was placed in the distal left common carotid artery and an emboli prevention device (*arrow* in **E**) was passed through the ICA origin stenosis but was kept lower than usual to prevent disruption of the distal stenosis by the filterwire tip. Following stenting and angioplasty and removal of the filter there was no residual stenosis in the ICA (*arrow* in **F**). A hydrophilic soft-tipped 0.014-in. wire was then passed carefully through the stent and into a Sylvian branch of the MCA and a 2.5-mm coronary balloon was used to predilate the lesion (*arrow* in **G**). There was marked recoil of the lesion following angioplasty so a 3 × 8 mm chromium cobalt stent was deployed in the cavernous ICA at nominal inflation pressure. This resulted in restoration of normal MCA flow (*arrow* in **H**) as well as complete resolution of the stenosis (*arrow* in **I**). The patient began to have neurologic recovery immediately and returned to a normal neurologic state within 24 h. He received an oral clopidogrel load and aspirin immediately after the intervention.

few reported in the literature have had severe underlying stenoses, either of the intracranial or extracranial vessel *(29)*. In these patients the symptomatic lesions likely contain a vulnerable plaque that has caused either intraplaque hemorrhage or plaque rupture with platelet activation leading to thrombosis. Such lesions may have a high propensity for reocclusion, both early and delayed, and therefore stenting may allow both early recanalization as well as definitive treatment of the causative lesion, reducing the risk of reocclusion. Adequate platelet inhibition is critical in these cases and such patients should be treated with GP IIb/IIIa antagonists during the procedure, and as soon as possible after the intervention they should also receive clopidogrel and aspirin to prevent early stent thrombosis. This approach should not be considered as a standard approach but in the select patients it has been the authors' experience that it can be safely performed.

Clot Extraction

Mechanical embolectomy, or clot removal, is an emerging alternative to thrombolysis in IS. In some circumstances, pharmacological thrombolysis, even IA thrombolysis may be contraindicated (e.g., active systemic bleeding) or associated with a high risk of ICH (e.g., recent head injury or neurosurgery). By physically removing the clot, thrombolytics and even anticoagulants may not be needed, or their doses may be greatly reduced. Furthermore, a major limitation of thrombolysis is the speed of recanalization due to the fact that not all thrombi can be pharmacologically thrombolysed; therefore, a complementary mechanism for recanalization is critical.

Although several devices are under investigation for this purpose, until August of 2005 there were no approved devices designed for acute stroke treatment *(30,31)*. Since August 2005, the FDA approved the MERCI (Mechanical Embolus Removal in Cerebral Ischemia) Clot Retriever to "remove blood clots from the brain in patients experiencing an ischemic stroke." The MERCI retriever system includes a flexible nickel-titanium wire that assumes a helical shape once it is passed through the tip of a microcatheter. In practice, this device is passed through a microcatheter distal to the thrombus, and the catheter is removed; the clot is then trapped in the helix and withdrawn from the vessel under negative pressure applied through a balloon occlusion guide catheter (Fig. 3). The decision to approve the MERCI retriever was based on the data from the intention-to-treat MERCI trial. A total of 114 patients suffering an occlusion of the MCA were treated. The recanalization rate of the target vessels was 53.5%, but serious device-related events occurred in 3.5% of patients. The overall study mortality at 90 d was 39%, but among patients in whom embolectomy was unsuccessful the mortality was nearly 61%. Good outcome, defined as a modified Rankin Score ≤2 at 90 d, was achieved in 25% of patients in the MERCI trial, which is similar to the percentage of patients with a good outcome in the placebo arm of PROACT II. Probably for this reason, and the fact that there was no concomitant control arm to the study, the FDA approved the device for the "removal of clots" and not for stroke therapy. Currently, there is no evidence that using the Merci Retriever will improve outcome in patients with IS.

Other devices are commercially available that can be used for the purpose of embolectomy but they are all snares designed for the removal of foreign bodies. Nonetheless we and others have used these devices to successfully remove thrombi in patients with acute ischemic stroke *(32)*. One such device is the GooseNeck (MicroVena Corp.) snare, which is essentially a lasso. Snaring should be considered in patients who have cardioembolism because such emboli are less likely to be affixed to an underlying plaque (unpublished data). The technique of snaring involves the passage of a microwire and microcatheter through the occlusion. The wire is then exchanged for the GooseNeck, which is slightly oversized for the occluded artery. The lasso of the snare is deployed just distal to the occluded segment by withdrawal of the microcatheter; then the snare and microcatheter are withdrawn together into the thrombus. The snare is engaged into the thrombus and the microcatheter is advanced slightly to tighten the snare, but not so tightly as to tear through the thrombus. Finally the microcatheter and snare are withdrawn

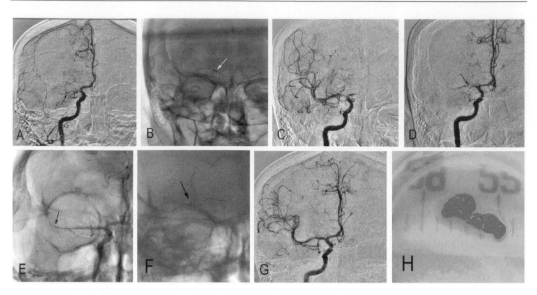

Fig. 3. Mechanical embolectomy. An 82-yr-old woman developed depressed awareness and left hemiparesis during a coronary artery intervention shortly after receiving a GP IIb/IIIa antagonist. Immediate four-vessel cerebral angiography revealed a proximal right middle cerebral artery (MCA) occlusion (*black arrow* in the **A** [AP angiogram]). The anterior cerebral artery was patent and supplied a few pial collaterals to the MCA (*white arrow* in **A**). A microwire was passed through the occlusion and a 2-mm coronary balloon was inflated (*white arrow* in **B**) within the proximal MCA resulting in TIMI 2 flow (**C**). Immediately after withdrawal of the balloon the vessel reoccluded (**D**) and remained so despite repeat inflations. The guide catheter was exchanged for a 7 Fr balloon-occlusion guide which was placed in the proximal ICA. A Merci® retriever, through a microcatheter placed just distal to the distal end of the thrombus (*arrow* in **E**), was then deployed (*arrow* in **F**). The snare was then retracted into the distal third of the thrombus and then the balloon of the guide catheter was inflated to occlude antegrade blood flow into the ICA. While negative pressure was applied to the lumen of the guide with a 60-cc syringe the microcatheter and snare were withdrawn simultaneously and slowly into the guide catheter. The guide catheter was then removed and flushed. Repeat angiography revealed complete MCA recanalization (**G**). The snare contained a gelatinous heterogeneous thrombus (**H**).

as a unit into the guide catheter while negative pressure is applied within the guide catheter to facilitate thrombus removal and decrease the likelihood of distal embolization. Retrograde flow is induced by applying negative pressure within the guide, which is greatly facilitated by the use of a balloon-occlusion guide catheter that can be inflated gently within the ICA to occlude all antegrade flow. A similar procedure can be performed with a balloon guide in the subclavian artery or, if large enough, the VA in cases of VB occlusion. When successful, this technique can lead to very rapid recanalization and excellent clinical outcomes with a very low risk of complications.

The disadvantage of the technique is that lesion wire access is lost and often the guide catheter has to be completely removed if the retrieved thrombus becomes lodged within the guide lumen. For this last reason the placement of a sheath in the common carotid artery or subclavian is very helpful since it permits rapid recanalization of the target vessel. In addition these devices have the potential to cause arterial perforation, dissection, or distal embolization. The stiffer MERCI retriever device and other nitinol devices may be more likely to cause injury than the lasso-type snare.

Periprocedural Medical Management

Maintaining patients' airway, breathing, and circulation is mandatory in the rush to recanalize the occluded vessel. Although, most patients are able to breathe spontaneously (patients with diffuse brainstem ischemia notwithstanding), those with a depressed level of consciousness may hypoventilate or be at risk for aspiration. These patients should be intubated and mechanically ventilated prior to beginning the intervention, despite the fact that the neurologic exam and the ability to communicate with the patient are lost. The delay induced by intubation is critical regarding the initiation of recanalization; however, the necessity to stop in mid-procedure for an emergency intubation is a situation to be prevented. Our approach is to perform intubation only when absolutely necessary, and done in the angiography suite so that there is no delay in initiating the intervention. Not sedating patients permits monitoring for a response to treatment and early detection of possible complications. For example, headache is potentially an important sign of vascular irritation and intracerebral bleeding. Its occurrence during an intervention always requires patient reevaluation and reassessment of the operative technique and equipment position, particularly the wire. If a headache resolves with simple measures and there is no vessel perforation on angiography and no clinical deterioration then the intervention can be continued. If a patient's headache or, in the case of nonverbal patients, severe agitation persist then strong consideration should be given to termination of the procedure in order to obtain a CT scan or at least a thorough angiographic and clinical reevaluation.

Blood pressure (BP) control is the most important periprocedural clinical factor. Under ischemic conditions the cerebral arteries maximally vasodilate to maintain cerebral blood flow (CBF) in the optimal range (i.e., cerebral autoregulation). A direct result of this vasodilatation is that CBF becomes linearly proportional to the mean arterial pressure (MAP). Therefore, cerebral ischemia can be potentiated by iatrogenic or spontaneous declines of MAP resulting in decreased CBF below the critical levels for tissue survival *(33)*. Similarly, excessive elevations of MAP may lead to marked elevations of CBF and particularly if recanalization is successful, the risk of reperfusion injury and hemorrhage will be increased. The optimal range for BP varies for each patient but in general MAP should be maintained below the 135 mmHg (185/110 mmHg) threshold for patients receiving thrombolytics but above 110 mmHg (150/90 mmHg) *(34)*. β-Blockers are very useful, and safe, in controlling BP but nitroprusside should be used for persistently and severely elevated blood pressures. Although nitroglycerin is effective, it can cause headache, which can mimic or mask the headache of ICH.

In general it is preferable not to drop arterial blood pressures before recanalization is achieved unless they are significantly elevated. If complete recanalization is achieved then pressures can be lowered into the normal to high–normal ranges. In certain circumstances where the risk of ICH may be high (e.g., long duration of ischemia, large doses of thrombolytics or GP IIb/IIIa antagonists were given, or a long standing arteriosclerotic lesion is treated, etc.) blood pressures should be lowered into the low normal or occasionally into hypotensive ranges. It is critical to keep in mind that the prevention of ICH is the single most important task following any cerebral intervention. Intracerebral hemorrhage has no effective treatment and is fatal in up to 80% of cases.

Further, we recommend giving all patients oxygen via a nasal cannula or nonrebreather face mask if needed during the procedure. Supplemental oxygen increases brain-tissue oxygenation and is generally safe. Although there is some concern that high oxygen levels may worsen reperfusion injury, we feel that preserving the ischemic penumbra is essential.

The management of poststroke and ICH patients can be complex and is best performed with the assistance of an experienced neurointensivist and stroke neurologist. For this purpose, after the procedure all patients should be sent to a neurologic intensive care unit for monitoring. Frequent neurologic checks should be performed, at least every 15 min. Particular attention should be paid to the occurrence of headache, the worsening of deficits, or the development of a decreased level of consciousness, all of which could be the signs of ICH. If any of the above develops, an urgent CT scan of the brain should be obtained. The management of ICH following thrombolysis is quite difficult and the prognosis is greatly worsened if ICH develops. If ICH is present, any residual doses or effects of anticoagulants, thrombolytics, or antiplatelets should be reversed if possible. Neurosurgical consultation should be obtained immediately but it is unclear if there is in fact a role for neurosurgical intervention in this setting *(35,36)*.

CONCLUSION

Endovascular treatment of acute ischemic stroke remains very complex, with the continuous need to balance between the drive to achieve rapid recanalization and the risk of intracranial bleeding. Management of these patients requires a thorough understanding of the intracranial cerebral vasculature and the pathophysiology of stroke. Nonetheless, a variety of tools and pharmacological agents are available and excellent clinical results can be achieved with a thoughtful approach to the patients with ischemic stroke.

REFERENCES

1. American Heart Association. Heart Disease and Stroke Statistics—2005 Update. American Heart Association 2005.
2. Caplan LR. TIAs: we need to return to the question, 'What is wrong with Mr. Jones?' Neurology 1988;38:791–793.
3. Abciximab in acute ischemic stroke: a randomized, double-blind, placebo-controlled, dose-escalation study. The Abciximab in Ischemic Stroke Investigators. Stroke 2000;31:601–609.
4. Thrombolytic therapy with streptokinase in acute ischemic stroke. The Multicenter Acute Stroke Trial—Europe Study Group. N Engl J Med 1996;335:145–150.
5. Furlan A, Higashida R, Wechsler L, et al. Intra-arterial prourokinase for acute ischemic stroke. The PROACT II study: a randomized controlled trial. Prolyse in Acute Cerebral Thromboembolism. JAMA 1999;282:2003–2011.
6. Tissue plasminogen activator for acute ischemic stroke. The National Institute of Neurological Disorders and Stroke rt-PA Stroke Study Group. N Engl J Med 1995;333:1581–1587.
7. Moskowitz M, Caplan L. Thrombolytic treatment in acute stroke: review and update of selective topics. Cerebrovascular Diseases: Ninteteenth Princeton Stroke Conference: Boston: Butterworth-Heinemann, 1995.
8. del Zoppo GJ, Ferbert A, Otis S, et al. Local intra-arterial fibrinolytic therapy in acute carotid territory stroke. A pilot study. Stroke 1988;19:307–313.
9. del Zoppo GJ, Poeck K, Pessin MS, et al. Recombinant tissue plasminogen activator in acute thrombotic and embolic stroke. Ann Neurol 1992;32:78–86.
10. Katzan IL, Masaryk TJ, Furlan AJ, et al. Intra-arterial thrombolysis for perioperative stroke after open heart surgery. Neurology 1999;52:1081–1084.
11. Brott T, Adams HP, Jr., Olinger CP, et al. Measurements of acute cerebral infarction: a clinical examination scale. Stroke 1989;20:864–870.
12. Adams HP, Jr., Brott TG, Furlan AJ, et al. Guidelines for thrombolytic therapy for acute stroke: a supplement to the guidelines for the management of patients with acute ischemic stroke. A statement for

healthcare professionals from a Special Writing Group of the Stroke Council, American Heart Association. Circulation 1996;94:1167–1174.

13. Hacke W, Ringleb P, Stingele R. [How did the results of ECASS II influence clinical practice of treatment of acute stroke]. Rev Neurol 1999;29:638–641.

14. Barr JD. Cerebral angiography in the assessment of acute cerebral ischemia: guidelines and recommendations. J Vasc Interv Radiol 2004;15:S57–S66.

15. Furlan AJ. Acute stroke therapy: beyond i.v. tPA. Cleve Clin J Med 2002;69:730–734.

16. Lee DH, Jo KD, Kim HG, et al. Local intraarterial urokinase thrombolysis of acute ischemic stroke with or without intravenous abciximab: a pilot study. J Vasc Interv Radiol 2002;13:769–774.

17. Abou-Chebl A, Bajzer CT, Krieger DW, Furlan AJ, Yadav JS. Multimodal therapy for the treatment of severe ischemic stroke combining GP IIb/IIIa antagonists and angioplasty after failure of thrombolysis. Stroke 2005;36:2286–2288.

18. Hacke W, Kaste M, Fieschi C, et al. Intravenous thrombolysis with recombinant tissue plasminogen activator for acute hemispheric stroke. The European Cooperative Acute Stroke Study (ECASS). JAMA 1995;274:1017–1025.

19. del Zoppo GJ, Sasahara AA. Interventional use of plasminogen activators in central nervous system diseases. Med Clin North Am 1998;82:545–568.

20. Qureshi AI, Ali Z, Suri MF, et al. Intra-arterial third-generation recombinant tissue plasminogen activator (reteplase) for acute ischemic stroke. Neurosurgery 2001;49:41–48; discussion 48–50.

21. Arnold M, Schroth G, Nedeltchev K, et al. Intra-arterial thrombolysis in 100 patients with acute stroke due to middle cerebral artery occlusion. Stroke 2002;33:1828–1833.

22. Figueroa BE, Keep RF, Betz AL, Hoff JT. Plasminogen activators potentiate thrombin-induced brain injury. Stroke 1998;29:1202–1207; discussion 1208.

23. Yokogami K, Nakano S, Ohta H, Goya T, Wakisaka S. Prediction of hemorrhagic complications after thrombolytic therapy for middle cerebral artery occlusion: value of pre- and post-therapeutic computed tomographic findings and angiographic occlusive site. Neurosurgery 1996;39:1102–1107.

24. Collet JP, Montalescot G, Lesty C, et al. Disaggregation of in vitro preformed platelet-rich clots by abciximab increases fibrin exposure and promotes fibrinolysis. Arterioscler Thromb Vasc Biol 2001;21:142–148.

25. Sacco RL, Kargman DE, Gu Q, Zamanillo MC. Race-ethnicity and determinants of intracranial atherosclerotic cerebral infarction. The Northern Manhattan Stroke Study. Stroke 1995;26:14–20.

26. Ringer AJ, Qureshi AI, Fessler RD, Guterman LR, Hopkins LN. Angioplasty of intracranial occlusion resistant to thrombolysis in acute ischemic stroke. Neurosurgery 2001;48:1282–1288; discussion 1288–1290.

27. Nakano S, Iseda T, Yoneyama T, Kawano H, Wakisaka S. Direct percutaneous transluminal angioplasty for acute middle cerebral artery trunk occlusion: an alternative option to intra-arterial thrombolysis. Stroke 2002;33:2872–2876.

28. Qureshi AI, Siddiqui AM, Suri MF, et al. Aggressive mechanical clot disruption and low-dose intra-arterial third-generation thrombolytic agent for ischemic stroke: a prospective study. Neurosurgery 2002;51:1319–1327; discussion 1327–1329.

29. Li S, Miao Z, Zhu F, et al. Combined intraarterial thrombolysis and intra-cerebral stent for acute ischemic stroke institute of brain vascular diseases. Zhonghua Yi Xue Za Zhi 2003;83:9–12.

30. Bellon RJ, Putman CM, Budzik RF, Pergolizzi RS, Reinking GF, Norbash AM. Rheolytic thrombectomy of the occluded internal carotid artery in the setting of acute ischemic stroke. AJNR Am J Neuroradiol 2001;22:526–530.

31. Gomez CR, Misra VK, Terry JB, Tulyapronchote R, Campbell MS. Emergency endovascular treatment of cerebral sinus thrombosis with a rheolytic catheter device. J Neuroimaging 2000;10:177–180.

32. Chopko BW, Kerber C, Wong W, Georgy B. Transcatheter snare removal of acute middle cerebral artery thromboembolism: technical case report. Neurosurgery 2000;46:1529–1531.

33. Ahmed N, Nasman P, Wahlgren NG. Effect of intravenous nimodipine on blood pressure and outcome after acute stroke. Stroke 2000;31:1250–1255.

34. Adams HP, Jr., Brott TG, Crowell RM, et al. Guidelines for the management of patients with acute ischemic stroke. A statement for healthcare professionals from a special writing group of the Stroke Council, American Heart Association. Circulation 1994;90:1588–1601.

35. Juvela S, Heiskanen O, Poranen A, et al. The treatment of spontaneous intracerebral hemorrhage. A prospective randomized trial of surgical and conservative treatment. J Neurosurg 1989;70:755–758.

36. Batjer HH, Reisch JS, Allen BC, Plaizier LJ, Su CJ. Failure of surgery to improve outcome in hypertensive putaminal hemorrhage. A prospective randomized trial. Arch Neurol 1990;47:1103–1106.

III CHALLENGING CASE ILLUSTRATIONS AND PEARLS

16 Case: Left Carotid Artery Stenting with a Challenging Type III Aortic Arch

Jacqueline Saw, MD

CONTENTS

HISTORY

A 65-yr-old man underwent left endarterectomy 2 yr ago for symptomatic left carotid artery stenosis. Upon follow-up with duplex ultrasound, he was found to have asymptomatic restenosis 80–99% involving the left common carotid artery (CCA). His past medical history includes long-standing hypertension, hyperlipidemia, and prior three-vessel coronary artery bypass surgery. On physical examination, he had a left carotid bruit, and normal neurologic examination. Given his prior history of left endarterectomy, he was felt to be at high risk for redo endarterectomy for restenosis. Thus, he was referred for left carotid stenting.

DIAGNOSTIC ANGIOGRAPHY

The patient had a type III aortic arch with normal great vessel branching (Fig. 1). He had a 90% stenosis involving the distal left CCA (Fig. 2). The left internal carotid artery (ICA) has no significant disease, but the origin of the left external carotid artery (ECA) had an 80% stenosis. The left ICA supplied the left middle cerebral artery (MCA), but only partially filled the left anterior cerebral artery (ACA) because of competitive filling via the anterior communicating artery from the right ACA (Fig. 3). Given this underlying anatomy, a difficult carotid stenting procedure is anticipated.

CAROTID STENTING PROCEDURE

With the steep type III aortic arch and disease involving the origin of the ECA, it will be difficult to advance a standard guide or sheath into position. Anticipating this challenge, we proceeded with intervention using a modified 9 Fr AL1 guide (see Fig. 3)

From: *Contemporary Cardiology: Handbook of Complex Percutaneous Carotid Intervention*
Edited by: J. Saw, J. E. Exaire, D. S. Lee, and S. Yadav © Humana Press Inc., Totowa, NJ

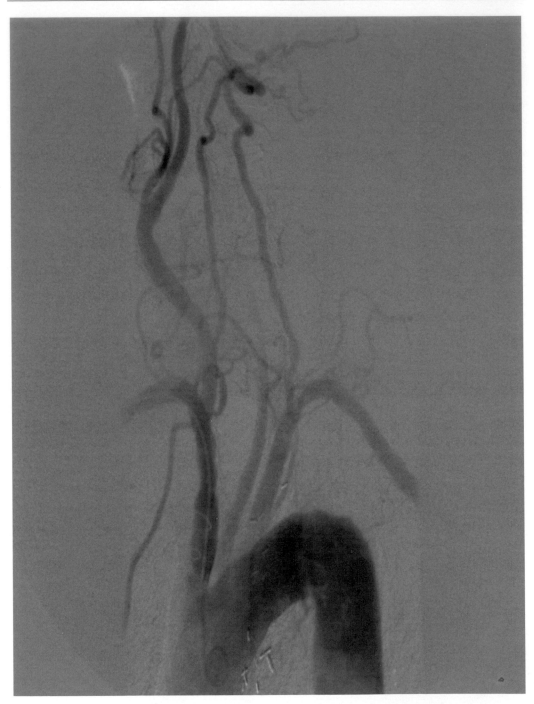

Fig. 1. Aortic arch angiogram showing a type III arch (Movie 1).

positioned at the left CCA ostium. A 5 Fr 125-cm length VTK catheter was telescoped within the AL1 guide, and used to engage the left CCA origin (Fig. 4). The AL1 guide was then advance into position, engaging the origin of the CCA. The VTK catheter was then withdrawn.

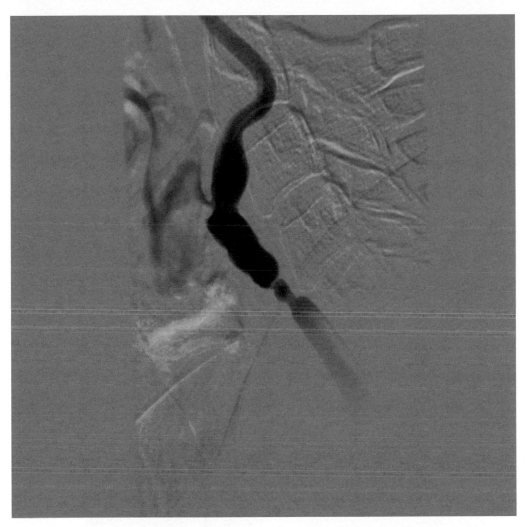

Fig. 2. Carotid angiogram showing 90% stenosis of the distal left internal carotid artery, and 80% ostial left external carotid artery stenosis (Movie 2).

This setup provided sufficient support to advance an emboli protection device (EPD) into the ICA. The FilterWire EX™ device was successfully maneuvered across the CCA stenosis into the ICA, and deployed in the cervical ICA (Fig. 5). To facilitate delivery of the stent, we placed a 0.014-in. buddy wire into the ECA. We first introduced a 300-cm length Balance Middle Weight (BMW, Guidant, Indianapolis, IN) into the ECA (Fig. 6), and then exchanged out using a 4.0 × 20 mm Maverick²™ balloon (Boston Scientific, Natick, MA) (Fig. 7) into an Ironman wire (Guidant, Indianapolis, IN). Predilatation of the distal CCA lesion was performed using this balloon. We then advanced a 9.0 × 40 mm Precise™ stent (Cordis, Warren, NJ) into the distal CCA (Figs. 8 and 9) and successfully deployed it. Postdilatation was performed with a 6.0 × 40 mm Aviator™ balloon (Cordis, Warren, NJ) (Fig. 10).

Final bifurcation angiography showed good apposition of stent with minimal residual stenosis of the distal CCA (Fig. 11). Final intracranial angiography after retrieval of the FilterWire EX™ device showed good filling of both the left ACA and MCA,

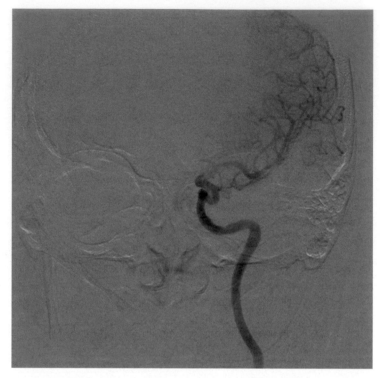

Fig. 3. Intracranial angiography showing normal filling of the left middle cerebral artery, but only minimal filling of the left anterior cerebral artery (Movie 3).

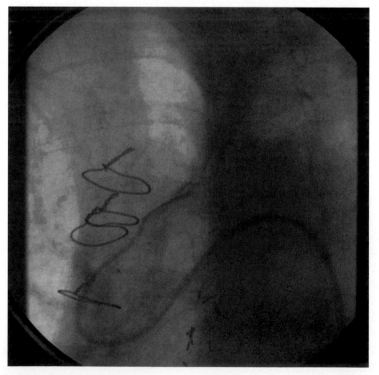

Fig. 4. Cine demonstrating the guide position with the type III aortic arch.

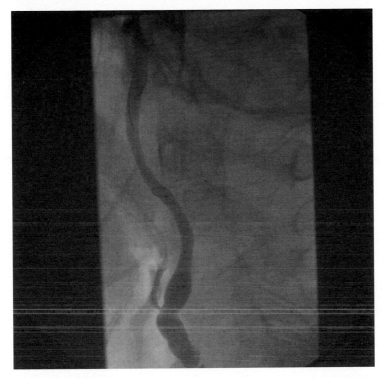

Fig. 5. Angiogram demonstrating the FilterWire EX™ device placed in the internal carotid artery.

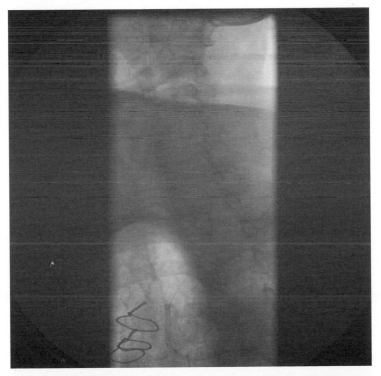

Fig. 6. Advancing the Balance Middle Weight wire into the external carotid artery for additional support.

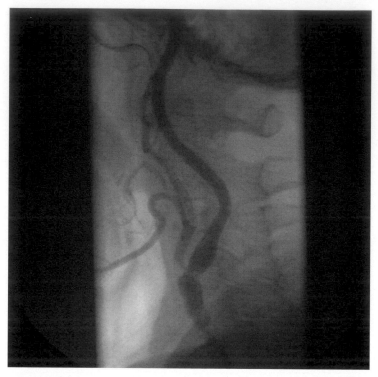

Fig. 7. An over-the-wire balloon is advanced into the external carotid artery, to enable exchange of the Balance Middle Weight wire for an Ironman wire (Movie 7).

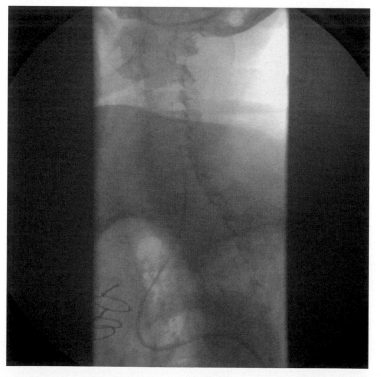

Fig. 8. Cine showing advancing of the self-expanding stent into position (Movie 8).

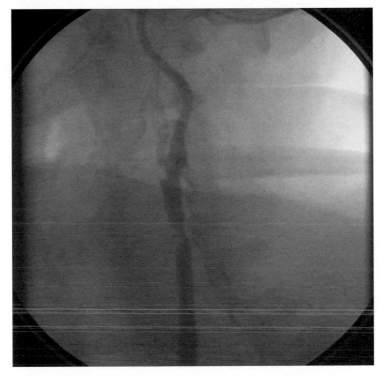

Fig. 9. After predilatation of the distal common carotid artery stenosis (Movie 9).

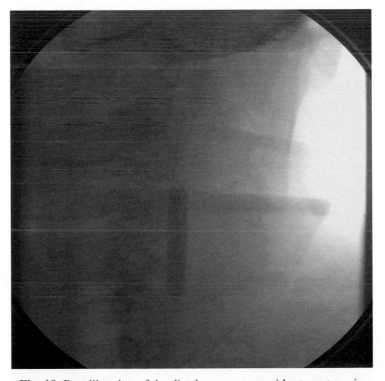

Fig. 10. Postdilatation of the distal common carotid artery stenosis.

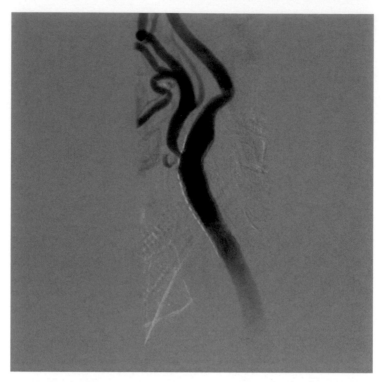

Fig. 11. Final carotid bifurcation angiography after carotid stenting (Movie 11).

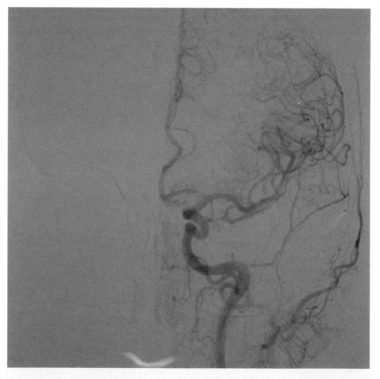

Fig. 12. Final intracranial angiography showing normal filling of the anterior and middle cerebral arteries (Movie 12).

without any evidence of embolization (Fig. 12). The patient tolerated the procedure well without any complications.

LEARNING POINTS

1. In the setting of type III aortic arch, typically a guide approach is preferable to a sheath approach. With this technique, a 0.035-in. guidewire can be advanced into the ECA and used as a support to advance the guide into distal CCA. However, when there is ostial disease involving the ECA, it is not advisable to cross the ECA with the 0.035-in. guidewire or with a catheter, which may disrupt the ostial ECA plaque causing embolization into the ICA. Thus, in the setting of type III arch with ostial ECA disease, an alternative guide approach is to just place the guide (e.g., modified AL1 guide) at the origin of the CCA.

2. With this approach, as the guide is only engaging the ostium of the CCA, the operator should consider using a 0.014-in. buddy wire in the ECA (e.g., Ironman) as a support to advance the self-expanding stent into position. As the Ironman has a stiff body, we tend to cross into the ECA first with a BMW wire, before exchanging out via an over-the-wire balloon with the Ironman.

17 Case: Stenting of a Tortuous Left Internal Carotid Artery

J. Emilio Exaire, MD

CONTENTS

HISTORY

A 56-yr-old man presented with a history of transient ischemic attacks suggesting left mid-cerebral artery (MCA) territory. He had symptoms of right arm and leg weakness, as well as slurred speech. His past medical history included hypertension and hyperlipidemia, as well as three-vessel coronary artery disease. A head computed tomography (CT) scan was performed urgently and reported to be normal. A carotid duplex ultrasound revealed a 60–79% stenosis of the left internal carotid artery (ICA). After neurologic evaluation, he was referred for carotid artery stenting because he was thought to be at high risk for carotid endarterectomy given his coronary anatomy.

DIAGNOSTIC ANGIOGRAPHY

The patient had a type II aortic arch with normal origin of the supra-aortic vessels. The right ICA was normal angiographically, giving rise to the right MCA and anterior cerebral artery (ACA), with a patent anterior communicating artery. The left vertebral artery was normal in caliber without stenosis. A minor 20% basilar artery stenosis was found. The posterior communicating arteries were absent bilaterally. The left ICA had a 95% lesion with severe tortuosity at about the lesion site with a 180° turn (Fig. 1).

CAROTID ARTERY STENTING PROCEDURE

After heparin (100 U/kg) was provided to achieve an activated clotting time (ACT) close to 300 s, a long (125 cm) JR4 catheter was used to selectively engage the left common carotid artery (CCA). Using a roadmap, a stiff-angled Glidewire® (Terumo Medical, Somerset, NJ) was advanced through the JR4 catheter into the left external carotid artery (ECA). The stiff-angled Glidewire® was then withdrawn and a 6-cm tip

From: *Contemporary Cardiology: Handbook of Complex Percutaneous Carotid Intervention*
Edited by: J. Saw, J. E. Exaire, D. S. Lee, and S. Yadav © Humana Press Inc., Totowa, NJ

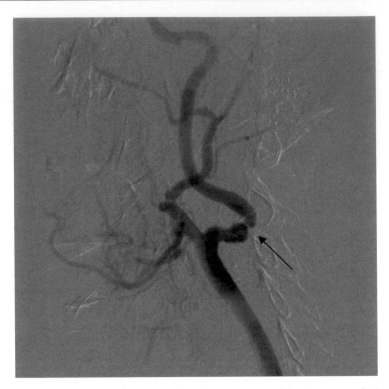

Fig. 1. Baseline carotid angiogram showing the left internal carotid artery stenosis *(arrow)* and the severe angulation at the site.

Amplatz Super Stiff™ (Boston Scientific, Natick, MA) wire was advanced through the JR4 catheter; the JR4 catheter was then withdrawn. The sheath was upsized to a short 8 Fr sheath and the long JR4 catheter was used to telescope an 8 Fr H1 guide catheter (Cordis, Warren, NJ). After the guide catheter was advanced, both the JR4 and the stiff-angled Glidewire® were withdrawn.

We then attempted to cross the lesion with an AngioGuard XP™ (Cordis, Warren, NJ) device. However, because of the critical stenosis and severe tortuosity, this filter device could not be delivered. A 300-cm 0.014-in. Balance Middle Weight (BMW wire, Guidant Corporation, Indianapolis, IN) was used as a buddy wire, and it crossed the lesion easily. The BMW wire was advanced into the petrous portion of the left ICA, somewhat straightening the angulation of the ICA. Despite this, the AngioGuard XP™ device was unable to negotiate the tortuous ICA. Therefore, an unprotected predilatation with a 2.0 × 20 mm Maverick²™ (Boston Scientific, Natick, MA) over-the-wire balloon was performed (Fig. 2). Following this, another attempt to cross with the AngioGuard XP™ again was unsuccessful. At this point, the over-the-wire balloon was advanced into the petrous segment of the left ICA over the BMW wire. The BMW wire was then exchanged to a long (300 cm) 0.014-in. Ironman wire (Guidant, Indianapolis, IN), but resulted in pseudostenosis of the ICA. We were then able to advance the AngioGuard XP™ to the pre-petrous left ICA and deployed it successfully (Fig. 3). The Ironman wire was left in position to provide support for advancing other catheter equipments (i.e., balloon and stent).

The lesion was further predilated with a 4.0 × 20 mm CrossSail® (Guidant, Indianapolis, IN) balloon. An 8.0 × 40 mm Precise™ (Cordis, Warren, NJ) stent was

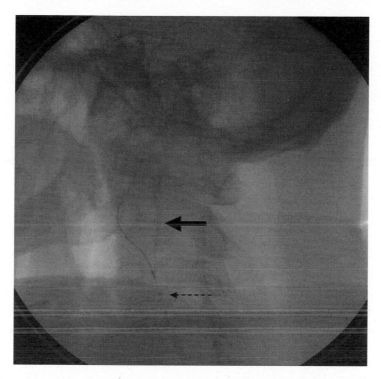

Fig. 2. Predilatation with a 2.0 × 20 mm Maverick²™ balloon was performed *(bold arrow)*. The undeployed AngioGuard XP™ *(dashed arrow)* was advanced into the external carotid artery to provide support.

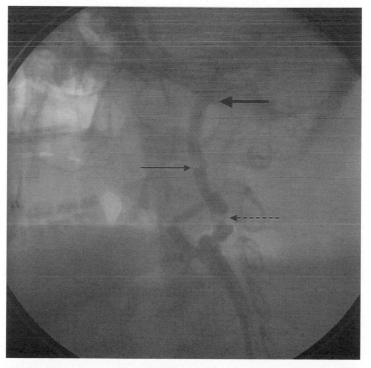

Fig. 3. Pseudostenosis *(arrow)* of the internal carotid artery beyond the original lesion *(dashed arrow)* was present with the AngioGuard XP™ *(bold arrow)* device in place.

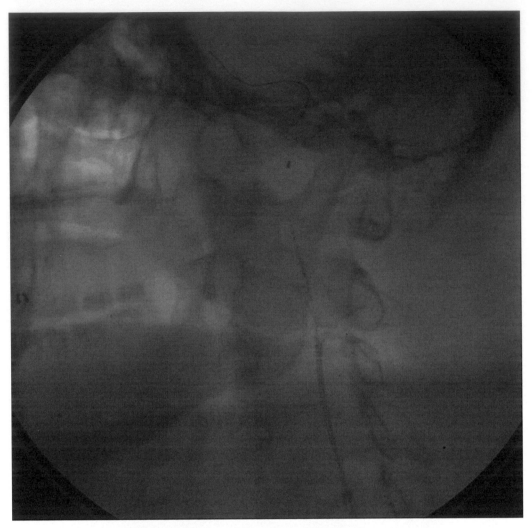

Fig. 4. Self-expanding stent deployment (Movie 4).

successfully advanced into the lesion (Fig. 4), extending into the left CCA. Prior to the stent deployment, the Ironman wire was withdrawn. Postdilation was performed using a 5.5/20 mm Viatrac® (Guidant, Indianapolis, IN) balloon. The angiogram revealed 10% residual stenosis with slow-flow. Thus, before retrieving the AngioGuard XP™ device, several aspirations using an Export catheter (Medtronic, Minneapolis, MN) were performed. The final intracranial angiography demonstrated brisk flow without distal embolization (Fig. 5).

LEARNING POINTS

1. Severe angulation of the ICA may adversely affect crossing the stenosis with an emboli protection device (EPD). If the EPD does not advance, a "buddy-wire" technique may help to straighten out the vessel angulation. A soft- or medium-bodied 0.014-in. coronary wire may be attempted first. Sometimes, an extra support wire (e.g., Ironman) is necessary to provide enough support and straighten the vessel. As in our patient, the

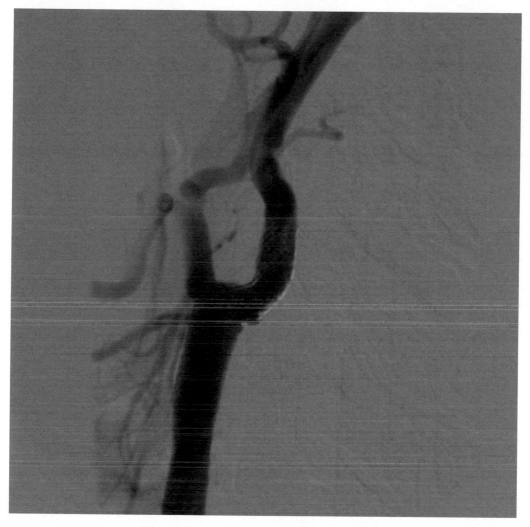

Fig. 5. Final angiography of the bifurcation (Movie 5).

use of an extra support wire may result in pseudostenosis. Therefore, an anatomical reference to mark the area to be treated is desirable. Intracranial flow may be compromised with pseudostenosis, thus crossing the lesion with the EPD should be performed expediently.

2. Predilating the lesion with a 2.0-mm coronary balloon after an unsuccessful attempt at EPD delivery is reasonable if the stenosis is very severe.

3. Slow-flow during the procedure may provoke neurologic symptoms. This is usually due to the EPD filter being overwhelmed with plaque and thrombus embolization. If the EPD is collapsed at this point, small debris may travel to the intracerebral circulation. Aspiration with an Export catheter or multipurpose catheter will remove the stagnant column of blood, which contains the suspended debris. This helps reduce distal embolization.

18

Case: Stenting of a Critical Internal Carotid Artery Stenosis With String Sign

Jacqueline Saw, MD

CONTENTS

HISTORY
DIAGNOSTIC ANGIOGRAPHY
CAROTID STENTING PROCEDURE
LEARNING POINTS
REFERENCES

HISTORY

A 60-yr-old man presented with a history of transient ischemic attack (TIA) 2 mo ago, in which he experienced aphasia lasting 6 h. He also had a history of long-standing hypertension, hyperlipidemia, and a 14 pack-year smoking history. On physical examination, he had a soft right carotid bruit and a normal neurologic exam. A noncontrast head CT showed no abnormality. However, carotid duplex ultrasound demonstrated that his right internal carotid artery (ICA) had a 60–79% stenosis, and his left ICA was occluded. After evaluation by a neurologist and a vascular surgeon, it was felt that carotid revascularization was appropriate. However, he was considered to be at high risk for right carotid endarterectomy because of the contralateral occlusion, and also because of the high location of the right ICA stenosis. Therefore, he was referred for carotid artery stenting.

DIAGNOSTIC ANGIOGRAPHY

The patient had a type II aortic arch with normal great vessel branching. He had a 50% stenosis in the proximal right ICA. The right ICA supplied the right anterior and middle cerebral arteries (ACA and MCA), with contralateral filling of the left ACA via an anterior communicating artery (ACOM), and also filling of the right posterior cerebral artery (PCA) via a posterior communicating artery (PCOM). With the diagnostic 5 Fr JR4 in the proximal left common carotid artery (CCA), the left ICA appears occluded (Fig. 1). However, advancing the catheter into the carotid bifurcation showed that the left ICA was subtotally occluded (99% stenosis), with a trickle of flow through the

From: *Contemporary Cardiology: Handbook of Complex Percutaneous Carotid Intervention*
Edited by: J. Saw, J. E. Exaire, D. S. Lee, and S. Yadav © Humana Press Inc., Totowa, NJ

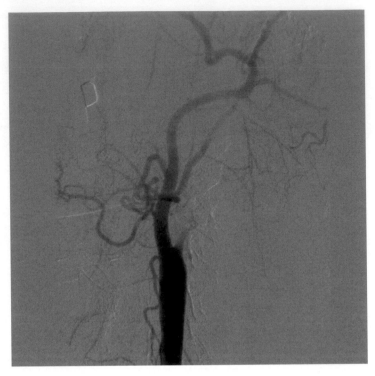

Fig. 1. With the diagnostic 5 Fr JR4 in the proximal left common carotid artery, the left ICA appears occluded (Movie 1).

stenosis (string sign) (Fig. 2). The distal left ICA filled via collaterals from the ophthalmic artery through the external carotid artery, and also from very slow antegrade flow through the subtotal proximal stenosis (Fig. 3). With this anatomy, this patient was at high risk of a left hemispheric stroke, particularly because he already had a recent TIA from this carotid territory. Therefore, we proceeded to percutaneous revascularization of this critical left ICA stenosis.

CAROTID STENTING PROCEDURE

An 8 Fr sheath was placed in the right common femoral artery. Using a telescoping technique, an 8 Fr H1 guide (Cordis, Warren, NJ) was advanced into the distal left common carotid artery (CCA) over a 125-cm 5 Fr JR4 catheter. Initial attempts to cross the subtotal left ICA occlusions with a 0.014-in. Synchro wire (Boston Scientific, Natick, MA) was unsuccessful, as the angle of the H1 guide was deflecting the wire from the stenosis. Therefore, the H1 guide and femoral sheath was exchanged to an 8 Fr 70-cm Raabe sheath. This facilitated entry across the subtotal occlusion with the Synchro wire. The wire is advanced freely into the petrous portion of the ICA (Fig. 4). A coronary 2.0 × 20 mm Maverick2™ (Boston Scientific, Natick, MA) over-the-wire balloon was tracked over this wire into the high cervical ICA (Fig. 5), and intraluminal confirmation was performed by contrast injection through this balloon (Fig. 6). We proceeded to balloon dilatation of the proximal subtotal occlusion at 8 atm, which created a sufficient channel to enable crossing the stenosis with an emboli protection device. The AngioGuard XP™ (Cordis, Warren, NJ) device was used, which easily traversed the

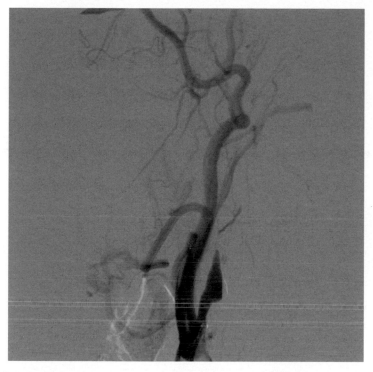

Fig. 2. Advancing the JR4 catheter into the carotid bifurcation and injecting contrast at this location showed the presence of a string sign of the left internal carotid artery (Movie 2).

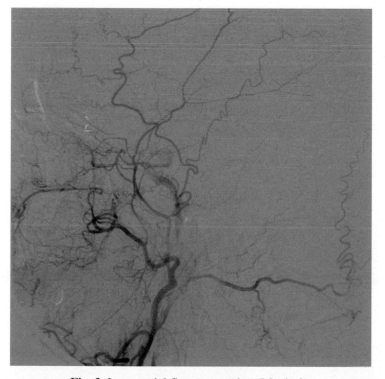

Fig. 3. Intracranial flow prestenting (Movie 3).

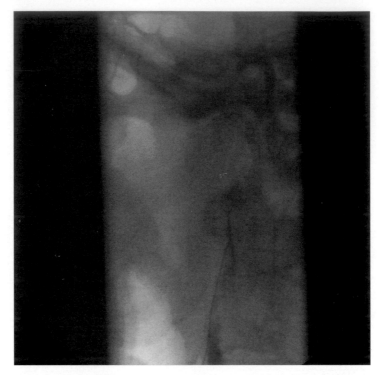

Fig. 4. The 0.014-in. Synchro wire was advanced freely into the petrous portion of the left internal carotid artery (Movie 4).

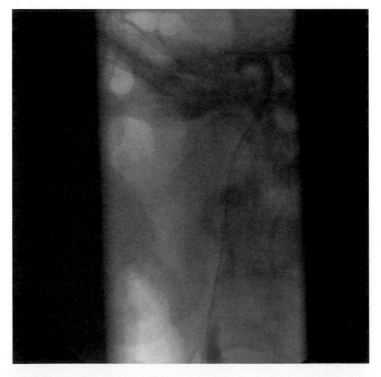

Fig. 5. A coronary 2.0 × 20 mm Maverick²™ over-the-wire balloon was tracked over the 0.014-in. Synchro wire into the high cervical internal carotid artery (Movie 5).

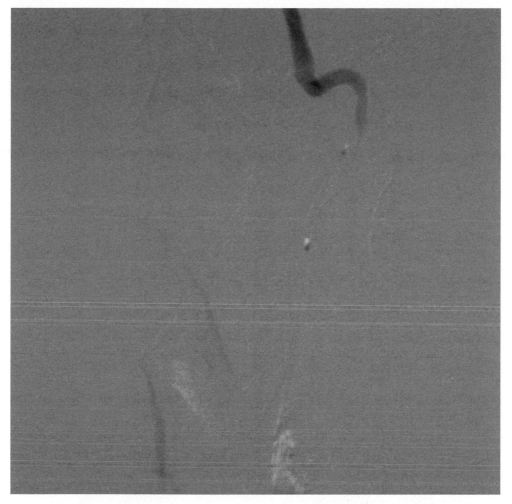

Fig. 6. Intraarterial luminal confirmation was performed by contrast injection through the Maverick^{2TM} over-the-wire balloon (Movie 6).

stenosis, and was deployed in the straight segment of the ICA before the petrous bone (Fig. 7). Because of the long-segment of proximal stenosis, an 8.0 × 40 mm Precise^{TM} (Cordis, Warren, NJ) nitinol self-expanding stent was chosen and deployed across the carotid bifurcation (Fig. 8). Postdilatation was performed using a 6.0 × 30 mm Aviator^{TM} (Cordis, Warren, NJ) balloon (Fig. 9) at 10 atm. An excellent result was obtained, with minimal residual stenosis and good flow distally (Fig. 10). Intracranial angiography demonstrated filling of the left ACA and MCA via the patent left ICA (Fig. 11). The patient tolerated the procedure very well with no new neurologic symptoms, and was discharged home the following day.

LEARNING POINTS

There are several learning points from this case illustration.

1. The absence of a carotid bruit does not signify the lack of a severely obstructive carotid artery lesion. In a prospective evaluation of carotid bruits among 145 patients, the

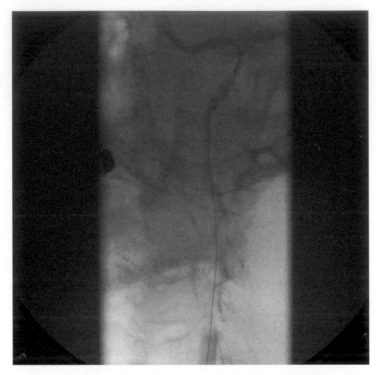

Fig. 7. The AngioGuard XP™ device easily traversed the stenosis (with the Synchro wire left in as a buddy wire), and was deployed in the straight segment of the internal carotid artery before the petrous bone (Movie 7).

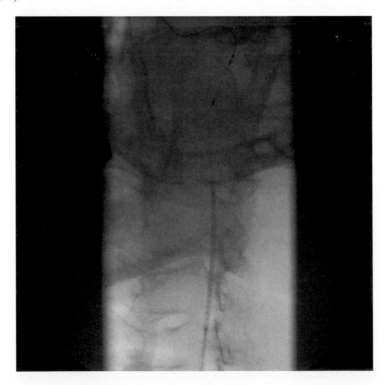

Fig. 8. An 8.0 × 40 mm Precise™ nitinol self-expanding stent was deployed across the carotid bifurcation (Movie 8).

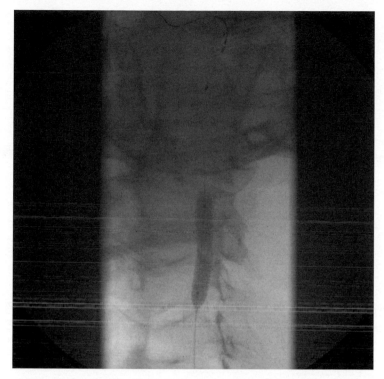

Fig. 9. Postdilatation was performed using a 6.0 × 30 mm Aviator™ balloon.

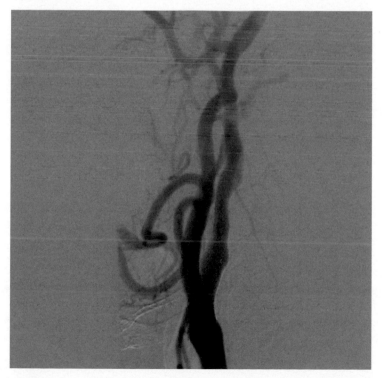

Fig. 10. Excellent angiographic result was obtained, with minimal residual stenosis and good flow distally (Movie 10).

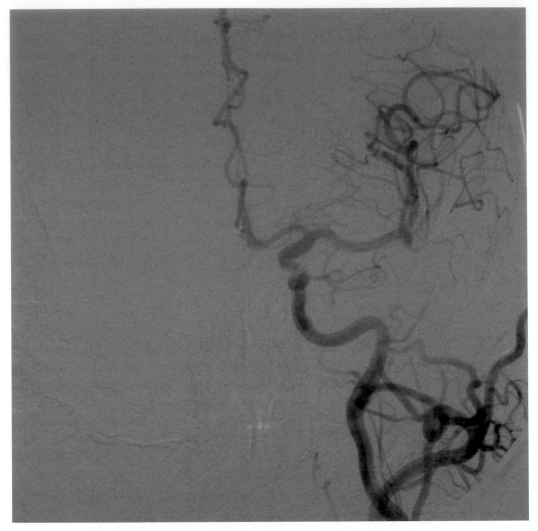

Fig. 11. Final intracranial angiography demonstrating filling of the left anterior and middle cerebral arteries via the patent left internal carotid artery (Movie 11).

sensitivity of carotid auscultation in identifying a significant (70–99% stenosis) CCA or ICA stenosis was only 56%, with a specificity of 91% *(1)*. Similarly, the presence of a carotid bruit does not necessarily signify a severe carotid lesion. For instance, in this same study, the positive predictive value of a carotid bruit was only 27% for diagnosing a significant CCA or ICA stenosis *(1)*. Therefore, confirmation with a noninvasive imaging test is necessary.

2. The carotid "string sign" represents an angiographically long tapered narrowing of the ICA, usually close to the carotid bifurcation. It occurs distal to a critically severe atherosclerotic lesion because of decrease perfusion pressure beyond the stenosis, leading to subsequent collapse of the distal ICA *(2)*. Despite the misleading angiographic appearance, the artery distal to the proximal stenosis is typically not diseased, rendering this vessel amenable to carotid revascularization of the proximal lesion. However, care should be taken to rule out other infrequent, but potential causes of "string signs," such as dissection or subtotal thrombosis *(3)*. This case is an example in which duplex

ultrasound may be misleading, which in this case, incorrectly surmised that the left ICA was occluded, precluding carotid revascularization for this vessel. It is recommended that results from duplex ultrasound be confirmed with an additional test (e.g., conventional angiography, magnetic resonance angiography) before the decision of revascularization.

3. When evaluating an ICA occlusion, it is important to advance the diagnostic catheter closer to the occlusion to allow a better assessment of the anatomy. In this case, without advancing the JR4 into the carotid bifurcation, we would not have clearly identified the "string sign." In addition, it is also important to evaluate the intracranial circulation in the setting of an ICA occlusion, particularly evaluating where collaterals originate from (e.g., external carotid artery, vertebral artery, circle of Willis), and whether the ICA fills retrograde or antegrade from collaterals.

4. Interventionalists should be versatile in using both the guide and sheath approaches for carotid stenting. In this case, although intuitively a guide approach would have given us more support to advance equipments through a critically stenotic lesion, this approach impeded wire crossing because of the innate angulation of the guide. For this case, a long straight sheath actually facilitated wire access, without compromising much support.

5. Predilatation of this critical stenosis was necessary before crossing with an emboli protection device. Using an over-the-wire balloon was also advantageous as it allowed us to confirm through contrast injection that we were in the true lumen of the ICA.

REFERENCES

1. Magyar MT, Nam EM, Csiba L, Ritter MA, Ringelstein EB, Droste DW. Carotid artery auscultation—anachronism or useful screening procedure? Neurol Res 2002;24:705–708.
2. Sekhar LN, Heros RC, Lotz PR, Rosenbaum AE. Atheromatous pseudo-occlusion of the internal carotid artery. J Neurosurg 1980;52:782–789.
3. Mehigan JT, Olcott Ct. The carotid "string" sign. Differential diagnosis and management. Am J Surg 1980;140:137–143.

19

Case: Stenting of a Carotid Endarterectomy Patch Restenosis and Aneurysm

J. Emilio Exaire, MD

CONTENTS

HISTORY

A 60-yr-old woman with a history of right carotid artery endarterectomy (CEA) 4 yr ago and a repeat CEA 2 yr ago developed restenosis of the proximal and distal clamp sites requiring carotid stent 1 yr ago. She received a 6 × 20 mm Precise™ (Cordis, Warren, NJ) stent to the distal CEA site and an 8 × 20 mm Precise™ stent to the proximal CEA site. At the time of that intervention, the venous patch used for the CEA was noted to be mildly dilated and ectatic. She subsequently developed re-restenosis and a pulsatile mass in the right neck with compression of the right internal jugular artery 1 yr later.

DIAGNOSTIC ANGIOGRAPHY

The patient had a type I aortic arch with normal origin of the great vessels. Using a stiff-angle tip Glidewire® (Terumo Medical, Somerset, NJ) that was positioned into the right common carotid artery (CCA) a JR4 catheter was advanced over-the-wire. A selective angiogram revealed a large aneurysm between the previously placed proximal and distal stents (Fig. 1). The proximal stent also had moderate 50% focal restenosis; the external carotid artery (ECA) had an ostial lesion. The intracerebral circulation was normal (Fig. 2). Given the presence of a large aneurysm and two prior surgical interventions (making repeat surgery high risk owing to the presence of scar tissue), we proceeded to exclude the aneurysm using a stent graft. We also intentionally coiled the right ECA to prevent retrograde flow from sustaining the aneurysm sac.

From: *Contemporary Cardiology: Handbook of Complex Percutaneous Carotid Intervention*
Edited by: J. Saw, J. E. Exaire, D. S. Lee, and S. Yadav © Humana Press Inc., Totowa, NJ

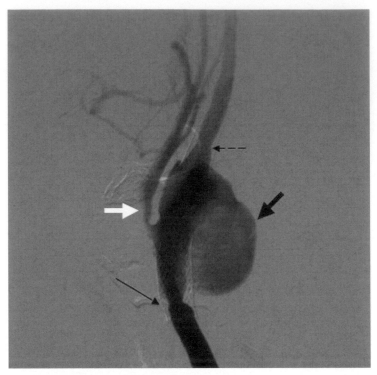

Fig. 1. The aneurysm is shown with the black bold arrow. The proximal stent has a focal moderate restenosis *(black arrow)*. The distal stent has mild restenosis *(black dashed arrow)*. The external carotid artery has an ostial lesion *(white arrow)*.

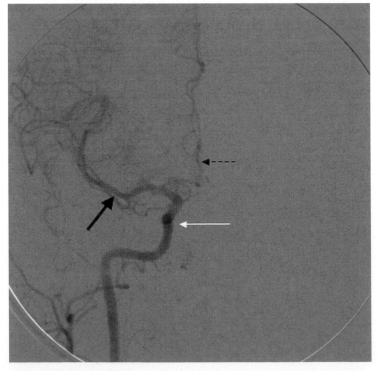

Fig. 2. Normal intracerebral angiogram before the intervention. *White arrow*: distal right internal carotid artery. *Black dashed arrow*: anterior cerebral artery. *Black bold arrow*: middle cerebral artery.

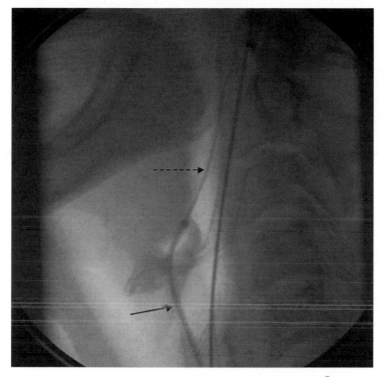

Fig. 3. The *dashed arrow* shows the position of the stiff-angled Glidewire® in the external carotid artery; the *arrow* shows the diagnostic JR4 catheter inside the external carotid artery. A 1- to 1.5-cm gap from the origin of the vessel to the desired place where the coils are to be deployed decreases the risk of coil embolization.

CAROTID STENTING PROCEDURE

The Glidewire® was advanced into the petrous portion of the internal carotid artery (ICA) and a 5 Fr diagnostic JR4 catheter was advanced over-the-wire. This wire was withdrawn and a 1-cm tip Amplatz Super Stiff™ (Boston Scientific, Natick, MA) wire was advanced through the JR4 catheter. The JR4 diagnostic catheter was then withdrawn and an 8 Fr JR4 guide was advanced into the CCA. The stiff-angled Glidewire® was advanced into the ECA and the 5 Fr diagnostic JR4 catheter was advanced over-the-wire (Fig. 3). The Glidewire® was then withdrawn, and using contrast injections from the JR4 guide to gauge positioning, selective coiling of the ECA was performed. Four coils were necessary to achieve complete occlusion of the right ECA (two 5-mm Cook coils followed by two 5- to 3-mm tapering Cook coils) (Fig. 4). At this point, a FilterWire EX™ (Boston Scientific, Natick, MA) was deployed in the prepetrous ICA (Fig. 5).

The JR4 catheter was then withdrawn from the right ECA. An 8 × 50 mm Viabahn™ (Gore Medica, Flagstaff, AZ) stent graft was then advanced over the Amplatz Super Stiff™ wire and positioned extending from the right CCA into the right ICA (Fig. 6). The stent was deployed (Fig. 7) and postdilated with a 7 × 20 mm OptaPro™ (Cordis, Miami, FL) balloon (Fig. 8). The final result was excellent with minimal residual leak into the aneurysm, and flow to the ECA was excluded (Fig. 9). Postprocedure, the patient complained of jaw claudication, but fortunately that resolved after a few days. The neck mass receded soon after the intervention. A month later, a repeat angiogram showed excellent coverage of the lesion without any leak (Fig. 10).

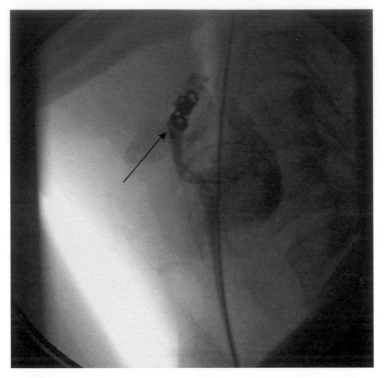

Fig. 4. After deploying four coils *(arrow)*, the flow to the external carotid is completely occluded.

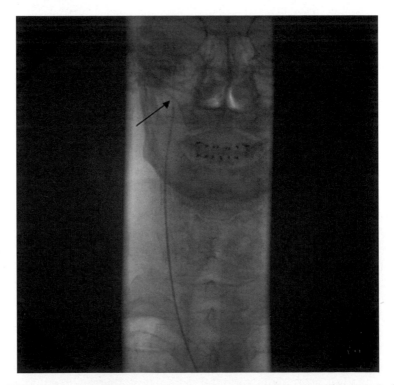

Fig. 5. Filter Wire placement in the prepetrous segment of the internal carotid artery before the stent graft is deployed.

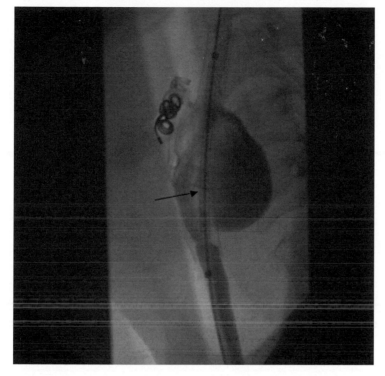

Fig. 6. The stent graft is positioned *(arrow)* so as to cover the whole length of the aneurysm.

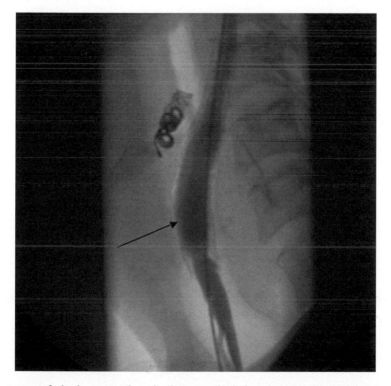

Fig. 7. After stent graft deployment, there is almost no leak, but the apposition of the stent is not ideal *(arrow)*.

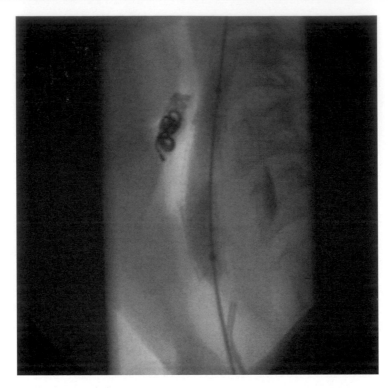

Fig. 8. A 7 × 20 mm OptaPro™ balloon is used for postdilation.

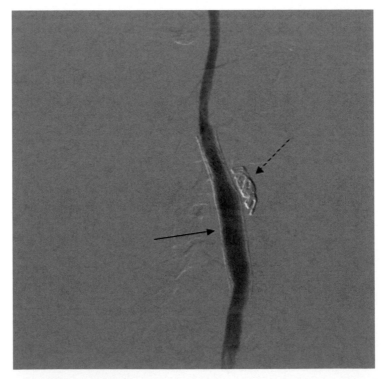

Fig. 9. Final angiography result. Notice the absence of flow into the external carotid artery *(dashed arrow)* and the almost inexistent leak into the aneurysm *(arrow)*.

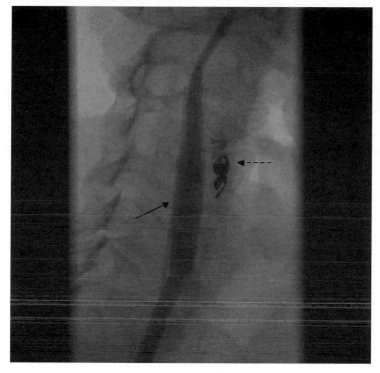

Fig. 10. Repeat angiography 1 mo later demonstrating no leak from the external carotid artery *(dashed arrow)* or the internal carotid artery *(arrow)*.

LEARNING POINTS

1. Aneurysm of a carotid endarterectomy patch is a rare complication usually presenting as a pulsatile neck mass. Isolated case reports have shown successful treatment with stent grafting *(1,2)*.
2. Once covered with the stent graft, the aneurysm may still have two potential sources of blood: antegrade through the CCA and retrograde through the vast collateral system of the ECA. Therefore, it is mandatory to exclude the flow in the ECA (e.g., using coils as in our patient) simultaneous with placement of an appropriately sized stent graft with percutaneous interventions.
3. Jaw claudication is uncommon with percutaneous carotid stenting. In our patient, it was necessary to completely occlude flow of the ECA, which resulted in the jaw claudication. However, owing to the presence of extensive neck and face collaterals (from ipsilateral and contralateral flows), occlusion or severe stenosis of the ECA is usually well tolerated. In our patient, the jaw claudication resolved after a few days.
4. When deploying coils in the ECA, it is important to avoid placing a coil at the ostium of the ECA, as the risk of embolization is greater if positioned close to the bifurcation. Usually a 1-cm gap from the origin of the ECA to the desired place to deploy the coil is adequate.
5. Stent graft is usually more difficult to deliver compared to a regular self-expanding nitinol stent, thus a stiff wire is almost always necessary. Postdilation is also always performed because the stent graft may not be completely opposed to the vessel wall.

6. Following successful exclusion of the aneurysm, it is important to perform repeat
   follow-up imaging to ensure that the aneurysm leak is sealed. This may be done with
   conventional angiography or CT angiography.

REFERENCES

1. Mousa A, Bernheim J, Lyon R, et al. Postcarotid endarterectomy pseudoaneurysm treated with combined stent graft and coil embolization—a case report. Vasc Endovascular Surg 2005;39:191–194.
2. Martin ND, Carabasi RA, Bonn J, Lombardi J, DiMuzio P. Endovascular repair of carotid artery
   aneurysms following carotid endarterectomy. Ann Vasc Surg 2005;19:913–916.

20 Case: Carotid Stenting With Slow Flow and Distal Embolization

J. Emilio Exaire, MD

CONTENTS

HISTORY

A 77-yr-old man with asymptomatic severe left internal carotid artery (ICA) stenosis detected by carotid duplex ultrasound. He had a history of three-vessel coronary artery disease, coronary artery bypass graft surgery in 1971, and several percutaneous coronary interventions. He also had systemic hypertension and hyperlipidemia. The patient had persistent exertional anginal symptoms despite prior coronary interventions, and thus he was felt to be at high risk for surgical carotid endarterectomy. Therefore, he was referred for carotid artery stenting.

DIAGNOSTIC ANGIOGRAPHY

A type I aortic arch was found with normal origin of the supra-aortic vessels. The right ICA was normal, and gave rise to normal right anterior cerebral artery (ACA) and middle cerebral artery (MCA). There was absence of posterior communicating arteries (Fig. 1). Both the left and right vertebral arteries were normal in caliber without stenosis. A 90% ostial stenosis of the left ICA was demonstrated (Fig. 2). Following diagnostic angiography, we proceeded to stenting of this severe left ICA lesion.

CAROTID ARTERY STENTING PROCEDURE

Unfractionated heparin (100 U/kg) was administered to obtain an ACT close to 300 s. A 6 Fr 90-cm Shuttle sheath (Cook, Bloomington, IN) was advanced into the left common carotid artery (CCA) via a telescoping access. With this approach, a long 5 Fr 125 cm JR4 diagnostic catheter is passed within the Shuttle sheath, and the whole system is advanced over a stiff-angled Glidewire®. The JR4 is used to engage the left CCA and the Glidewire® is advanced just short of the lesion. The JR4 catheter is then

From: *Contemporary Cardiology: Handbook of Complex Percutaneous Carotid Intervention*
Edited by: J. Saw, J. E. Exaire, D. S. Lee, and S. Yadav © Humana Press Inc., Totowa, NJ

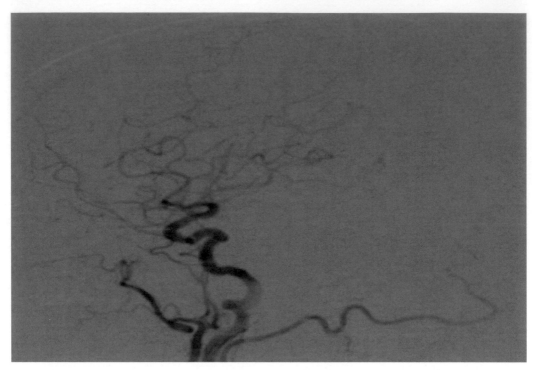

Fig. 1. Intracranial carotid angiography preprocedure in the lateral projection. Left anterior cerebral and middle cerebral arteries. Notice the absence of posterior communicating artery (Movie 1).

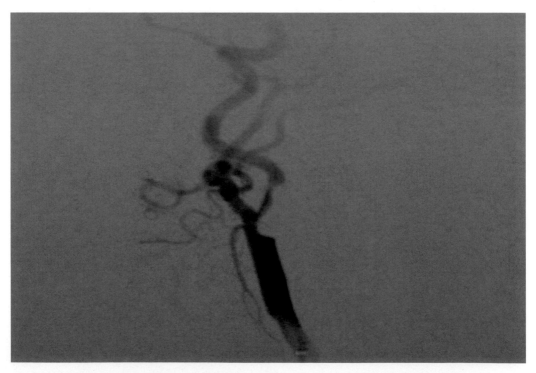

Fig. 2. Diagnostic carotid angiography of the bifurcation lesion (Movie 2).

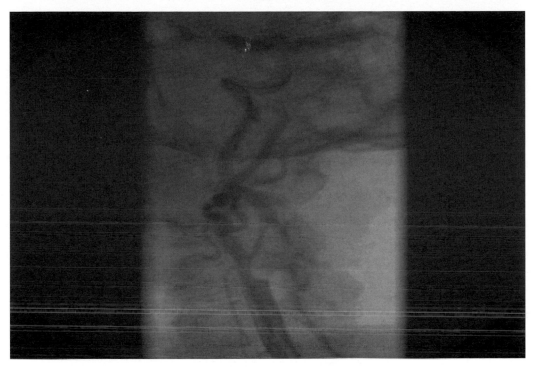

Fig. 3. AngioGuard XP™ placement (Movie 3).

advanced into the CCA and the Shuttle sheath is advanced over it. Once the sheath is in place, both the Glidewire® and the JR 4 are withdrawn. A 6-mm AngioGuard XP™ (Cordis, Warren, NJ) device was advanced into the prepetrous ICA and deployed without any complications (Fig. 3). The lesion was predilated with a 4.0 × 30 mm Maverick²™ (Boston Scientific, Natick, MA) balloon. After this, an 8.0 × 30 mm Precise™ (Cordis, Warren, NJ) nitinol stent was deployed. Postdilatation with a 5.5 × 30 mm Aviator™ (Cordis, Warren, NJ) balloon was performed (Fig. 4).

At this point, the patient complained of facial pain, and then developed aphasia and right hemiparesis. The postdilatation angiography showed slow flow into both the ICA and external carotid artery (ECA) (Fig. 4). At this point, suctioning with an Export catheter of the PercuSurge® GuardWire™ system (Medtronic, Minneapolis, MN) was performed. The AngioGuard XP™ was then collapsed and withdrawn. After filter retrieval, the patient remained aphasic and hemiparetic. Intracerebral angiograms following filter retrieval showed a distal MCA embolization in the M3 segment (Fig. 5). At this point, the patient received intraarterial abciximab (half bolus, 0.125 mg/kg) through the Shuttle sheath. Because of the distal nature of the MCA embolization, we did not proceed to further intracranial interventions. We waited with the patient in the angiography suite for approx 30 min. Repeat angiography was performed (Fig. 6) showing improved intracranial flow with partial resolution of the embolus. Within this timeframe, the patient's symptoms improved, he was no longer aphasic, and had very mild residual weakness on his right side. The patient was then transferred to radiology for an emergent computed tomography (CT) head scan to rule out intracranial bleeding. Another repeat CT scan 24 h later was also negative for intracranial bleed. Overnight, the hemiparesis resolved. The patient was finally discharged 72 h following the procedure without any neurologic deficit.

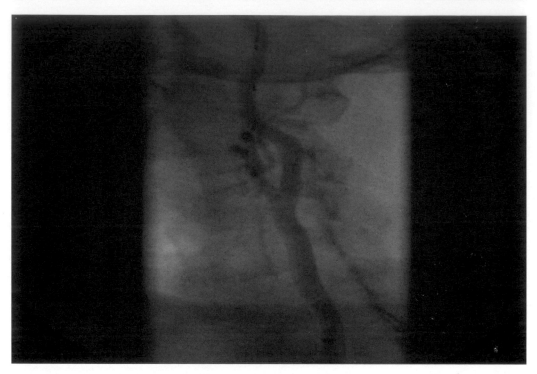

Fig. 4. Bifurcation angiogram following stent postdilatation. Note the slow flow and the hazy appearance of the AngioGuard XP™ filter due to plaque embolization (Movie 4).

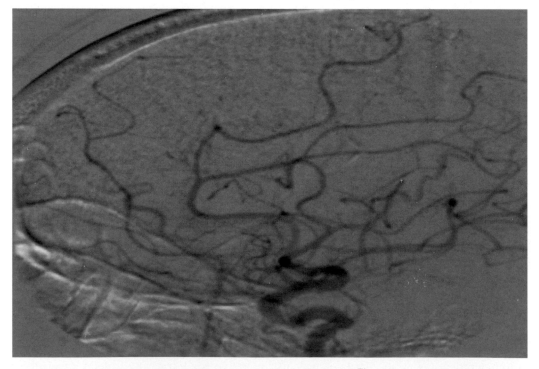

Fig. 5. Intracranial carotid angiography following AngioGuard XP™ retrieval. Notice the slow flow at the M3 segment of the middle cerebral artery. The contrast stains the affected area (Movie 5).

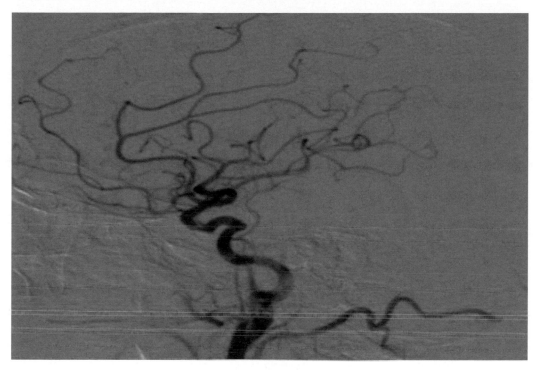

Fig. 6. After intraarterial abciximab, the intracranial flow and neurological symptoms slowly improved (Movie 6).

LEARNING POINTS

1. Distal embolization occurs frequently with carotid stenting, especially during stent postdilatation. With the use of filter emboli protection device (EPD), distal emboliza-tion fill up the filter basket, leading to slow flow. This can result in cerebral ischemia with neurologic symptoms. If the EPD is collapsed at this point in the presence of slow flow, the embolic debris may travel downstream into the intracranial circulation. Therefore, aspiration with either a multipurpose catheter or an Export catheter would remove the stagnant column of blood that contains the liberated debris. This helps to reduce distal embolization upon retrieval of the EPD.

2. In our patient, the plaque burden overwhelmed the EPD and a small embolic debris traveled to the MCA. The overall risk of minor stroke during carotid artery stenting is about 1%. If the embolus is in the proximal segments of the MCA (M1 or M2 seg-ments), an attempt should be made to retrieve it with a snare device, or perform balloon angioplasty to improve flow. If the embolus is lodged in the distal segments (M3 and M4) a conservative approach is recommended, as the patient's prognosis is usually good, and spontaneous resolution of symptoms typically occurs. However, intraarterial abciximab and/or tPA may be required if symptoms do not spontaneously improve, to reduce thrombus formation or thrombolyse clot superimposed on the embolized plaque. This approach is associated with a higher risk of intracerebral hemorrhage, and the patient should be watched closely for this.

3. A CT head scan should be performed immediately and in the next 24 h to rule out bleeding. If the patient recovers within the following 24 h, the prognosis is excellent.

21 Case: Acute Stroke Intervention With a Large Thrombotic Burden

Jacqueline Saw, MD

CONTENTS

HISTORY

A 69-yr-old man presented with new-onset atrial fibrillation, complaining of shortness of breath. His past medical history is significant for coronary artery disease, ischemic cardiomyopathy (ejection fraction 15%), diabetes mellitus, and hypertension. He was admitted to hospital and started on intravenous heparin. The day after admission, he developed right hemiplegia with deviation of his eyes to the left. Immediate noncontrast brain computed tomography (CT) showed remote left cerebellar infarct but no evidence of acute intracranial abnormality. However, brain magnetic resonance imaging (MRI) showed extensive cortical and basal ganglia subacute infarction involving two thirds of the left middle cerebral artery (MCA) territory. Therefore, he underwent urgent cerebral angiography at 6 h after symptom onset.

DIAGNOSTIC ANGIOGRAPHY

A 5 Fr Vitek catheter was used for cerebral diagnostic angiography. There was a large thrombus in the distal left internal carotid artery (ICA), with slow antegrade flow into the left anterior cerebral artery (ACA), and complete occlusion of the M1 segment of the left MCA (Figs. 1 and 2). We proceeded to immediate percutaneous intervention to salvage neurologic function.

PERCUTANEOUS INTRACRANIAL INTERVENTION

A 0.035-in. stiff-angled Glidewire® (Terumo Medical) was advanced via the Vitek catheter into the proximal left ICA. The Vitek was advanced over this wire into the proximal left ICA. The Glidewire® was then exchanged for a 0.035-in. 6-cm tip Amplatz Super Stiff™ (Boston Scientific, Natick, MA) wire for more stable support. The Vitek catheter was removed and a 7 Fr 90-cm Shuttle sheath (Cook, Bloomington, IN) was

From: *Contemporary Cardiology: Handbook of Complex Percutaneous Carotid Intervention*
Edited by: J. Saw, J. E. Exaire, D. S. Lee, and S. Yadav © Humana Press Inc., Totowa, NJ

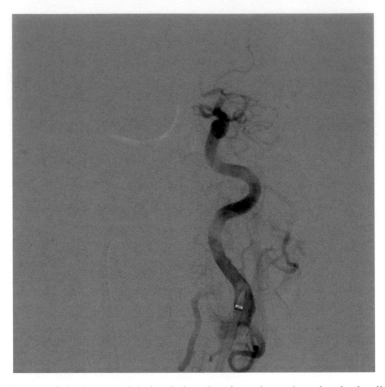

Fig. 1. PA projection of the intracranial circulation showing a large thrombus in the distal left internal carotid artery, with slow antegrade flow into the left anterior cerebral artery, and complete occlusion of the M1 segment of the left middle cerebral artery (Movie 1).

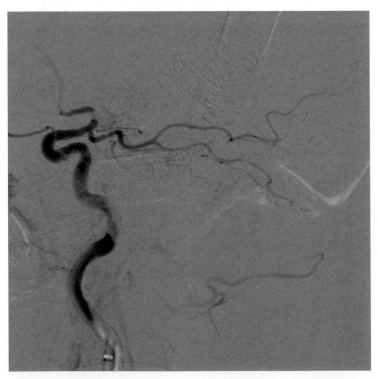

Fig. 2. Lateral projection of the intracranial circulation showing the large thrombus in the distal left internal carotid artery (just beyond the posterior communicating artery) (Movie 2).

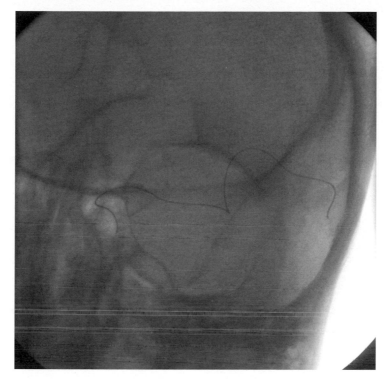

Fig. 3. The occluded left middle cerebral artery was crossed with a Synchro wire, and a 2.0 × 9.0 mm Maverick²™ balloon was inflated in the M1 segment.

advanced into the proximal left ICA. The stiff angled Glidewire® was then advanced into the distal ICA just beyond the petrous portion of the ICA. A 6 Fr MPD Envoy® (Cordis, Miami, FL) guide was then inserted through the Shuttle sheath and positioned just beyond the petrous portion of the left ICA. This setup allowed a stable support for intracranial intervention.

A 0.014-in. long Synchro wire (Boston Scientific, Natick, MA) was used to cross the occluded M1 segment of the left MCA, supported by an over-the-wire 2.0 × 9.0 mm Maverick²™ (Boston Scientific, Natick, MA) balloon. This balloon was advanced into the occluded M1 segment and inflated at 6 atm (Fig. 3). The balloon was then exchanged to a RapidTransit™ (Cordis, Miami, FL) catheter over the Synchro wire. Intra-arterial Retavase (3 mg) and abciximab (5 mg) was administered through the RapidTransit™ catheter, and also through the Shuttle sheath (1 mg of Retavase and 5 mg of abciximab). Despite these maneuvers, flow was still occlusive to the MCA territory (Fig. 4). We then exchanged the Envoy® guide to a 7 Fr Concentric® balloon guide catheter (Concentric Medical, Mountain View, CA) into the proximal ICA through the Shuttle sheath. The balloon on the Concentric® guide was inflated to occlude the ICA. The RapidTransit™ catheter was reintroduced beyond the M1 occlusion, and a 4 mm Amplatz GooseNeck® snare (Ev3) was advanced through it. Once the snare was distal to the M1 occlusion (Fig. 5), the snare and the RapidTransit™ catheter was removed in unison, while simultaneously aspirating through the side port of the Concentric® balloon guide. We retrieved a large thrombus through this maneuver. This step was repeated once more, and another large thrombus was retrieved. These maneuvers finally eradicated the M1 occlusion with good distal intracranial flow (Figs. 6 and 7).

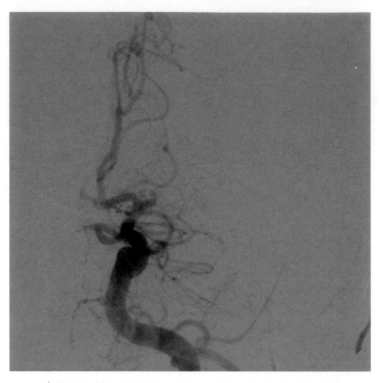

Fig. 4. After intraarterial thrombolysis, flow to the anterior cerebral artery is improved, but the M1 segment of the middle cerebral artery is still occluded (Movie 4).

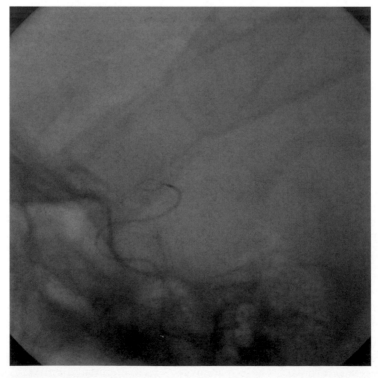

Fig. 5. A RapidTransit™ catheter was introduced beyond the M1 occlusion, and a GooseNeck® snare was advanced through it.

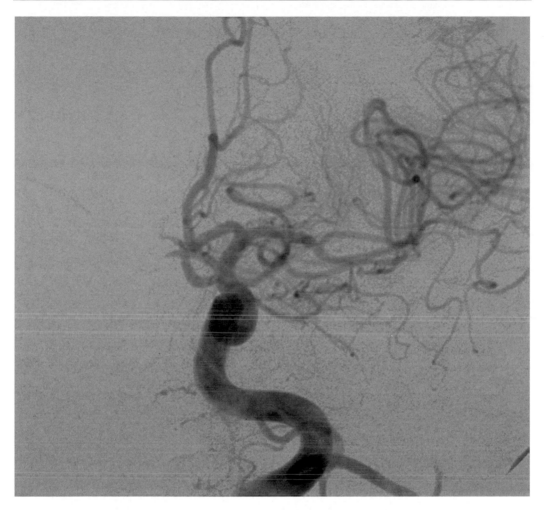

Fig. 6. Final intracranial angiography in the PA projection after mechanical embolectomy, showing normalization of intracranial flow (Movie 6).

The patient tolerated this procedure well, and was transferred to the intensive care unit for recovery. He survived the hospitalization; however, he had persistent right hemiparesis on discharge.

LEARNING POINTS

1. This patient had an embolic MCA stroke, which is cardiac in origin, either from the left atrium (due to the new-onset atrial fibrillation), or from the left ventricle (given the ischemic cardiomyopathy with ejection fraction of 15%) (see Fig. 1 in Chapter 1). Emergent head CT scan is necessary, ideally complemented with CT or MR angiography if available. Options for treatment for an acute embolic cerebral event include intravenous thrombolytic or percutaneous intervention. In our patient, the large territory involvement suggested very proximal involvement of an MCA, and thus the percutaneous approach is appropriate.
2. For percutaneous acute stroke treatment due to thrombotic embolism, administration of a thrombolytic agent is a key therapeutic element. Intraarterial administration of

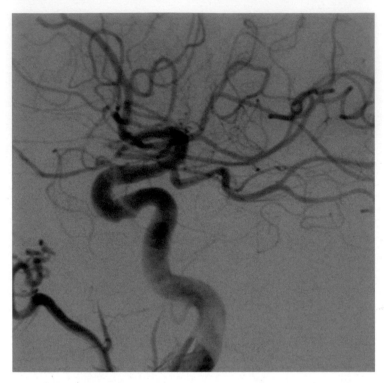

Fig. 7. Final intracranial angiography in the lateral projection showing normalized intracranial flow (Movie 7).

thrombolytic and glycoprotein (GP) IIb/IIIa inhibitors is best achieved with a catheter positioned in proximity of the thrombus (some operators place catheter proximal to, some place it within the thrombus, and others place it distal to the thrombus). Please see Chapter 15 for details of drug choices and doses.

3. Mechanical embolectomy can be used adjunctively with intraarterial thrombolysis, especially in the presence of large thrombus burden (as in our patient). A snare (e.g., GooseNeck®) is often used for emboli of cardiac origin. It is introduced through a catheter (e.g., RapidTransit™) placed distal to the embolus, the snare is then pushed out of the catheter tip into the distal vessel, which opens up the snare's loop. The snare and catheter is then pulled back as a unit into the thrombus, and then the snare is retrieved partially by pulling it part way into the catheter. This closes up the loop and captures the thrombus. The snare and catheter is then pulled back together as a unit into the guide catheter.

4. For this patient, we used a Concentric® balloon guide which allowed inflation of a balloon in the ICA to occlude antegrade flow, thus reducing the risk of distal embolization during snare retrieval. Retrieval was also done simultaneously with aspiration through the side port of the Concentric® balloon guide to help capture the thrombus and prevent embolization. The Merci® Retrieval System (Concentric Medical, Mountain View, CA) is now available in the United States, which has a 0.014-in. nitinol guidewire with five helical loops distally to capture emboli.

5. Another option of percutaneous acute stroke treatment is the use of 0.014-in. guidewire and coronary angioplasty balloon to disrupt the clot, which can open up the arterial lumen expediently, but may cause embolization downstream. Fortunately, the emboli that are liberated and propagated downstream tend to be smaller than the initial thrombus, and thus may lodge in smaller distal arteries with fewer neurologic deficits.

22

Case: Left Internal Carotid Artery Stenting in a Bovine Aortic Arch

David S. Lee, MD

HISTORY

A 78-yr-old Caucasian man presented with left eye amaurosis fugax that resolved within 3–4 min. He had a past history of myocardial infarction, coronary artery bypass surgery in 1987, ischemic cardiomyopathy with ejection fraction 25–30%, and permanent pacemaker insertion for sick-sinus syndrome. His risk factors include hyperlipidemia and hypertension; he quit smoking 16 yr ago. He denied chest pain, shortness of breath, palpitations, or other neurologic symptoms. He has NYHA Class II congestive heart failure. His carotid duplex ultrasound showed moderate bilateral internal carotid artery (ICA) stenosis 60–79% (left ICA PSV 239 cm/s, EDV 62 cm/s, ratio 4.87; right ICA PSV 174 cm/s, EDV 46 cm/s, ratio 1.75). Thus, he was referred for further evaluation and management for symptomatic left ICA stenosis.

Given his ischemic cardiomyopathy with poor ejection fraction, he was considered high risk for carotid endarterectomy, and thus underwent carotid stenting. His asymptomatic right ICA stenosis would not qualify for revascularization at this time unless the severity of the stenosis was significantly underestimated by ultrasound. He was enrolled into a clinical trial protocol, and was started on full dose aspirin (325 mg po daily) and Plavix (75 mg po daily) 5 d prior to the procedure.

DIAGNOSTIC ANGIOGRAPHY

A 5 Fr short sheath was placed in the right common femoral artery. Subsequently, a straight pigtail catheter was advanced over a 0.035-in. 260-cm Wholey wire (Mallinckrodt,

From: *Contemporary Cardiology: Handbook of Complex Percutaneous Carotid Intervention*
Edited by: J. Saw, J. E. Exaire, D. S. Lee, and S. Yadav © Humana Press Inc., Totowa, NJ

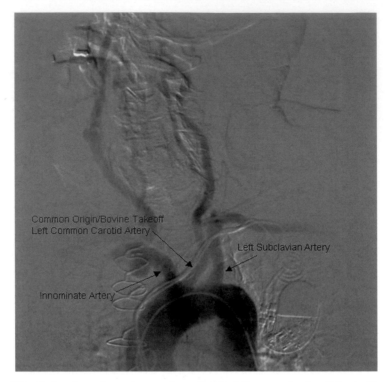

Fig. 1. Aortic arch angiogram in an LAO oblique projection (Movie 1).

Hazelwood, MO) into the aortic arch. An arch aortogram was then performed in an LAO oblique projection (Fig. 1). Subsequently, a long JR4 catheter (125 cm) was used to selectively engage the innominate artery. An innominate artery angiogram was then performed. Using roadmapping (trace subtraction angiography), a stiff-angled Glidewire® (Terumo Medical, Somerset, NJ) was advanced into the right common carotid artery (CCA) and the JR4 catheter was advanced over this stiff-angled Glidewire® into the right CCA. A right CCA angiogram (Fig. 2) with cerebral angiogram was then performed (Fig. 3). As can be seen, the right CCA has an aneurysm. In addition, the right anterior cerebral artery (ACA) supplies flow across the anterior communicating artery (ACOM) to the left ACA.

Subsequently, the JR4 catheter was then brought back to the origin of the innominate artery and used to selectively engage the bovine/common origin left CCA. Using roadmapping and the stiff-angled Glidewire®, the JR4 catheter was advanced into the left CCA. A left CCA angiogram (Figs. 4 and 5) with cerebral angiogram was then performed (Fig. 6). Diagnostic angiography is always performed prior to intervention, either at the same time or on a previous day. The ease of which the diagnostic catheters can be advanced into position will predict the ease or difficulty of sheath or guide placement for the intervention. In this case, the angulation of the arch (type I) was not so severe that a JR4 diagnostic catheter could be advanced into the bovine takeoff of the left CCA. If the angle had been sharper, a Vitek or Simmons catheter may have been necessary. Usually, a Vitek catheter is preferred over a Simmons if the catheter needs to be advanced into either the distal CCA or the external carotid artery (ECA). Cerebral angiography should be performed prior to intervention. Cerebral angiography provides information about the

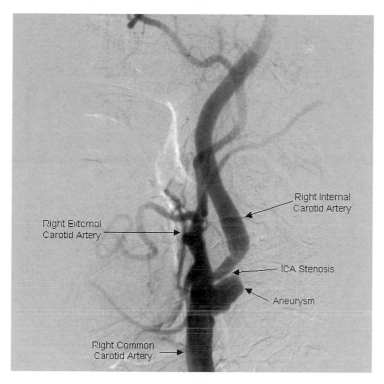

Fig. 2. Right common carotid artery angiogram.

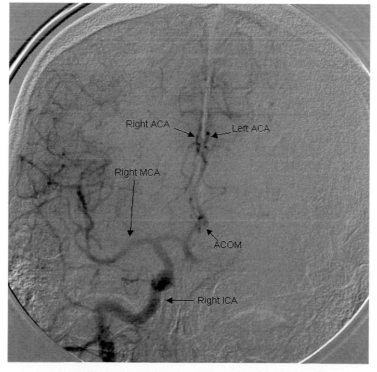

Fig. 3. Right cerebral angiogram in the PA projection.

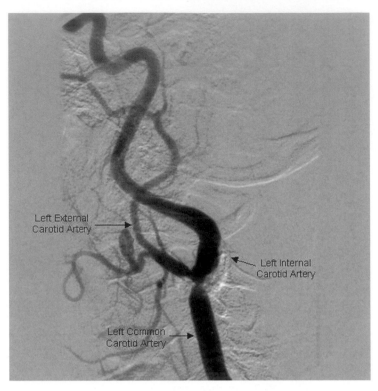

Fig. 4. Prestenting left common carotid artery angiogram in the LAO projection (Movie 4).

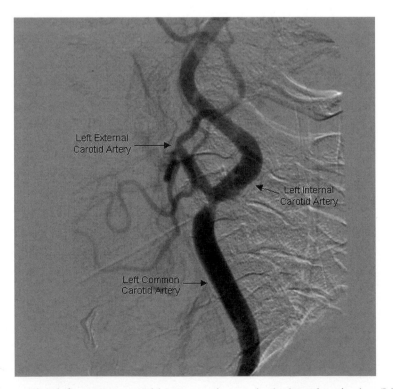

Fig. 5. Prestenting left common carotid artery angiogram in the lateral projection (Movie 5).

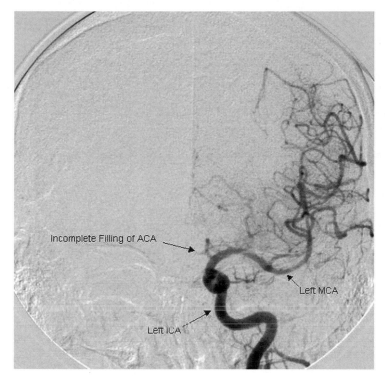

Fig. 6. Prestenting left cerebral angiogram in the PA projection (Movie 6).

distal circulation beyond the carotid artery, about the adequacy of collaterals, and provides a baseline for comparison if the neurologic status changes after the procedure.

ANGIOGRAPHIC FINDINGS

1. Type I aortic arch with bovine/common origin of the left CCA.
2. Mild disease in the innominate artery.
3. The right CCA has mild disease. The proximal right ICA has a 60% narrowing with severe ulceration of the carotid bulb. The right ICA fills the right middle cerebral artery (MCA) and ACA, and fills the contralateral ACA via a patent ACOM into the left A1 segment.
4. Left CCA has significant tortuosity in its proximal half. The distal left CCA has a severe 60–70% with slightly hazy stenosis just prior to the origins of the left ECA and ICA. The left ICA fills the left MCA and ACA. Competitive filling is seen in the left ACA system.

THE CHALLENGE

Performing a left carotid intervention in a bovine takeoff of the left CCA increases its complexity primarily from the viewpoint of increased angulation and tortuosity. Figure 7 shows a type I arch. The worst angulation of the takeoff of the left CCA from the arch is 90° in this case. Figure 8 shows a bovine arch in which the angulation is more severe and similar to a type III arch. As a catheter is advanced over a wire, the orientation of the tip of the catheter directs its force. The more that the tip of the catheter

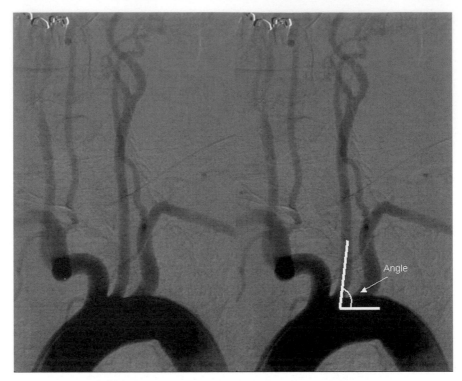

Fig. 7. Example of a type 1 aortic arch angulation.

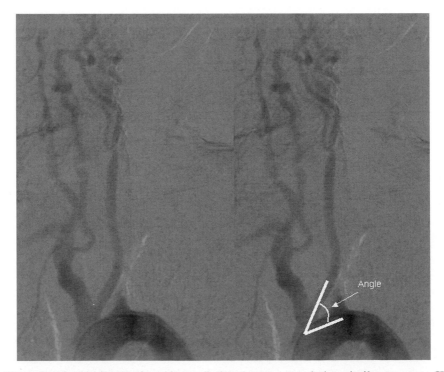

Fig. 8. Example of a bovine aortic arch angulation (greater angulation similar to a type III aortic arch).

lines up with the direction that you want it to go and where the wire is, the easier it is to advance the catheter. If the directions of forces are significantly different, then the amount of purchase the wire has distally as well as the stiffness of the wire compared to the pliability of the catheter or guide will determine how easily it can be advanced, vs the likelihood that the entire system will be prolapsed out of the artery of interest. A guide or sheath that has an angulated tip can be rotated into the origin of the artery making it easier to advance. Therefore, in more angulated situations, either a guide (e.g., H1 guide) or a sheath with a catheter-based introducer (e.g., Shuttle Select [Cook Incorporated, Bloomington, IN] with JB1 slip-catheter) will be easier to position than a sheath with a straight tapered introducer. Aside from the angulation/tortuosity issues, intervention in the left carotid artery of a bovine takeoff is not more complicated or difficult than usual.

GUIDE CATHETER APPROACH

In this case, a telescoping system using a 125-cm 5 Fr JR4 diagnostic catheter telescoped through an 8 Fr H1 guide was utilized to position the guide within the left CCA. Initially this system was advanced over a Wholey wire into the aortic arch. The JR4 catheter was used to engage the origin of the left CCA. Using roadmapping, a stiff angled Glidewire® was advanced into the mid-left CCA. Using a technique known as bootstrapping, the JR4 catheter was advanced slightly into the proximal to mid-thirds of the left CCA. Subsequently the H1 guide was carefully advanced over the JR4 and Glidewire® and rotated to engage the origin of the left CCA. As the guide turns and engages the origin of the artery, there is a tendency for the diagnostic catheter and wire to jump forward. Especially in this setting with a distal CCA stenosis, care must be taken to prevent the wire or worse the diagnostic catheter from advancing through the lesion. Once the guide has engaged the origin, the wire can be slightly advanced, then the diagnostic catheter followed by the guide into the proximal third of the CCA. Once the diagnostic catheter is near the junction of the mid- and distal thirds of the CCA, the guide can be gently advanced, with gentle torquing into the mid-CCA. As the angulation and tortuosity straighten from the positioning of the guide, care must be taken to not let the diagnostic catheter or wire migrate too far distally. With the guide in position, the diagnostic catheter and wire can slowly be withdrawn. Once these are removed, the guide catheter will be more compliant and may "fall back," which more accurately is the relaxation of the catheter conforming to the tortuosity of the vessel and arch. Assuming that the guide is in a stable position, the intervention can then proceed.

CAROTID INTERVENTION

The 5 Fr short sheath was exchanged for an 8 Fr sheath. A total of 6000 U of unfractionated heparin were administered, and a peak activated clotting time (ACT) of 298 s was obtained. A telescoping setup and the bootstrapping technique was used to get an 8 Fr H1 guide in position (as described in the preceding text). Once in position, a 6-mm AngioGuard XP™ (Cordis, Warren, NJ) emboli protection device was then passed across the distal left CCA stenosis and deployed in the prepetrous portion of the extracranial left ICA. Subsequently, the lesion was dilated with a 4.0 × 20 mm CrossSail® balloon (Guidant, Indianapolis, IN) at 12 atm (Fig. 9). The lesion was then stented using an 8.0 × 20 mm Precise™ stent (Cordis, Warren, NJ). The stent was then postdilated with a 6.0 × 20 mm Aviator™ balloon (Cordis, Warren, NJ) at 10 atm. The

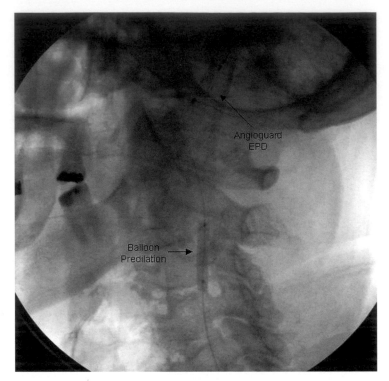

Fig. 9. Balloon predilation of the left internal carotid artery stenosis. The position of the AngioGuard XP™ emboli protection device (EPD) is shown.

initial stenosis was 60–70% and the final stenosis was 10% after stent deployment and postdilation. There was no slow flow noted throughout the procedure. The AngioGuard XP™ device was then captured using the retrieval sheath. Final left CCA angiogram (Fig. 10) with cerebral angiogram (Fig. 11) was then performed, and the guide catheter was brought back to the origin of the left CCA and the final left CCA angiogram was performed. A right common femoral artery angiogram was then performed and with confirmation of the sheath above the femoral bifurcation and below the iliac brim, an 8 Fr Angio-Seal was deployed in the right common femoral artery.

POSTINTERVENTION COURSE

The patient was monitored in-hospital overnight. He had no complications. His blood pressure was well controlled with systolic blood pressure readings in the 120s. The postprocedure neurology evaluation showed no new changes. Follow-up carotid duplex ultrasound the following morning showed improvement in the velocities on the left ICA (PSV 97 cm/s, EDV 31 cm/s, ratio 1.16) with estimated stenosis of 20–39%.

LEARNING POINTS

1. The angulation of the left CCA off of the innominate artery in a bovine arch means that the overall angle from the aortic arch to the proximal left CCA is usually much sharper. In the worst cases, it is <45°, making it the equivalent of a type III arch. In the event that a type III arch is already present, the bovine takeoff makes sheath or guide positioning much more difficult, if not nearly impossible. Interventionalists early in their

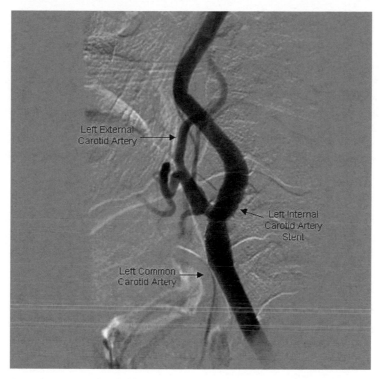

Fig. 10. Poststenting left common carotid artery angiogram (Movie 10).

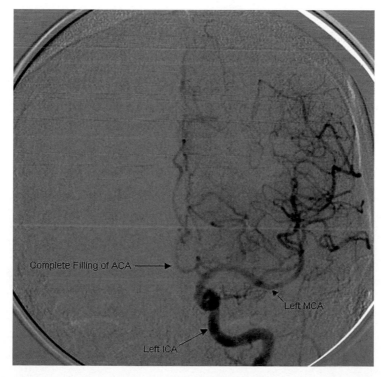

Fig. 11. Poststenting left cerebral angiogram in the PA projection (Movie 11).

experience will likely not want to perform these types of cases until they have acquired more experience.

2. Typically the worse the angulation, the more that a guide will be preferred to a sheath. A telescoping system with a 5 Fr 125 cm JR4 or Vitek diagnostic catheter telescoped through an 8 Fr H1 guide is probably the best system to access sharply angulated and tortuous vessels. The introduction of the Shuttle Select system by Cook Incorporated with various slip catheters, including the JB1, JB2, and Vitek, means that in most cases, the angulated artery can also be accessed using the smaller diameter sheath system.

23

Case: Right Carotid Artery Stenting via Right Brachial Artery Approach

David S. Lee, MD

CONTENTS

HISTORY

A 68-yr-old Caucasian man with a history of atrial fibrillation, myocardial infarction in 1994 (with subsequent ejection fraction of 30%), and thoracic aortic aneurysm who underwent coronary artery bypass grafting and thoracic aneurysm repair in 1999. His cardiac risk factors include hyperlipidemia and hypertension; he quit smoking years ago. In 2003, he was diagnosed with a type B aortic dissection extending from just beyond his left subclavian artery into his common and external iliac arteries bilaterally. The dissection was managed medically, and he was discharged home on medical therapy. He was subsequently referred for further evaluation. In 2004, his aortic artery slowly increased in size (aortic isthmus went from 5.1 cm to 5.7 cm, and mid-thoracic aorta from 3.1 cm to 4.0 cm). He subsequently presented with interscapular back pain and severe hypertension. Repeat CT scan revealed that his aortic isthmus had increased to 7.1 cm. His blood pressure and pain were controlled, and he underwent presurgical evaluation.

His carotid duplex ultrasound showed severe right internal carotid artery (ICA) stenosis 80–99% (PSV 452 cm/s, EDV 141 cm/s, ratio 10.3), with only mild disease on the left ICA 20–39% (PSV 88 cm/s, EDV 27 cm/s, ratio 1.2). With this severe asymptomatic right ICA stenosis, his risk of perioperative stroke with cardiothoracic surgery for his enlarging aortic aneurysm was increased. His treatment options included staged carotid endarterectomy followed by aortic surgery, combined carotid endarterectomy with aortic surgery, carotid angioplasty ± stenting followed by aortic surgery, or aortic surgery

From: *Contemporary Cardiology: Handbook of Complex Percutaneous Carotid Intervention*
Edited by: J. Saw, J. E. Exaire, D. S. Lee, and S. Yadav © Humana Press Inc., Totowa, NJ

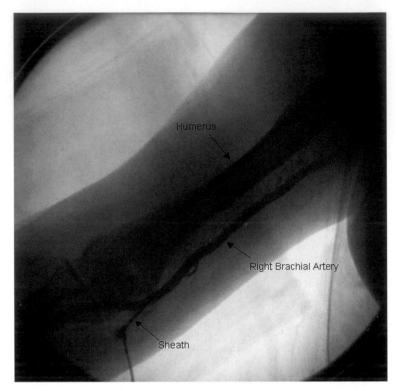

Fig. 1. Brachial arteriogram (Movie 1).

alone without carotid revascularization. Following extensive discussion between the cardiothoracic surgeon, the vascular surgeon, the neurologist, and the cardiologist, the decision was made to proceed with carotid revascularization prior to aortic surgery to decrease the perioperative stroke risk from the aortic surgery.

The least morbid approach for carotid revascularization was thought to be percutaneous carotid intervention. If a reasonable result was obtained by balloon angioplasty alone without dissection, then the plan was not to place a stent such that surgery could be expedited. Stenting would be performed only in the setting of a suboptimal result after angioplasty. If this were the case, then his aortic surgery would have to be delayed by one month (due to the need for antiplatelet therapy), which was agreed on by the surgeons. Femoral access was contraindicated because of his extensive type B aortic dissection. He therefore underwent diagnostic carotid and cerebral angiography with potential right ICA stenting via a brachial artery approach.

DIAGNOSTIC PROCEDURE

A 5 Fr arterial sheath was placed in the right brachial artery (Fig. 1). A 5 Fr JR4 diagnostic catheter was then advanced over a 0.035-in. 260-cm Wholey wire (Mallinckrodt, Hazelwood, MO) into the innominate artery. It was exchanged for a 5 Fr Pigtail catheter, and an innominate artery angiogram was performed (Fig. 2). The pigtail was then exchanged for the 5 Fr JR4 which was used to selective engage the right common carotid artery (CCA). A right CCA angiogram was then performed (Fig. 3) followed by a cerebral angiogram (Fig. 4).

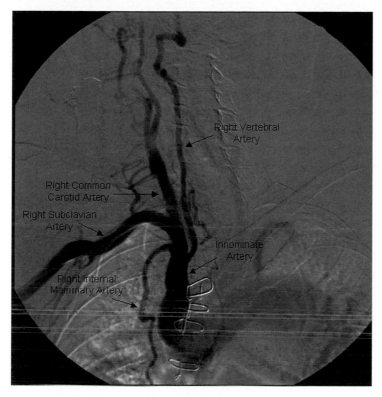

Fig. 2. Innominate artery angiogram (Movie 2).

ANGIOGRAPHIC FINDINGS

The right CCA has mild disease. The proximal right ICA has a 90% stenosis. The right external carotid artery (ECA) has minimal disease. The right middle cerebral artery (MCA) territory has delayed filling with only flash filling of the A1 segment of the anterior cerebral artery (ACA).

THE CHALLENGE

When carotid artery stenting is not possible via femoral access, typically this is either due to distal abdominal aortic occlusion or dissection, or severe diffuse peripheral arterial disease in the distal aorta, iliac, and femoral arteries. Femoral access is the preferred route for carotid intervention because of the size of the femoral arterial vessels and the route to the carotid bifurcation. The size of the common femoral artery, external iliac artery, and the common iliac artery typically allows the use of 6–9 Fr size sheaths without too much difficulty. Distal ischemia and distal embolization are usually better tolerated by the lower extremity than the upper extremity. The route to the carotid bifurcation, while angulated, typically does not involve sharp angles or tortuosity throughout its course. The exception to this is the type III and bovine arch, but even these difficult anatomic cases are more easily dealt with using a femoral approach.

When femoral access is not possible, the alternative routes of access are the radial, brachial, and axillary routes. Direct carotid injection is only of historical interest. Of these three routes, the brachial artery offers the best balance between size and complications.

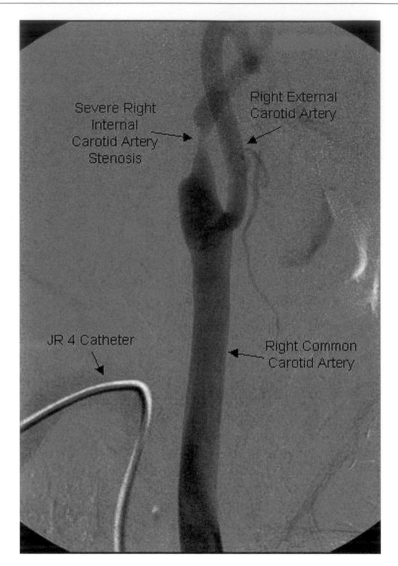

Fig. 3. Right common carotid artery angiogram (Movie 3).

The radial artery can be used successfully and case reports of radial artery access for carotid intervention have been described; however, the largest size that typically can be used in the radial artery is 6 Fr. The radial artery also has a much higher likelihood of spasm. For carotid intervention, the axillary approach should be avoided if at all possible. Overall, the brachial route is preferred.

In brachial access especially for the left carotid artery, typically the contralateral side away from the diseased carotid artery is used for access. The degree of difficulty in reaching the carotid bifurcation is dependent on the arch anatomy. The greater the degree of angulation, the more difficult the access will become. For type III arches and the right carotid artery, access can be considered from either the right or left brachial arteries depending on which route has better angulation (Fig. 5). In certain cases, a guide can be used from the brachial artery and used to engage the origin of the CCA. A buddy wire in the ECA can also be used for additional support.

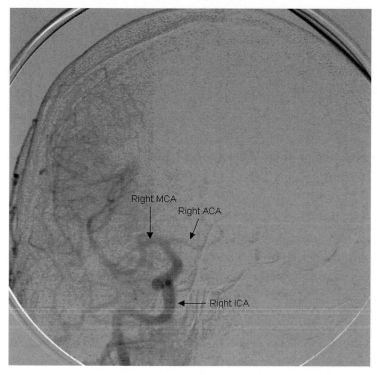

Fig. 4. Prestenting right cerebral angiogram in the PA projection (Movie 4).

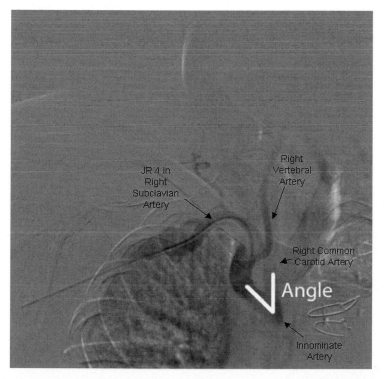

Fig. 5. Right subclavian artery—right common carotid artery angulation (Movie 5).

INTERVENTIONAL APPROACH

Most commonly, a sheath system is used rather than a guide to limit the access size in the brachial artery. Initially a short sheath is placed in the brachial artery. A 5 Fr diagnostic catheter is used to access the right or left CCA. Depending on the angulation and tortuosity of the arch, a JR4 catheter, a Vitek Catheter, or a Simmons Catheter can all be utilized. Assuming that the distal CCA is free of significant disease, a stiff angled Glidewire® (Terumo Medical, Somerset, NJ) can be advanced into the ECA. If the tortuosity is significant, the diagnostic catheter can be advanced into the ECA and the Glidewire® exchanged for a Amplatz extra-stiff or super-stiff wire. Care must be taken when advancing this extremely stiff wire as it may potentially prolapse out the entire system into the aortic arch. Once the wire is in position, the diagnostic system can be exchanged for a sheath. The typical sheath is straight with a stiff dilator. Often, it can be very challenging to advance the sheath, particularly into the origin and proximal CCA. If the dilator is too stiff, it can be exchanged for a diagnostic catheter, although the transition between the diagnostic catheter and tip of the sheath is not smooth and has the potential to cause a proximal antegrade dissection. An Ansel sheath also can be used. The Ansel sheath has several variants with different degrees of angulation proximally. In more tortuous cases, the Ansel sheath can be more easily advanced than the typical straight sheath. The newest development that will assist interventionalists using brachial access was the recent release of the Shuttle Select system (Cook, Bloomington, IN) with several compatible slip catheters including the H1, JB1, JB2, Vitek, and Simmons. This system has the advantage of shaped catheters for access along with a 6 Fr sheath size with a pliable tip.

INTERVENTIONAL PROCEDURE

In this patient, the right brachial artery was accessed to perform carotid stenting on the right ICA. A 5 Fr JR4 was used to engage the origin of the right CCA. Subsequently, A 260-cm stiff-angled Glidewire® was advanced into the right ECA using trace subtraction angiography. The JR4 catheter was carefully removed and the 5 Fr arterial sheath was removed. A 6 Fr 80-cm Shuttle sheath was then used with the sheath dilator in place to carefully advance the sheath into the origin of the right CCA. The dilator was removed and the 5 Fr JR4 diagnostic catheter was advanced over the Glidewire® beyond the origin of the Shuttle sheath. The JR4 was then carefully torqued and rotated into the mid-CCA and the Shuttle sheath was carefully advanced over the JR4 into the mid-CCA. Subsequently, the JR4 catheter was withdrawn into the sheath and the JR4 and Glidewire® were removed (Fig. 6).

A Filterwire EZ™ was then advanced through the sheath and deployed in the prepetrous portion of the right ICA. A 5.5 × 20 mm Viatrac® (Guidant, Indianapolis, IN) balloon was then positioned across the stenosis (Fig. 7). It was then dilated at 6 ATM (Figs. 8 and 9). It was dilated a second time to 8 ATM to improve the residual stenosis. However, after the second inflation, a dissection flap was possibly seen in the RAO view (Fig. 10). Therefore, a lateral carotid angiogram was performed which confirmed the dissection at the edges of the lesion (Fig. 11). Therefore, a tapered 7–10 mm × 40 mm AccuLink™ stent was then deployed across the ICA stenosis back into the right CCA. The stent was post-dilated with a 6.0 × 20 mm Aviator™ (Cordis, Warren, NJ) balloon. The Filterwire EZ™ was retrieved using the retrieval sheath. Final postintervention carotid angiography (Fig. 12) and cerebral angiography (Fig. 13) were then performed. Improvement of cerebral blood flow was observed after stent placement.

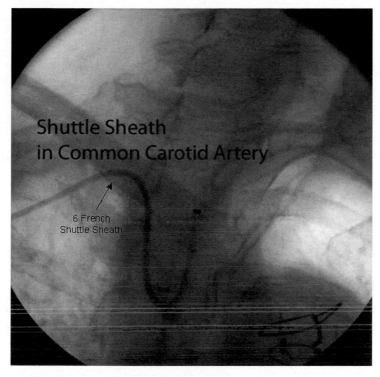

Fig. 6. Shuttle Sheath in position in right common carotid artery with marked angulation.

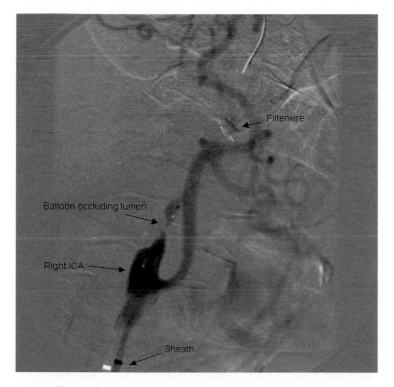

Fig. 7. Balloon positioning for predilatation (Movie 7).

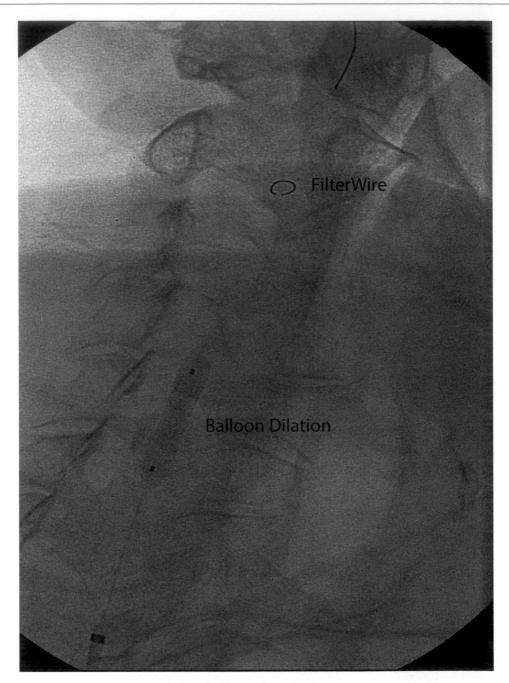

Fig. 8. Balloon predilatation.

POSTINTERVENTION COURSE

The patient was monitored overnight. He had no complications. His blood pressure was well controlled with systolic blood pressure readings in the 120 s. The postprocedural neurology evaluation showed no new changes. Approximately 5 wk later, the patient underwent successful open distal aortic arch and descending thoracic aortic replacement with an aortobifemoral aortic graft without complications.

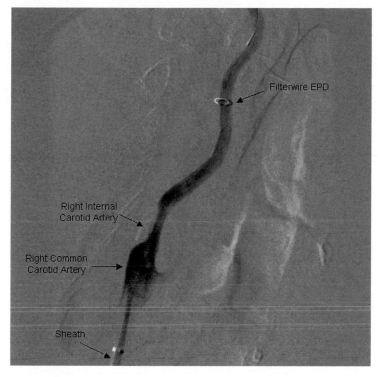

Fig. 9. Following first balloon predilatation (Movie 9).

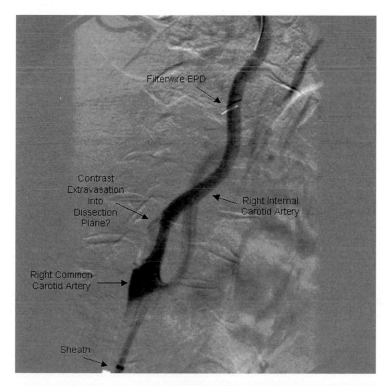

Fig. 10. Following second balloon predilatation (dissection flap seen) in the RAO projection (Movie 10).

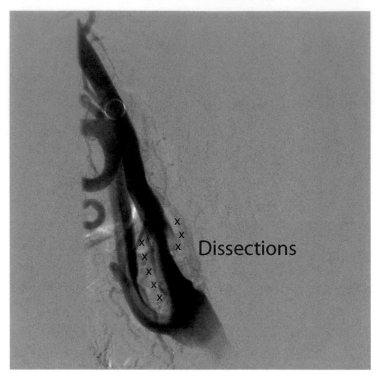

Fig. 11. Lateral angiogram reveals dissection flaps following balloon predilatation (Movie 11).

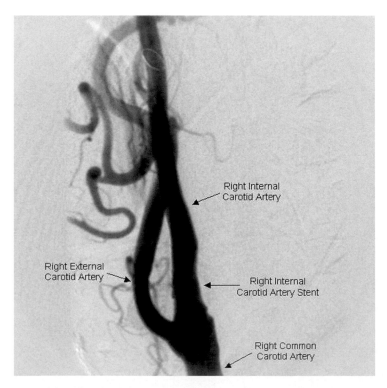

Fig. 12. Poststenting right carotid angiogram (Movie 12).

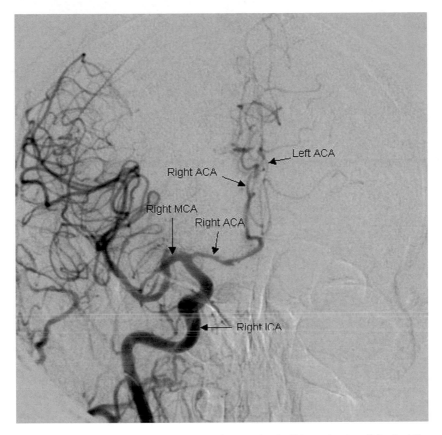

Fig. 13. Poststenting right cerebral angiogram in the PA projection (Movie 13).

LEARNING POINTS

1. Try to use femoral approach if possible, even if this necessitates an iliac artery intervention prior to carotid intervention. Obviously in certain instances, such as Type B dissection of the aorta and distal aortic occlusion or bilateral occlusion of both common and external iliac arteries may require the arm approach.
2. Use brachial rather than radial approach. Radial artery is more prone to spasm given the need for larger sheath size and length. Care must be taken when accessing the brachial artery. Try to limit sheath size to 6 Fr if possible.
3. Typically if intervening on the left carotid artery, contralateral brachial access will be preferred. Accessing the same side usually increases the angulation and tortuosity from left brachial access for LICA intervention. For the right carotid artery, which brachial artery to access depends on the angle of takeoff of the innominate from the aortic arch compared to the angle of the right subclavian artery to the right CCA.
4. Use of an Ansel sheath and now the Shuttle Select sheath may improve ability to position sheath in the distal common carotid artery.
5. In many instances, the use of a buddy 0.014-in. guidewire in the ECA may be beneficial to improve stability of the system during intervention.

6. Be cognizant of sheath position when advancing the stent. The stiffness of the stent often causes the sheath position to fall, which also may affect the emboli protection device position.
7. Take an angiogram of the sheath being withdrawn from the CCA to ensure that no damage has been done to the CCA.

ACKNOWLEDGMENT

I thank Deepak Vivek for his assistance in the preparation of this case.

24 Case: Ostial Innominate Artery Intervention

David S. Lee, MD

CONTENTS

HISTORY

A 65-yr-old Caucasian woman with risk factors of hypertension, dyslipidemia, and smoking had presented with a left-hemispheric stroke. She was well until the morning of the event, when she complained of several episodes of right-sided weakness and mild slurred speech. She presented to the Emergency Room approx 8 h after the onset of symptoms. At that point, she still had mild right arm and leg weakness, but her slurred speech had resolved. On physical examination, her strength was 4/5 on both right upper and lower extremities, decreased sensation, and brisk reflexes on the right. Her NIH stroke scale score was 1. She was treated with aspirin and clopidogrel and underwent urgent magnetic resonance imaging (MRI) and magnetic resonance angiography (MRA).

The MRI did not show any acute ischemic changes. However, the MRA revealed severe ostial innominate artery stenosis and possibly occluded or severely stenosed left subclavian artery. The left carotid bifurcation is anomalously high. There was no significant stenosis in either carotid bifurcation. The visualized cervical right vertebral artery is patent but no cervical left vertebral artery is seen. In the intracranial circulation, the M1 segment of the left middle cerebral artery (MCA) is likely occluded. The distal vertebral and basilar arteries are very small in caliber but this is likely at least in part developmental as there is a fetal origin of each posterior cerebral artery (PCA), with a hypoplastic right P1 segment and apparently absent left P1 segment.

Duplex ultrasound showed turbulent signals in the right common carotid artery (CCA) and the left subclavian artery suggestive of more proximal stenosis. The flow

From: *Contemporary Cardiology: Handbook of Complex Percutaneous Carotid Intervention*
Edited by: J. Saw, J. E. Exaire, D. S. Lee, and S. Yadav © Humana Press Inc., Totowa, NJ

in the left vertebral artery was retrograde and suggestive of left subclavian steal syndrome.

Thus, this patient had severe ostial/proximal stenoses or occlusions of her innominate artery and her left subclavian artery. The etiology of her left MCA stroke was not clear. There was evidence of atrial fibrillation or other arrhythmias. A transesophageal echocardiogram was performed that showed normal left ventricular function, and no cardiac source for embolism. She did have aortic atheroma that was moderately diffuse. There was no significant stenosis of the left carotid artery.

The decision to proceed to angiography and potential intervention was reached but not without some controversy. Her cerebral circulation was at risk given her likely occluded left subclavian artery, severely diseased innominate artery, and a recent stroke with likely occlusion of the proximal MCA. The benefit innominate intervention to improve cerebral blood flow via her right internal carotid artery (ICA) and right vertebral artery, as well as decreasing her stroke risk from the innominate stenosis, was balanced against the risk of procedural complications, including the possibility of hemorrhagic conversion of her stroke. Her minimal deficit was suggestive of either incomplete occlusion of her MCA or significant collateral flow. Improving collateral flow at this point after her stroke would likely be beneficial. After long discussion among the neurologists and interventionalists involved in her care, a decision was made to proceed to angiography and intervention of her innominate artery.

DIAGNOSTIC PROCEDURE

A 5 Fr short sheath was placed in the right common femoral artery using the modified Seldinger technique. The patient was given 2500 U of unfractionated heparin intraarterially. A 5 Fr angled pigtail catheter was then advanced over a long Wholey wire into the aortic arch. Central pressure was elevated at 240/130 mmHg. An arch aortogram was performed in the left anterior oblique projection (Fig. 1). A 5 Fr JR4 catheter was then used to selectively engage the origin of the innominate artery. The innominate artery angiogram (Fig. 2) with cerebral angiogram was then performed (Fig. 3). The JR4 catheter was then used to selectively engage the left CCA. Under roadmapping angiography and using a floppy Glidewire®, the JR4 catheter was advanced into the distal third of the left CCA. A left CCA angiogram was then performed (Fig. 4), followed by cerebral angiogram (Fig. 5).

ANGIOGRAPHIC FINDINGS

1. Type 3 aortic arch.
2. A 90% ulcerated proximal innominate artery stenosis with a 100 mmHg gradient between central and brachial pressures.
3. The right CCA and ICA only have mild disease. There was poor cortical filling into the right anterior cerebral artery (ACA) and MCA territories. There was a fetal PCA.
4. The right subclavian artery and vertebral artery only have mild disease. The intracranial right and left vertebral artery are small in caliber and merge to form a small basilar artery. There was poor filling of the basilar artery.
5. The left CCA and ICA have mild disease. There was a patent anterior communicating artery (ACOM) with filling of the contralateral ACA. There was also fetal PCA arising from the left ICA. The M1 segment of the MCA is occluded, and the MCA territory

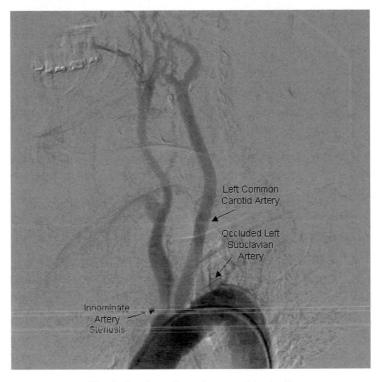

Fig. 1. Aortic arch angiogram (Movie 1).

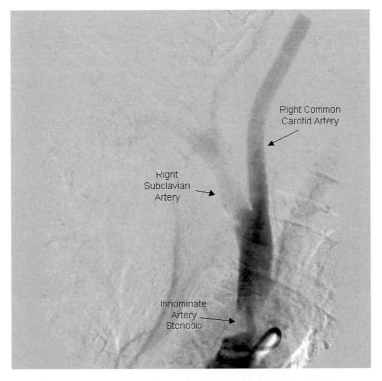

Fig. 2. Innominate artery angiogram in the lateral projection.

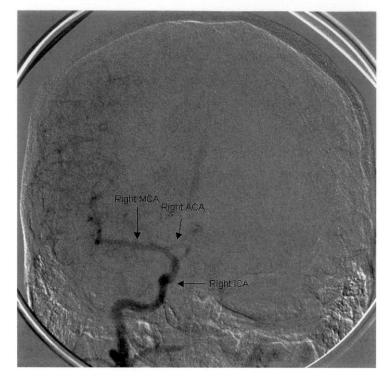

Fig. 3. Right cerebral angiogram in the PA projection (Movie 3).

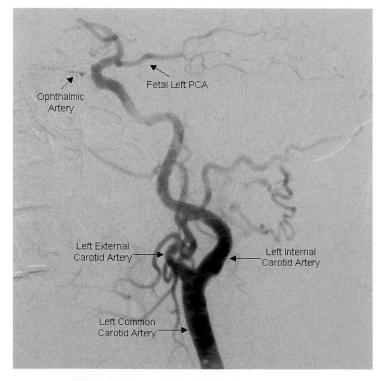

Fig. 4. Left common carotid artery angiogram.

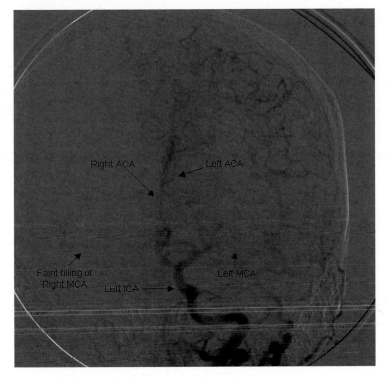

Fig. 5. Left cerebral angiogram in the PA projection (Movie 5).

fills via abundant pial collaterals from the left ACA and the left PCA. With the exception of the left MCA territory, there is normal cortical filling.

6. The left subclavian artery is occluded at its origin. The left subclavian artery fills via retrograde flow from the left vertebral artery, which fills via collaterals from the occipital branch of the left external carotid artery (ECA).

THE CHALLENGE

Ostial stenoses of the innominate or left common carotid arteries present difficulty primarily from achieving stable guide position in the aortic arch. If the lesion is not ostial, guide placement and stability is much easier. Ostial innominate stenosis intervention tends to be more challenging than ostial left CCA stenosis. The guide choice depends primarily on the angulation in the arch, the distance of the vessel origin from the peak of the arch, and the depth or diameter of the aortic arch. Guide choices include an H1, JR4, Multipurpose, and Amplatz guides. Sheaths are not good choices in this setting given their inability to position stably close to the ostium. Often, a preexisting guide (e.g., Amplatz) must be individually shaped using a sterile paper clip and boiling water or a heat gun (Fig. 3 in Chapter 10). Once the guide is in position in the aortic arch, a 0.014-in. buddy wire in the ECA can assist in stabilizing the guide in position. Another issue that must be kept in mind, especially for the innominate artery, is the diameter of the stent needed. If the origin/proximal innominate artery or CCA are large (≥8 mm), then larger guides (≥9 Fr) will be needed to accommodate the appropriate stent size.

The second challenge for treatment of ostial stenoses is the placement of an emboli protection device (EPD). Innominate artery intervention does provide an advantage, as

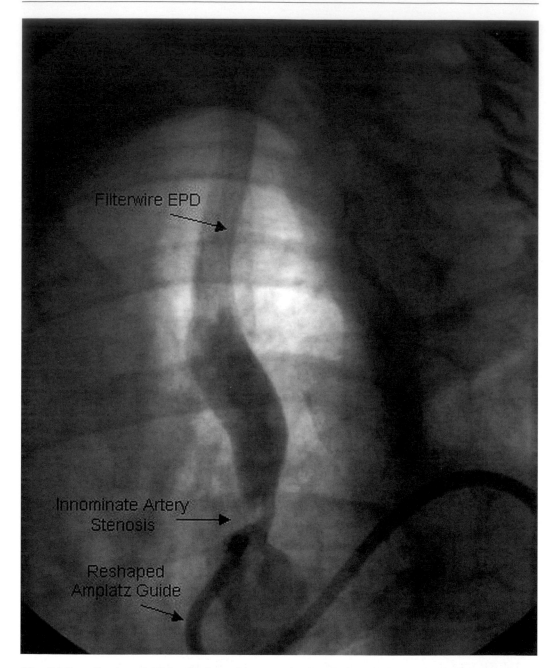

Fig. 6. Manually-shaped AL1 guide in position, proximal to the innominate artery stenosis (Movie 6).

an EPD can be placed in the ICA from a right brachial approach, rather than through the guide itself, resulting in better stability of the EPD. This option is obviously not available when treating the ostial left CCA.

Usually placement of the balloon or stent is not as complicated given the proximal location of the stenosis. However, care must be taken to be aware of guide position and EPD position as the device is being maneuvered into position. Not infrequently, there can be inadvertent substantial movement of both guide and EPD.

INTERVENTIONAL PROCEDURE

The 5 Fr sheath was exchanged for a 9 Fr short sheath. A 9 Fr system was utilized to accommodate an 8-mm diameter balloon-expandable stent. A 9 Fr H1 guide was advanced into the aortic arch over a 0.035-in. 260-cm Wholey wire (Mallinckrodt, Hazelwood, MO) using a telescoping system with a 5 Fr 125 cm JR4 catheter. The H1 guide was then used to selectively engage the origin of the innominate artery. However, because of the unfavorable angle, this catheter was subsequently removed, and a 9 Fr AL1 guide was shaped using a heating gun (Fig. 3 in Chapter 10). The 5 Fr 125 cm JR4 catheter was telescoped through this AL1 guide, and this was advanced over the Wholey wire into the aortic arch. The Wholey wire and JR4 were subsequently removed, and the AL1 guide was then used to selectively engage just the origin of the innominate artery proximal to the stenosis (Fig. 6). An additional 3500 U of unfractionated heparin were administered, and an ACT of 251 was achieved.

A long FilterWire EZ™ (Boston Scientific, Natick, MA) was then used to carefully cross the innominate stenosis and was deployed in the prepetrous portion of the right ICA. Angiography confirmed good apposition of the EPD in the right ICA (Fig. 7). Predilatation was then performed with a 5.0 × 15 mm Aviator™ balloon (Cordis, Warren, NJ) at 8 atm (Figs. 8 and 9). Subsequently, an 8.0 × 15 mm Genesis stent (Cordis, Warren, NJ) was then positioned across the stenosis (Fig. 10), and deployed at 10 atm (Fig. 11). The lesion was then postdilated using an 8.0 × 20 mm OptaPro balloon (Cordis, Warren, NJ) at 10 atm for two inflations (Fig. 12). Post-stenting innominate artery angiograms (Fig. 13) with cerebral angiograms were then performed (Fig. 14). The filter EPD was retrieved, and final angiograms done. The AL1 guide was disengaged from the innominate artery, and was removed over a 0.035-in. J wire. The 9 Fr sheath was removed and hemostasis was achieved with manual compression after administering 20 mg of Protamine.

POSTINTERVENTION COURSE

The patient was monitored overnight. She had no complications from the procedure. Her blood pressure in her right arm was significantly elevated after the innominate stent was placed. Her blood pressure was controlled with intravenous metoprolol and oral medications with systolic blood pressures in the 160–180 range overnight. She was eventually discharged to a rehabilitation facility for physical and occupational therapy prior to returning home.

LEARNING POINTS

1. The two main challenges in this setting are: (a) stable guide position near the origin of the vessel (and stenosis) without engaging the plaque/lesion and (b) placement and stability of the EPD in the ICA.
2. Typically a guide rather than a sheath is used in this setting as the sheath will have little purchase in the aortic arch and provide limited support.
3. The guide choices depend primarily on the vessel requiring intervention (ostial innominate or left CCA), tortuosity and angulation of the aortic arch, and the diameter or girth of the aortic arch. Typically, an 8 or 9 Fr guide is used. Examples include an H1, JR4, Multipurpose, and Amplatz guides. Sometimes, the AL1 guide has to be shaped

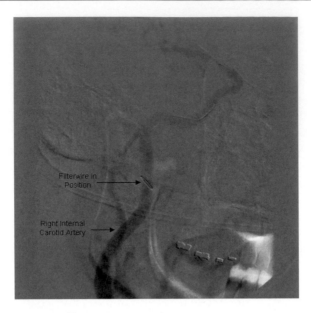

Fig. 7. FilterWire EZ™ emboli protection device in the internal carotid artery.

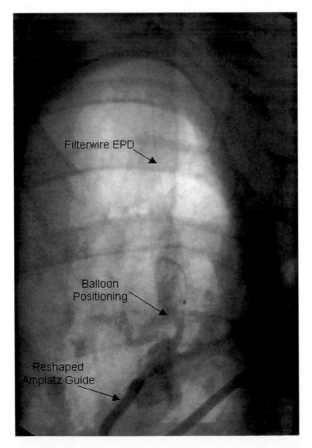

Fig. 8. Balloon positioning for predilatation of innominate artery lesion (Movie 8).

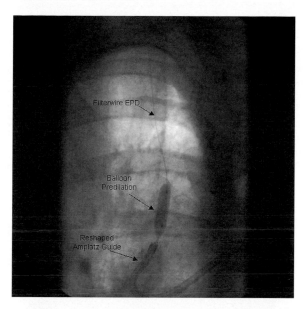

Fig. 9. Balloon predilatation of the ostial innominate artery lesion.

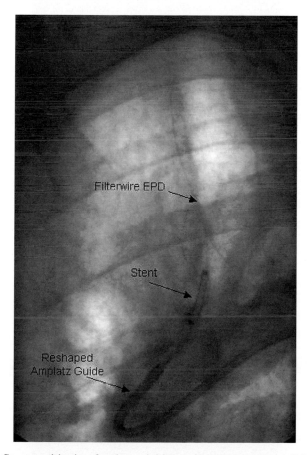

Fig. 10. Stent positioning for the ostial innominate artery lesion (Movie 10).

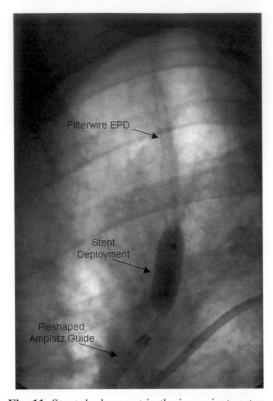

Fig. 11. Stent deployment in the innominate artery.

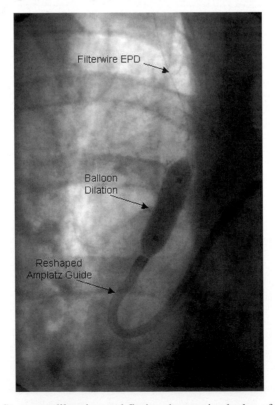

Fig. 12. Stent postdilatation and flaring the proximal edge of the stent.

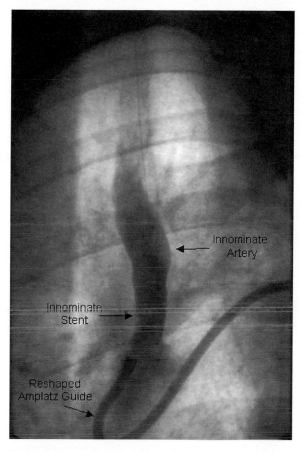

Fig. 13. Poststent angiogram of the innominate artery (Movie 13).

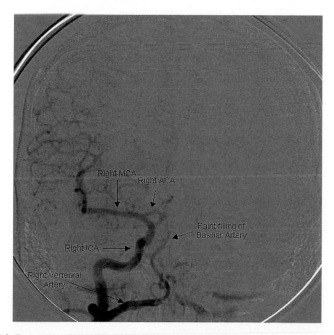

Fig. 14. Poststent right cerebral angiogram in the PA projection (Movie 14).

using a sterile paper clip and a heat gun into a configuration that is better fit for the arch angulation. The French size of the guide will depend on availability and the stent diameter required.

4. For positioning and radial strength, a balloon-expandable stent is typically preferred for an ostial position.

5. A 0.014-in. buddy wire is often helpful in providing extra stability.

6. The innominate artery provides more than one option for EPD placement. Because of the tendency of the guide to shift or move during balloon and stent positioning, more stable placement of the EPD can be obtained by placing it via a right brachial access into the right ICA. This option is obviously not available for left CCA stenosis.

INDEX